Empires of the Senses

Empires of the Senses

Bodily Encounters in Imperial India and the Philippines

ANDREW J. ROTTER

OXFORD
UNIVERSITY PRESS

OXFORD
UNIVERSITY PRESS

Oxford University Press is a department of the University of Oxford. It furthers the University's objective of excellence in research, scholarship, and education by publishing worldwide. Oxford is a registered trade mark of Oxford University Press in the UK and certain other countries.

Published in the United States of America by Oxford University Press
198 Madison Avenue, New York, NY 10016, United States of America.

Library of Congress Cataloging-in-Publication Data
Names: Rotter, Andrew Jon, author.
Title: Empires of the senses : bodily encounters in imperial India
and the Philippines / Andrew J. Rotter.
Description: New York, NY : Oxford University Press, [2019] |
Includes bibliographical references and index.
Identifiers: LCCN 2019002163 (print) | LCCN 2019005111 (ebook) |
ISBN 9780190924713 (updf) | ISBN 9780190924720 (epub) |
ISBN 9780190924706 (hardcover :alk. paper)
Subjects: LCSH: India—Civilization—1765–1947. |
Philippines—Civilization—20th century. | Senses and
sensation—India—History. | Senses and sensation—Philippines—History.
Classification: LCC DS428 (ebook) | LCC DS428.R68 2019 (print) |
DDC 954.03/5—dc23
LC record available at https://lccn.loc.gov/2019002163

1 3 5 7 9 8 6 4 2

Printed by Sheridan Books, Inc., United States of America

to Sam David Rotter Stevenson

CONTENTS

ACKNOWLEDGMENTS

I've been at this for a while, and in the course of reading and writing about two empires and five senses and more about sewers and leprosy than is healthy for most people, I have accumulated a great number of debts. I acknowledge too few of them here.

I was in the audience at Colgate University some years ago when Mark Smith gave a guest lecture about race and the senses in the American South. His talk was so arresting and provocative that it got me thinking about material I had run across even more years ago on how India smelled to the British when they arrived there in the nineteenth and twentieth centuries. Mark became a correspondent, and he has inspired and encouraged my work. Lizzie Collingham fed us in Duxbury and talked with me about Indian food. She writes like a dream about everything interesting. Chris Capozzola and Josh Gedacht gave me excellent advice about working in Manila, and Chris offered gentle and helpful criticism of a talk I gave at MIT. Trading notes with Mary Lui at the Rizal Library at Ataneo de Manila University was great fun. Paul Kramer has over the years read my work with a penetrating eye and commented on it with extraordinary grace. I've been encouraged in the project, through its ups and downs, by Jyoti Balachandran, Brooke Blower, Mark Philip Bradley, Susan Carruthers, Jay Cook, Nick Cullather, David Engerman, Lloyd Gardner, Kristin Hoganson, Aftab Jassal, Terri Keeley, Melanie Kiechle, Menachem Kogman, Prakash Kumar, Yanek Mieckowski, Michael Peletz, Andrew Preston, and Kelly Shannon, by Colgate and Cambridge University students at a joint seminar generously hosted by Andrew Preston at Cambridge in 2014, and by the stellar participants in the Society of Historians of American Foreign Relations Summer Institute in 2013. Audiences at Colgate, Ben-Gurion University (with thanks to Katrin Kogman-Appel and Ruth Ginio), the London School of Economics (Matthew Jones, twice), MIT (Jeff Ravel), and, by teleconference, the University of Texas-Austin (Mark Lawrence), were good enough to listen to me talk about latrines, cholera, and William Howard Taft's underwear, and to offer sharp questions and comments.

Colgate, my home institution, has treated me with great generosity for many years. My colleagues in the history department have made it a joy to climb the hill to the office each day (though perhaps not so much in December); my thanks to Antonio Barrera, Dan Bouk, Alan Cooper, Ray Douglas, Faye Dudden, Xan Karn, Rob Nemes, David Robinson, and Heather Roller for their stimulating and supportive presence. Other Colgate faculty members have been wonderful interlocutors, especially Tim Byrnes and Georgia Frank. I am grateful to the Research Council, and its chairs Lynn Staley, Judith Oliver, and Rick Braaten, for a senior faculty leave, research support, and a book subvention. My dean-provosts, most recently Doug Hicks and Tracey Hucks, have always been enormously encouraging. And many thanks to my Colgate-supported student assistants: Hannah Fuchs, Max Johnson, Annie Morrow, Jack Schnettler, and Julia Smaldone.

Thanks, too, to the archivists and librarians who endured with the patience of Job my questions about their collections and my requests for material. Archives and libraries are not organized for the benefit of someone researching the senses, so helping me required even more than the usual degree of imagination. Much gratitude to the professionals at the Library of Congress Manuscript Division, National Archives II in College Park, Maryland; libraries at Harvard, Syracuse, Princeton, and Colgate Universities; the American Philosophical Society in Philadelphia; the Center for Advanced Study at Princeton (whose crack librarians treated a trailing spouse with great kindness); the Bancroft Library at the University of California, Berkeley; Cornell University and the University of Michigan Libraries (which generously loaned me microfilm from their collections); the US Military History Institute in Carlisle, Pennsylvania; the Center for South Asia at Cambridge University; the British Library; the National Archives of India in Delhi; and the American History Collection at the Rizal Library, Ateneo de Manila University.

Lesley Chapman, Visual Resources Curator at Colgate, worked brilliantly and patiently through my many questions concerning images for the book, tracking down high resolution versions of pictures I had found, finding other and better pictures, and tracing them all to their sources. When I started this project, I knew that I wanted to publish it with Oxford University Press. I got lucky. As so many historians know, one shouldn't miss an opportunity to work with Susan Ferber. Susan still line edits (with a blue pencil, I think), and her care of the manuscript and its author have left me in awe. And her advice was always exactly right; for instance: "You don't need this example—this paragraph is already revolting enough." It has been a pleasure to work with her.

When I was starting out in the academy, I heard lots of talk about "intellectual community." It took some time for me to realize what it was, and to understand that I had one. I learned that an intellectual community, or mine anyway, was not just about mutual advice and support for scholarly projects but also friendship that existed beyond arguments made in articles and books and, in some cases, in spite of disagreements with them. So my intellectual community—also known as "my friends"—includes Naoko Shibusawa, Petra Goedde, Andrew Preston, Rob Nemes, Liz Marlowe, Jerry and Kathy Eisman, Valerie Weller, Faye Dudden, and Marshall Blake, and four men who have for many years inspired me with their work: Frank Costigliola, Carl Guarneri, Richard Immerman, and Walt LaFeber.

As always, my greatest debt is to my family. My father, Roy, died before the book was finished, but I think he would have liked it, especially the parts about medicine and food. My mother, Muriel, is unlikely to read it, but if there is a bit of playfulness in it, that's her bit. Lorraine and Chandran Kaimal, my in-laws, continue to astonish and inspire me with their energy; my son-in-law, Dan Stevenson, is a humane and intellectually curious mathematician and a delight to be around. Daughters Sophie and Phoebe . . . well. They are loving, hilarious, smart, accomplished, and warm young women who are deeply committed to social justice. Then there is Padma. Always. The book is dedicated to the youngest family member: Sam Stevenson, born in August 2017, charismatic minifauna and a pure joy.

Empires of the Senses

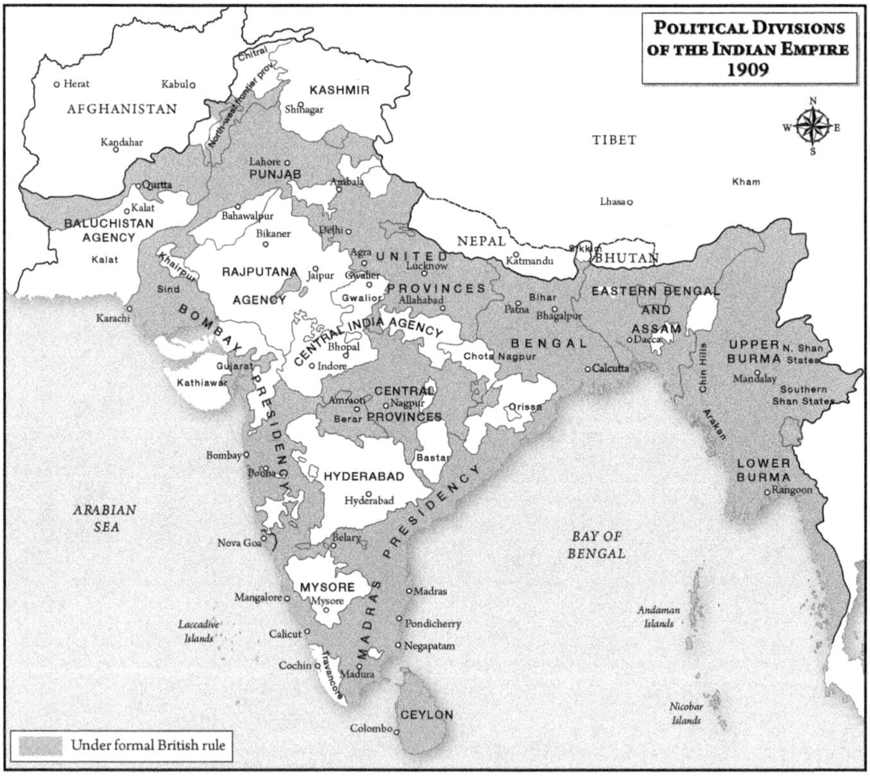

POLITICAL DIVISIONS OF THE INDIAN EMPIRE 1909

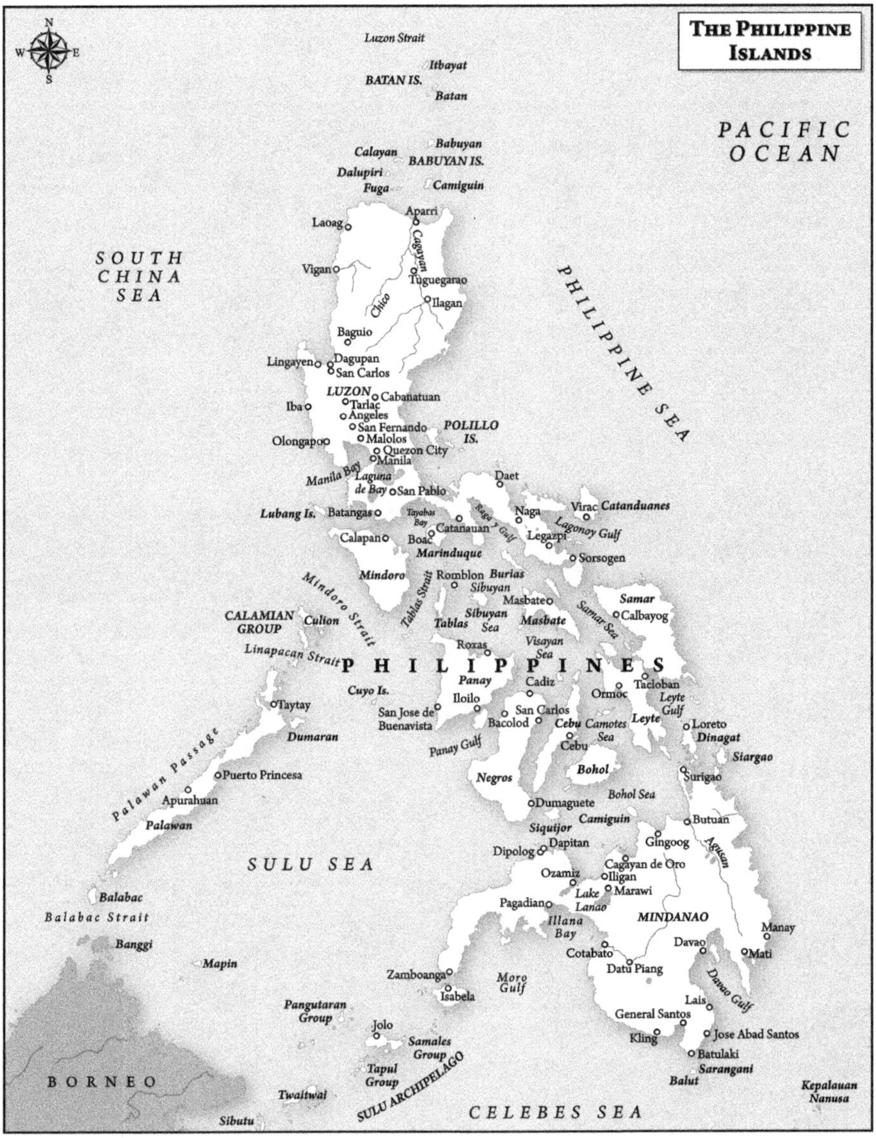
THE PHILIPPINE ISLANDS
PACIFIC OCEAN
SOUTH CHINA SEA
PHILIPPINE SEA
SULU SEA
CELEBES SEA
BORNEO
PHILIPPINES
Luzon Strait
Itbayat
BATAN IS.
Batan
Babuyan
Calayan
BABUYAN IS.
Dalupiri
Fuga
Camiguin
Aparri
Laoag
Cagayan
Vigan
Tuguegarao
Chico
Ilagan
Baguio
Lingayen
Dagupan
San Carlos
LUZON
Cabanatuan
Iba
Tarlac
Angeles
San Fernando
POLILLO IS.
Olongapo
Malolos
Quezon City
Manila
Manila Bay
Laguna de Bay
San Pablo
Daet
Lubang Is.
Batangas
Tayabas Bay
Catanauan
Ragay Gulf
Naga
Virac
Catanduanes
Lagonoy Gulf
Legazpi
Calapan
Boac
Marinduque
Sorsogen
Mindoro
Romblon
Burias
Sibuyan
Masbate
Samar
Mindoro Strait
Tablas Strait
Samar Sea
Calbayog
CALAMIAN GROUP
Culion
Tablas
Sibuyan Sea
Masbate
Roxas
Visayan Sea
Linapacan Strait
Panay
Cadiz
Tacloban
Ormoc
Leyte Gulf
Cuyo Is.
Iloilo
Taytay
San Jose de Buenavista
San Carlos
Bacolod
Cebu
Camotes Sea
Leyte
Loreto
Dinagat
Dumaran
Panay Gulf
Cebu
Siargao
Palawan Passage
Puerto Princesa
Negros
Bohol
Surigao
Apurahuan
Bohol Sea
Dumaguete
Palawan
Camiguin
Butuan
Siquijor
Dipolog
Dapitan
Gingoog
Agusan
Ozamiz
Cagayan de Oro
Iligan
Balabac
Lake Lanao
Marawi
Pagadian
Balabac Strait
Illana Bay
MINDANAO
Manay
Banggi
Davao
Mati
Cotabato
Mapin
Datu Piang
Zamboanga
Moro Gulf
Davao Gulf
Isabela
Lais
Pangutaran Group
General Santos
Jolo
Samales Group
Kling
Jose Abad Santos
Batulaki
Tapul Group
Sarangani
Balut
Twaitwai
SULU ARCHIPELAGO
Kepalauan Nanusa
Sibutu

Introduction

Embodied Empires

The forming of the five senses is a labor of the entire history of the world down to the present.

—Karl Marx, *Economic and Philosophic Manuscripts of 1844* (1932)

The senses, under the aegis and direction of the mind, give us a world.

—Yi-Fan Tuan, *Passing Strange and Wonderful* (1993)

Empire was many things. It involved economics, geopolitics, a desire for order and greatness, a craving for excitement and adventure. It also meant an encounter between authorities and subjects, an everyday process of social interaction, political negotiation, policing and schooling and healing. It meant violence, the imposition of control, and accommodation or resistance to it. All of these interactions were on some level intellectual, having to do with what people thought about each other. But they were also in significant ways mediated by the senses, by perceptions of others formed through seeing, hearing, touching, smelling, and tasting.

This book argues that all human relationships, including imperial ones, are shaped by all five senses; how we understand others, even more how we feel about them and thus how we act toward them, have a good deal to do with how we apprehend them through every sense. We have long assumed that how we see others, literally, and how we read the texts we generate about them, tell us all we need to know about our relations with them. Yet "the project of imperialism . . . could not be effected by sight alone," as historian Mark M. Smith has written. The entire human sensorium was engaged in the acts of making and accommodating and resisting empire.[1]

This study—the sensory history of the British in India from the formal imposition of their rule to its end (1857–1947) and the Americans in the Philippines from annexation to independence (1898–1946)—is unapologetically interested in life on empire's quotidian ground. It explores how the senses created mutual impressions of the agents of imperialism and their subjects, and in so doing illuminates connections between apparently disparate items, including the otherwise unremarkable comments (and complaints) found in memoirs and reports, the appearance of lepers, the sound of bells, the odor of excrement, the feel of cloth against skin, the first taste of meat spiced with cumin or of a mango. Men and women in imperial India and the Philippines apprehended each other through their sense organs and their skins. Anglo-Americans and Asians did not necessarily agree on the relative importance of their senses. They had different ideas from the start about what looked, sounded, smelled, felt, and tasted good or bad.

Both the British and the Americans saw themselves as the civilizers of what they judged to be backward societies, and they believed that a vital part of the civilizing process was to put the senses in the right order of priority and to protect them against offense or affront. Those lacking respect for the senses lacked self-control; they were uncivilized and thus unfit for self-government. Societies that looked shabby, were noisy and smelly, felt wrong, and consumed unwholesome food in unmannerly ways were not prepared to form independent polities and stand on their own. It was the duty of allegedly more sensorily advanced westerners to put the senses right before withdrawing the most obvious manifestations of their power. Indians and Filipinos had different ideas of what constituted sensory civilization, and to some extent they resisted British and American efforts to impose their versions on them. In the end, a synthesis of sorts would emerge that involved compromises between these nations' sensory regimes.

Empire was an embodied experience, for both its agents and subjects. People in imperial spaces not only think about each other; they meet each other hand to hand, face to face, body to body; they form through their senses impressions of others and have feelings about them. Their reactions are not always considered but may be instinctive, visceral, and above all emotional. People feel wonder at the seemingly different, mixed with fear—of bodily penetration, violation, pollution, or infection. Bodies are membranes, as scholar Laura Otis has argued, permitting osmosis that may be pleasurable or enlightening but also potentially distressing or threatening.[2] In their encounter with what they perceive as new and strange, people feel delight and alarm, hope and danger, arousal and disgust, exhilaration and terror. Imperial policy was shaped by laws approved in metropoles, but it was enacted on the ground, and the relationship between policy and practice was at all times reciprocal. Men and women—Britons and Indians, Americans and Filipinos—encountered each other every day, through their senses. They watched each other warily, glanced at each other, or averted their eyes out of deference, revulsion, or defiance. Britons and Americans fixed their gaze on their subjects and cataloged them by counting them and taking their pictures, while Indians and Filipinos might hope to fool or confound western eyes, hiding or deceiving with looks of feigned obedience or innocence. In India and the Philippines the Anglo-Americans heard what they regarded as discord, the jarring sounds of brass bands, shouting and spitting in the marketplace, the keening of mourners, and a babble of languages they could not understand. They hoped to impose new sonic regimes on their imperial outposts, trying first to get their subjects to quiet down, especially to lower the volume of the urban street, then to teach the most promising of them English, so they could be understood and thus better managed. Some Indians and Filipinos were willing to learn English and to make the language their own through a style of oratory they knew well, either to improve their positions or to confront the imperialists and demand their rights. Pungent smells entered western nostrils and signified to them Indians and Filipinos' lack of refinement, for who but an uncivilized people would tolerate the acrid odors of lanes and waterways, the reek of garbage, domestic animals, and human excrement? Yet who but a westerner, thought Indians and Filipinos, would go for days without bathing or spurn the olfactory delights of rose attar or coconut oil? The touched or felt environment of the tropics seemed to demand revision by the agents of empire. The skins of their subjects were rough—how else to explain the coarseness of their clothing and their apparent imperviousness to discomfort or lack of feeling?—while their land was rutted and broken, and the air they breathed heavy with heat and moisture and alive with insects. Worse, they conveyed by their touch or through contact with their bodily discharges contagious diseases, making proximity to them a frightening risk. Indians and Filipinos resisted the skin-to-skin demands of the interlopers, refusing, for example, to handle their dead as efficiently as the westerners liked, or spurning the intrusive touch of British or American doctors who wished to examine or inoculate them. What foods their subjects/masters ate, appalling in their appearance and taste, and how disgustingly they ate them! And yet not every new sight, sound, touch, smell, and taste offended its recipient. The westerners' most determined efforts to discipline Asian others by teaching them manners encountered not just resistance from those who preferred their own practices, but from Britons and Americans themselves, who found, often to their surprise, that there were delights to be had in opening their senses to their new environments and their people.

Empire was never a single project. It was instead an unwieldy cultural formation that included governance, and of which the senses constituted the most fundamental elements. To historian Jon Wilson, the British empire looks to have been "chaos"—there was, he says flatly, no "civilizing mission" in British India—but that is because he insists that such a mission could only have been characterized by consistency, unity, and single-mindedness by its rulers.[3] Both the Indian and Philippines empires looked chaotic because they were governed as federal structures, meaning that provincial or local control was by the twentieth century often conceded by central governments. India was too large and variegated for a small island to hold in its totality, and the Philippines was governed by Americans roughly as the United States was governed, with considerable local and state power. Still, there were in both places laws and requirements and sanctions laid down by central governments, in London and Calcutta then Delhi, in Washington and Manila. These concerned strategy, law and order, public works, public health, the creation of an education system, and other matters. And the empires were held together by everyday patterns: how rulers and subjects interacted, how they saw, heard, smelled, felt, and fed each other. The name of the cultural formation of empire was civilization.

The senses have been studied extensively by anthropologists and scholars of religion, but examinations of their history are vigorous and growing. Historians have adopted sense perception as a category of analysis, useful for the ways in which it allows us to apprehend differently (for example) the history of the body; social relations including understandings of race, class, and gender; and the history of the emotions. It enables the writing of history with more dimension and texture, giving it an instantiated, near-physical quality. Historians of the French *Annales* School have long argued that attention must be paid to senses other than vision, particularly in the study of European history prior to the eighteenth century. During the 1980s and 1990s, Alain Corbin published books on the social history of smell and sound. Constance Classen and David Howes, anthropologists by training, nevertheless ground their extensive scholarship on the senses in historical evidence. More than anyone else, Mark Smith has recast our understanding of the past in sensory terms, revealing how all the senses helped constitute US race relations, shaped the experience of the Civil War, and contributed broadly to the lived history of Europeans and Americans down the centuries. While sensory history has thus far touched only lightly on relations between people and nations, including the history of empire, the field seems a natural target for this kind of analysis.[4]

Several elements of sensory history seem especially worth noting. First, while the senses of course have a biological basis, they must be historicized. Take odor. Smells have chemical form: odor-producing molecules arrive and are recorded on the nerve endings inside the nostrils and produce reactions in all human brains. Yet smells have complicated meanings, which have shifted over time and depend on place. Humans have long distinguished between the civilized and the primitive on the basis of smell, the aesthetic and moral evaluation of which is learned through acculturation. None of the senses are stable or static. Because they cannot be fully explained by biology, the understanding of them varies from place to place.[5] As Norbert Elias argued, the European judgment of what (for example) stank changed with the Enlightenment, with its new definition of what was mannerly and therefore what it meant to be civilized.[6] Second, those who have thought about the senses have tended to rank them in order of importance. In *The Gutenberg Galaxy*, Marshall McLuhan claimed that with the invention of moveable type and the advent of the Enlightenment, vision emerged as the sense without peer, the sole "authenticator of truth," as hearing and especially the other three senses lost importance in text-based societies. Thus sight, McLuhan contends, carries a higher value than the other senses, and acuity of vision confers on those who have it civilization in its highest form.[7]

McLuhan's binary distinction between sight and the four other senses, known as "the Great Divide" theory, has been challenged for various reasons. Far from abandoning hearing and the others in favor exclusively of sight, humans everywhere have in fact continued to rely on all their senses, working together, to understand their surroundings. Taste without smell is unimaginable; touch is often triggered vicariously by the sight of an object that is sharp or rough. There is no evidence, according to historian Mark S. R. Jenner, "that if one sense grows in significance others must decline correspondingly"—sensory history is not a "zero sum game."[8] In addition, to rank seeing over all other senses is implicitly to demean other ways of evaluating the world. It may be true that humans rely more fully on the proximate or so-called lower senses—smell, touch, and taste—than on sight and hearing, senses that work at a distance, when social boundaries become blurred, as they do in imperial settings. Where sight and sound are unreliable markers of difference, other senses appear to become more acute.[9] In the end, it is better to attend to context, culture, and the balance of the senses through time and space.[10]

This book takes a comparative approach to the sensory experiences of the British Empire in India and those of the United States in the Philippines in order to de-provincialize exceptionalist national narratives. For many years, Americans regarded their experience with imperialism, in the Philippines and elsewhere, as a departure, an aberration, or not really imperial at all. Empire was something others did; if Americans expanded their territory it was the result of natural growth or a magnanimous desire to help others achieve similar freedom and virtues. Yet the British also told themselves throughout the nineteenth century that they were not imperialists, if the term was meant as a pejorative.[11] And, as the scholar Julian Go has observed, Americans were "well aware of the larger imperial field," especially the British presence in it, in which they undertook their efforts in the Philippines.[12] These were empires with interesting differences but crucial similarities, and considering them together offers insights into each in turn. There was also a transimperial exchange of information between the British in India and Americans in the Philippines. These empires were parallel undertakings with lateral connections. By the early twentieth century imperial agents were visiting each other's possessions and sharing ideas about how to address common problems, among them how to combat diseases such as malaria, cholera, and tuberculosis, what to do about lepers, how to manage sewage, how best to educate Indians and Filipinos, and more generally what to do with their puzzling and refractory Asian subjects.[13] European and American scientists, doctors, and sanitarians contributed to and read the same academic journals. In pursuit of their own comfort and welfare, Americans in the Philippines followed the British practice by creating a hill station to which to repair during the hottest season. Even critics of the US occupation found comparisons useful: in 1931, the anti-imperialist Senator Harry Hawes derided American officials in the islands as "imitators and champions of English satraps in India."[14]

Finally, Britons and Americans imagined themselves as part of a combined effort to civilize, in their own terms, others whom they regarded as backward in nearly every way. The British and Americans were linked by their shared understanding of a racialized Anglo-Saxonism; its self-proclaimed virtues, according to historian Paul Kramer, included "extraordinary purity and continuity, raging outward movement, and transformative power over land and people."[15] Both read avidly the work of Rudyard Kipling, the poet laureate of empire praised by American critics "as the greatest living English writer of fiction" at the end of the nineteenth century.[16] Soon after Admiral George Dewey defeated the Spanish fleet in Manila Bay in May 1898, Cecil Spring-Rice of the British Foreign Office wrote Theodore Roosevelt that the news of US annexation of the Philippines made him feel "as if a nightmare was over. It means possibly that our race and civilization is [*sic*] safe."[17] Roosevelt reciprocated the sentiment: the British, he said, had done "such marvelous things in India" that they could "gradually, as century succeeds century . . . transform the Indian population, not in blood, probably not in speech, but in government and culture, and thus leave [their] impress as Rome did hers on Western Europe."[18] A quarter century later, Lord Willingdon, formerly governor of the Madras and Bombay states, told the US Governor-General in the Philippines Leonard Wood that he hoped the Americans would stay on in the islands: "He is strongly of the opinion," Wood recorded, "that nothing could be more unfortunate for the English situation in India than for us to withdraw from here." Wood reassured his guest "that we had no intention of withdrawing."[19] In myriad ways, the British and Americans shared experiences of life in the tropics. They met with similar resistance, saw what they called beauty and monstrosity, heard sublime music and shrill cacophony, ate new foods that delighted or disgusted them, endured the same illnesses, felt the prickle of heat and humidity on their skins. Their noses wrinkled with pleasure and revulsion as they took in strong smells. In the heat and the wet their watches stopped; even time stood still.[20]

There was one other important similarity between the British and American empires, especially during the first decades of the twentieth century. In both cases, imperial policy was influenced by domestic changes, particularly the rise of social reform movements originating in Victorian Britain and emerging in the United States as Progressivism. Efforts to improve life in the metropoles—to change the habits of the poor and immigrants, to cleanse and beautify cities with parks, garbage collection, and the construction of modern sanitation systems, to reduce noise, to fight disease—were reflected in a variety of ways in India and the Philippines, and of course elsewhere in these empires. Even the reluctance to allow self-government by Asians was partly conditioned by fear of official corruption, of the kind progressives criticized in their own countries.[21] The process of reform also worked in reverse: solutions to problems tried first overseas might be applied to the metropoles too. And the racism of these empires was homegrown too: while Britons encountered far fewer people of color at home than Americans did, Indians who came to the United Kingdom experienced the kind of mistreatment that would have been familiar to African Americans.[22] These were empires formed from the inside out, and they were thus, for better or worse, sites of social experiment and innovation. The sensory stereotypes, preferences, and practices Britons and Americans brought with them to India and the Philippines had for years been rehearsed and refined at home; they were portable and powerful, well-sharpened instruments carried at times unthinkingly but always resolutely to imperial spaces.

The book—an extended essay really, but with a good number of footnotes—that follows is organized into chapters sense by sense, but also thematically and to some extent chronologically. It begins with a meditation on the senses and civilization, the concept that more than any other shaped thinking in imperial capitals about what empire meant and what it required. Self-government by their subjects was not the first thing on the minds of those who shaped empire. Yet the British eventually, and the Americans more quickly, came to understand that they could not formally control their colonies forever. Despairing of teaching the masses to behave properly, to learn English, to behave respectfully, and to lead clean lives, they focused on "civilizing" elite groups of Indians and Filipinos in order to prepare them for the responsibilities of eventual independence. Civilization meant rejecting the savage, the primitive, and the animal. It had gendered and class and religious meanings. It had emotional content. Above all, it was a racial concept, one that placed Anglo-Americans at the top of a naturalized hierarchy and men and women of color below. A crucial distinguishing feature of allegedly civilized whites was their respect for the five senses, something they claimed "uncivilized" people of color sadly lacked.

The next six chapters each take up a theme of empire in India and the Philippines by conveying an activity in process or an ongoing effort to achieve change. Chapter 2 concerns fighting. Both of these empires began with war. While the British East India Company had been in India since the late eighteenth century, only after a revolt by Indians beginning in 1857 did the British government establish formal rule over India as a colony, inserting its own officials into positions of authority and increasing the size of its army. The Americans came to the Philippines as part of their war against Spain in 1898, and while the Philippine front in that conflict at first cost little American blood, President William McKinley's announcement that the United States would annex the archipelago triggered three years of hard fighting with Filipinos determined to gain their independence. Britons and Americans tried to minimize the scope of these conflicts. To the British, the rising was the Sepoy Mutiny, a label that represented the struggle as undertaken only by a group of disgruntled Indian soldiers engaged in a convulsive but minor act. The Americans called the Philippines War an "insurrection," suggesting that it was a revolt against an established (American) government, though there existed in the islands no such thing when the fighting began in February 1899. Both of these conflicts established patterns of rule and instruments of colonial control that carried on for decades following their conclusions. And, as wars do, both provoked the direct engagement of Anglo-American and Asian bodies in ways that awakened and heightened the senses on all sides, initiating British and American campaigns to put Indian and Filipino senses right—in short, to bring civilization to people the westerners judged belligerent, primitive, and unmannerly.

Chapters 3 through 7 treat in turn each one of the five senses. Considering the senses separately prevents the jumbling together of perceptions that functioned in some measure independently of each other: each sense had its own value and valence in the pursuit of empire and its part in the quest to "civilize" Others. As chapter 3 shows, by the early twentieth century Britons and Americans insisted that sight was pre-eminent among the senses, and thus made it their first priority to reveal their subjects and make legible their social, political, and economic organization. As James Scott has argued, the state must "see" its constituents before it can rule them effectively. British and American governance relied on finding, counting, photographing, and making visually respectable their Indian and Filipino subjects—or at least the ones who might someday assume the responsibilities of governance themselves. The British and the Americans thus initially created in these colonies administrative units that were visible to them as rulers.[23]

Chapter 4 explores hearing, specifically efforts by the Anglo-Americans to remake the sonic environments of their possessions. Unnerved by the noise of the street and the indecipherability of Indian and Filipino speech, imperial officials sought first to get their subjects to quiet down—to cease their bell-ringing, cart-clattering, their high-pitched singing or discordant playing of instruments, the shouting of shopkeepers on market days—just as reformers back home were attempting to do with unruly lower classes and ethnic and racial minorities. If silence was seldom attainable, noise might be replaced by sound—that is, noise tamed and civilized. The ultimate goal of the British and Americans, elusive as it often seemed, was to educate some number of their elite subjects, training them in job skills and manners, but most pointedly teaching them to speak English. One could not know what an Indian soldier or a Filipino farmer was up to if one could not understand his language. Even if it was too much to hope that all Indians and Filipinos would learn English, if there were enough around who could understand and converse with their rulers and translate for the rest of their fellow citizens, it would make far easier the task of managing them all. Subjects must be made audible as they were legible.

Chapter 5 is the first of three chapters concerned with the pursuit of public health in India and the Philippines. Its concern is smell, perceptions of the odors of others' environments and bodies. When Britons and Americans arrived in India and the Philippines, they described themselves as under assault by odor. Some of the smells were pleasant, including flowers and the odors of the land at sunset in the Rajasthan desert or Manila's Luneta Park. Many more were noxious, and westerners at first ascribed to them directly some of the illnesses they suffered in the tropics. The land, they said, released miasmas, some of which were foul-smelling, others insidiously odorless, all borne on breezes into undefended noses. Westerners regarded bad smells as pathogenic. The perils were everywhere: marsh gases and the odors of hemp production, the smell of garbage or human bodies burning, the stink of rotting food or dead animals. Most prevalent and dangerous was human urine and especially excrement, left exposed and untreated in the open air or flowing in uncovered ditches and deposited in fields, rivers, or cisterns. Even as European and American cities were initiating their own sewage projects that carried human wastes underground and away from civilized noses, the builders of empire undertook similar sanitation programs in their imperial possessions. They attributed resistance to these plans to the stubborn primitivism of the "natives."

Touch—or rather, hapticity, the combination of touch (active) and feel (passive), through the fingertips and the skin—is the subject of chapter 6. The environments of the tropics felt wrong to the whites who entered them: the air was heavy on their skins, the land uneven underfoot, the allegedly coarse skins of the people who lived there rasped or oozed against their own on contact. "Native" bodies, claimed the foreigners, seethed with disease. The advent of the germ theory in the late nineteenth century came slowly. Yet over time, Britons and Americans who had been sure that the environments they had entered in Asia were pathological learned that mere inhalation of foul-smelling air would not kill them, though it likely indicated the presence of deadly substances. The pathogen itself was often a bacterium, and it could be absorbed only by direct contact, through an orifice or the open skin of an infected person or by ingestion of polluted food or water. Disease resided less in the land than in the people who inhabited it. This led the British after 1857 and the Americans immediately on their arrival in the Philippines to separate themselves as much as possible from their subjects. They created cantonments, tried to isolate themselves in their homes and offices, and went to hill stations when the weather turned uncomfortable. But they could never achieve full haptic isolation. They needed servants and soldiers. They would not resist sexual contact with Indians and Filipinos. Americans, and eventually the British too, realized that if they were in time to remove the formal trappings of their power from their possessions they would need to know their Asian counterparts haptically. To heal their illnesses they must touch them. The British would shake the hands of Indian politicians. The Americans would dance with Filipina women at the frequent *bailes* held in the Americans' honor. Again, revulsion and attraction characterized the sensory relationship between Anglo-Americans and their subjects.

The final chapter concerns taste, more broadly the act of consuming food and drink or the placing of substances in the mouth. Taste resides in the acculturated tongue of the taster. Confronted in their Asian colonies with unfamiliar foods and beverages, the British and Americans responded somewhat differently. The British in early nineteenth-century India opened themselves to the tastes of their new environment, often admitting that a diet of pulses and vegetables well cooked and spiced was desirable. Only after the Great Rebellion did the British grow suspicious of curry and rice. Like the treacherous sepoys, these foods seemed to threaten their bodies, causing them to lose control of their bowels and perhaps even poisoning them. They reverted to their own foods, imported from home or other colonies—though in the end, despite themselves, they could not fully jettison the flavors conjured by their Indian cooks. The first Americans, soldiers who came by the thousands to the Philippines, brought with them a suspicion of local practices, including foodways, and their rations were in any case prescribed for them by the army. Over time, as necessity required and the conflict abated, the Americans moved cautiously to consume Filipino food and drink, finding, for instance, that mangoes were irresistible. In the end, it was the sense of taste that proved most susceptible to synthesis, as Britons especially but Americans increasingly conceded that local foods were fresher and carried greater savor than imports from home.

The book concludes by contemplating the fate of these two imperia and the role of the senses in their formal end. The British and Americans did not disappear from India and the Philippines following independence but retained influence in their former colonies. India (and Pakistan) became members of the British Commonwealth, an association of Britain and most of its former colonies that recognize the monarch and consult together on a range of affairs. The United States kept large military bases in the Philippines and continued to dominate trade with the islands. But power devolved unquestionably to Indians and Filipinos. That it did was in part the result of a (reluctant) British and (somewhat less troubled) American recognition that elites in both nations had in some measure accomplished the sensory tasks their rulers had set for them. Leading Filipino men wore western clothes, and while this was not always the case in India, where the nationalists donned homespun *khadi* (cotton cloth woven by hand), at least most officials abjured Mohandas Gandhi's costume of a *dhoti* and a shirtless torso.[24] Paving roads and building railroads made travel quieter and smoother. Leaders in both nations spoke English, however accented, and so could be comprehended and negotiated with. Smells had been suppressed if not eliminated. Sewers were not ubiquitous, but the major cities had them, or parts of the cities did, and closed latrines existed even in some of the villages. Epidemic diseases such as cholera, smallpox, and malaria had declined in frequency and lethality. And, if the Americans accepted rather than delighted in Filipino cooking, the British embraced Indian food so much so that when they left India, a number of them brought their cooks back to Britain or became frequent diners at Indian restaurants there. In short, key Indians and Filipinos had adapted to the sensory regimes brought to them by their imperial rulers and had convinced their rulers to adapt to some extent to theirs. They no longer offended so grievously the standards of respectable behavior on which westerners, with no little hypocrisy, had insisted. They had become "civilized."

This book represents a new way to think about sensory, imperial, comparative, and international history. Its organization is something of a compromise between competing interests. Dividing the book into chapters dedicated to one sense at a time, for example, threatens the concept of intersensoriality, or the notion that no one sense does its work alone. As any attempt to consider the senses all at once, chapter by chapter, would have muddied the narrative, the book considers the senses collectively at its beginning and end, and, when relevant, includes the other senses in the intervening chapters that cover principally only one. Related to this challenge is that of analyzing change over time. It is hard to impose on empire's halting history a taxonomy of phases that explains in a linear fashion how matters evolved through time. A third challenge is the need to include in the analysis the sense perceptions not just those of the imperial powers but of Indians and Filipinos, and to treat all sides of their encounters with the balance they deserve. As often as possible, the book gives sensory presence to Indians and Filipinos, despite the limitations of the archival sources, and even if too often their words come through western interlocutors. While acknowledging this challenge is hardly the same as surmounting it, its recognition highlights how much work remains to be done on the subaltern sensorium. Finally, analysis on this scale—trying to represent the views of millions of Indians, Filipinos, Britons, and Americans—makes it impossible to speak of single cultures. While the book generalizes, it nevertheless distinguishes broadly among different constituencies in these four countries on the basis of class, caste, race, gender, religion, and maturity. For the most part, it focuses on the sensory culture of political elites. Britons and Americans concentrated their civilizing efforts on those Indians and Filipinos—the "enlightened" *bhadralok* and the *ilustrados*—for whom, whatever the westerners' doubts concerning their potential, there seemed at least some hope of achieving success.

The effort to "civilize" Indians and Filipinos by altering their sensory cultures was unquestionably about the exertion of power, by states and their agents, and about accommodation and resistance to it. The alleged dichotomy between causation and representation, and between culture and power, has been debated for years by foreign relations historians and others. The discussion, in my view, has gone the way of all attempts to posit binary oppositions in complex historical situations—that is, toward a reconciliation of perceived opposites, or the idea, in this case, that culture inheres in power and cannot be abstracted from it. Power was asserted, resisted, and transacted in thousands of encounters every day in India and the Philippines. Agency was contested. Overhanging all of these encounters stretched institutions of formal imperial authority: schools, prisons, hospitals, military compounds; the office of the Bombay Municipal Corporation; the leper colony established by the Americans on Culion Island in the Philippines. These were sites of power, wherein women and men were to be disciplined, altered, civilized. In all of them, the five senses of the parties were engaged.

Some of the key concepts deployed here require clarification. First, the terms "Selves" and "Others" are used to denote the perception that there were fundamental differences between Britons and Americans, on the one hand, and Indians and Filipinos, on the other. Although it traffics in binary oppositions without addressing complex historical circumstances, the descriptions of Selves and Others remain useful, if only because they—the descriptions, not the words—were frequently emphasized by men and women during the heyday of empire. Whatever the differences Anglo-Americans were willing to acknowledge among themselves, they were still (they claimed) more alike than different. They were civilized. Real difference was Otherness, characterized by alleged racial inferiority, tropic-induced indolence, a dangerous sexuality (despite male effeminacy), a penchant for violence, indifference to hygiene, and overall primitiveness. Others lacked respect for bodies, their own and those of others, and their manifest willingness to abuse and insult the senses made them uncivilized. Selves project onto Others their own most shameful traits and fantasies residing in the fraught categories of race, illness, and sexuality. When Selves made imperial subjects of Others, seeking to control their bodies and behaviors, they were in fact seeking self-control, a relief from their own anxiety.[25] The historian Francis Hutchins has written of "the Victorian predilection for ascribing to Indians precisely those traits which Victorians were taught to consider most reprehensible in their own lives," including savagery, lasciviousness, and childishness, and the Americans to whom Rudyard Kipling addressed his poem "The White Man's Burden" in 1899 might have recognized themselves as "Half devil and half child," and felt themselves challenged "To search your manhood / Through all the thankless years."[26]

Another binary concept that is imprecise yet unavoidable is the use of the words "West" (or "westerners") and "East" to characterize Europeans and Americans on one side and Asians on the other. These terms cannot actually represent the actual positions of east and west on a spherical globe, and they are also insidious in their assumption of Selfhood (the West) and Otherness (everywhere else). And yet these terms were used by these historical subjects frequently enough that it would seem forced to avoid them altogether. So while I do not accept their accuracy, they are occasionally a convenient shorthand. Even worse is the term "native," the use of which has become synonymous with profound condescension. When used in the writings of agents of empire, and quoted here, it therefore is placed it in quotation marks to highlight the period in which it appeared.

In the end, this book finds its footing in the interstices of what many foreign relations and imperial historians have long regarded as solid evidence. It concerns perception, feeling, bodies in contact, that elusive concept called culture, and of course the five senses. As the anthropologist Clifford Geertz put it: "No matter how much one trains one's attention on the supposedly hard facts of social existence, who owns the means of production, who has the guns, the dossiers, or the newspapers, the supposedly soft facts of that existence, what do people imagine human life to be all about, how do they think one ought to live, what grounds belief, legitimizes punishment, sustains hope, or accounts for loss, crowd in to disturb simple pictures of might, desire, calculation, and interest. Everyone, everywhere and at all times, seems to live in a sense-suffused world. . . . One can ignore such facts, obscure them, or pronounce them forceless. But they do not thereby go away. Whatever the infirmities of the concept of 'culture' . . . there is nothing for it but to persist in spite of them."[27] Above all, it was in the effort to "civilize" the subjects of empire, and the subjects' response to this effort, that we find most fully on display what "people imagine human life to be all about." The various meanings of the civilization concept in the nineteenth and early twentieth centuries captured the full range of the human sensorium, and its discussion will illustrate how the five senses shaped two empires over many decades. Let us open our eyes, ears, noses, hands, and mouths to a new apprehension of empire.

1

The Senses and Civilization

> If to be white and respectable meant to acquire behaviors that demanded restraint and civility, they also proscribed something else; racial and class "lower orders" did not share the prescribed attributes. Becoming adult and bourgeois meant distinguishing oneself from what was uncivilized, lower-class, and non-European.
>
> —Ann Laura Stoler, *Haunted by Empire* (2006)

> Colonialism minus a civilizational mission is no colonialism at all.
>
> —Ashis Nandy, *The Intimate Enemy* (1983)

When Britons came to India and Americans to the Philippines, they found all of their senses engaged, or "assaulted," as many of them said. The Britons' arrival, usually by ship into Bombay, was especially memorable. Even "before any land could be seen," recalled the British traveler Anne Bremner, "the hot air was filled with the smell of spices, until we eventually arrived in Bombay, where the thick aroma became part of the cacophony of noise from hordes of people, all shouting, pushing, and spitting red betel nut."[1] Margery Hall, a self-described "working girl from Birmingham" who arrived in 1938, wrote: "Bombay I remember well. It was the East's first assault upon my senses, and my memories are of heat, flies, noise, people, and horror of horrors the quayside, scarlet with blood so I thought. This turned out only to be millions of spits, mingled with betel nut."[2] "There is nothing in life that ever quite compares with the first discovery of the East, the genuine, flamboyant, garish East," concluded Major G. Horne. "Thus in wonder we had feasted our eyes on the new sights and harkened to the new sounds of that swirling colourful city half beautiful, half tawdry with its crowded streets and green gardens with thousands of crows wheeling and croaking above the trees and a railway station built very much like a cathedral in the grand Victorian style. . . . Here was gathered a kaleidoscope of colourful humanity . . . ; here also, amid the scents and sounds of browning *chapattis* and bubbling *ghi*, were the *charwalas*, the vendors of *pan* and dealers of rice and curries served on plates of banana leaves, the sellers of fruit and, as always, the wailing procession of beggars and the scurrying, scavenging 'pi' or *pariah* dogs."[3]

Then out of Bombay most of them went: to outposts in the Rajasthan desert, the mountains of the northwest, steamy Calcutta, the scrublands of Madras State in the south. Anne Bremner visited the coast near Portuguese Goa, where she encountered terrible roads that rattled her teeth, the distressing sight of men wearing only loincloths and "women in grubby cotton saris," and the "dreadful" smells of fermenting coconut and "filleted fish . . . nailed or hung from the trees, being dried for 'Bombay duck,'" a local delicacy.[4] Margery Hall followed her husband throughout north India, and while she delighted in the hill station at Simla—"the smell was of wood warmed by sun, pine and fir trees, spices, and light hilly air, so still and quiet that sound was almost an intrusion"—she recalled most vividly "the overwhelming heat of the plains in the hot weather; the strange smells, the strange people, causing the odd panic in me, and worms for breakfast! It was semolina porridge, and as I looked at it to add my sugar, I saw myriads of little cooked worms. It could almost be called worm porridge."[5] There were places in which the senses seemed to be intensified. For Mary Chenevix Trench, it was the train north toward a posting in Gilgit, in the Himalayas: "It was hot and dusty and every stop, night and day, rang with the yells of tea-boys and food vendors on the platform, while people shouted and struggled to get onto the train. By day I loved watching the people and the scenery and was suitably shocked by the way the train stopped at intervals in the country side in order that everyone (tho' not of course us in the first class carriage which included our own loo) might squat down in full view of us all. Meals were in a well appointed dining car but there is no doubt about it that English food in Indian trains and hotels is, or was, very nasty indeed. Greasy fried or watery scrambled eggs, stringy meat or chicken, bad vegetables and potatoes and no salads or raw fruit."[6] Viola Bayley visited Hindu women in purdah, away from the presence of men. There she found a baby "swaddled unbearably tightly [with] flies crawling round its eyes. I was told later that it was against custom to wash a baby during the first weeks. My nose could have apprised me of that fact! As I always found, the women were very friendly and one had to submit to having one's clothes fingered and commented on. Perhaps it was just as well that one didn't understand the language as the comments were obviously very frank."[7] Erica Farquharson and her husband attended a feast in their honor. "We were all garlanded and the smell of marigolds and tuberose, and the scratchy tinsel round my neck had to be endured and it was very hot," she recalled. "My eyes grew heavy with the heat, scent of flowers and glitter but we sat through it all and were polite until we could go home without offending our kindly, noisy, excitable hosts."[8]

The Indian bazaar was a particularly stimulating place, involving dazzling visual shifts in "an unplanned bricolage of structures," noise amounting to an ever-changing "symphony of diverse pitches, volumes, and tones," powerful aromas, attractive and far less so, constant physical contact with others' bodies, and confrontation with an array of foodstuffs, at once enticing and repulsive.[9] Deborah Dring found all her senses engaged in the market place: "Our parents always thought we'd catch something if we went down to the bazaar. But my brothers and I always looked upon the bazaar as being too exciting. All those lovely stalls covered with sticky sweets and silver paper and piles of fruit and those little flares they lit, the old boys sitting stitching clothes or boiling things in huge *dekshis*. I'll never forget the smell—partly a very strong spice, an incensy smell—and all that heat and the movements and the people and the colour. There was a little temple which had rows and rows of little brass bells all round. If you were a good Hindu you jingled all the bells as you passed, and I remember thinking, 'Now that's marvelous! If only I could go past and jingle a few bells.' But . . . the bazaar was a forbidden land when I was a child."[10]

There were fewer of these kinds of observations made by Americans in the Philippines, of whom there were never as many as there were Britons in India, and there were far fewer women, who were, as these accounts suggest, on the whole more eloquent in their sensory reminiscences than were men.[11] Yet the Philippines was nevertheless a shock to Americans' senses. Mary Fee came to the islands to teach in the first decade of the twentieth century. She arrived on the waterfront at Manila and took a horse-drawn cart, a *carromato*, into the city: "The carromato wheels were iron-tired, and jolted . . . . We rattled up [the] street." They pulled up at a church, just at noon: "Instantly there burst out such a clamor of bells as we had never before heard—big bells and little bells, brass bells and broken bells—and brass bands lurking in unknown spots seemed to be assisting. I do not know whether the Filipinos were originally fond of noise or whether the Spaniards taught them to be so. At any rate, they both love it equally well now." Then, to lunch: "We entered a stone-flagged lower hall where several shrouded carriages would have betrayed the use to which it was put had not a stable odor first betrayed it . . . It was a bare, cheerless apartment, hot in the unshaded light of a tropical noonday. The tables were not alluring. The waiters were American negroes. A Filipino youth, dressed in a white suit, and wearing his black hair in a pompadour, was beating out 'rag time' at a cracked piano." As for the food, "the vegetables were canned, the milk was canned, the butter was canned." Only the dessert was locally sourced—an "acid, flavorless banana and . . . gummy, sticky [guava] jelly."[12]

Like Deborah Dring, Grace Paulding found her senses fully engaged in the market, in her case in Mindanao. It was, she wrote, "by far the most barbaric and picturesque scene one could ever hope to look at. The dirt and smells were indescribable but, once you got used to that, it was a sight worth seeing and probably couldn't be duplicated anywhere else on earth."[13] When they believed they had effectively suppressed the movement for Philippine independence, American officers undertook to improve the health of their soldiers and the Filipinos whose bodies bore contagious diseases. They ordered a thorough examination of all schoolchildren, including "a study of the condition of sight, hearing, and examination for evidence of nasal obstruction, diseased tonsils, seriously defective teeth, disorders of nutrition . . . for enlarged glands, skin diseases"—all problems which threatened to prevent Filipinos from fully sensing their environment and the wishes of the Americans who now sought to control it.[14] Children were advised by the authors of a school textbook: "We need all our senses to examine things. . . . These senses are all controlled from the brain, and we can often, by use and attention, develop them, just as we can develop habits and train our muscles. We must therefore be careful (1) to take good physical care of our organs of sense; (2) not to dull our senses by alcohol, tobacco, tea, coffee, and injurious drugs; and (3) to train and develop the senses by using them correctly and for definite purposes."[15]

British and American senses told them many things about their hosts. Indians and Filipinos were, they thought, different from themselves, fundamentally Other. Opinion was divided over why that was so—the nature of Asians? The nature of all people of color? Their tropical environment?—but westerners believed that Indians and Filipinos were an exotic people, set apart by their habits and customs, the way they used their bodies, how they regarded and provoked the five senses. Westerners felt, for example, that their subjects loved "display," which meant the visual ostentation associated with bright colors and exaggerated performance, and that they also had a penchant for revealing too much of themselves. They made noise; they were boisterous, clamorous, excitable. Their felt environment was harsh, irritating to the skin or, because of their snakes, insects, and razor grass, a danger to western bodies—and yet their bodies, despite their apparent filthiness and coarseness, were alluring and might be touched, even penetrated. They reeked of stables and excrement and rotting fish; they were also fragrant and "incensy" and smelled bracingly of pine and "bubbling *ghi*." Like Mary Fee's banana, their food was "acid," "flavorless," "gummy"—and yet so often more tempting than the watery eggs on trains in India or the canned butter eaten by Americans in the Philippines. Frightening and attractive, dangerous and beguiling, appalling and charming, confounders of expectation and the ways of propriety and decency, Indians and Filipinos were, without question, regarded by their uninvited British and American guests as *uncivilized*.

Civilization was a concept with broad currency in nineteenth and twentieth century Europe and the United States. The word was used frequently in political discourse. Britons and Americans regarded civilization as having started with the Greeks and Romans, and saw themselves as its rightful heirs. When medieval Europeans embarked on "wars of colonization and expansion," according to Norbert Elias, they made contact with "lesser" Others, pagans and heretics representing barbarism. Fearful that as a result of these campaigns the

Catholic Church and "chivalrous society" were under threat, western Europeans embraced the concept of *civilité,* "an expression and a symbol of a social formation" that would distinguish themselves, the anxious guardians of "the West," from the soulless, fetid hordes they encountered on the frontier. Elias dates the rise of *civilité* to the 1530 publication of the treatise *De civilitate morum puerilium* (On civility in children) by Desiderius Erasmus. The treatise was popular—Elias finds 130 editions in a variety of languages—and it concerned "outward bodily propriety," manners, and the refinement of the senses and the sense organs. Civilized people had good manners, and knew to avoid offending the senses. It was particularly important not to disgust others. Erasmus insisted, for example, on proper care of the nose and its contents. There should be no mucous showing in the nostrils. Only peasants and sausage makers wiped their noses on their clothing or their caps; civilized people blew their noses into a cloth. It was acceptable to blow with one's fingers, but if the discharge hit the ground, "it must be immediately trodden away with the foot." Erasmus inspired others, among them the seventeenth-century diplomat Antoine de Courtin, who advised: "You should avoid yawning, blowing your nose, and spitting. If you are obliged to do so in places that are kept clean, do it in your handkerchief . . . and do not look into your handkerchief afterward." Advice on decorum in seeing and smelling came from the Florentine Enlightenment writer Giovanni Della Casa: "It does not befit a modest, honorable man to prepare to relieve nature in the presence of other people; nor to do up his clothes afterward in their presence. . . . For the same reason, it is not a refined habit, when coming across something disgusting in the street, as sometimes happens, to turn at once to one's companion and point it out to him. It is far less proper to hold out the stinking thing for the other to smell, as some are wont, who even urge the other to do so, lifting the foul-smelling thing to his nostrils and saying, 'I should like to know how much that stinks,' where it would be better to say, 'Because it stinks do not smell it' "—though Della Casa has not yet reached the point of refusing to touch "the thing." Scrupulousness came also to the consumption of food. Civilized people washed their hands before eating. "It is not very decorous to offer something half-eaten to another," wrote Erasmus, and "it shows little elegance to remove chewed food from the mouth and put it back on the [platter]. If you cannot swallow a piece of food, turn round discreetly and throw it somewhere." Much later, in 1859, an anonymous author prescribed the use of a fork, since to eat with the fingers was "cannibal." These and other manners would be invoked by the British and Americans in their empires, where they observed, with alarm and disgust, their violation by their allegedly uncivilized subjects.[16]

While the definition of civilization evolved in the years following the Enlightenment, it retained that part of its meaning concerning manners and thus the senses. In his *Reflections on the French Revolution* (1790), Edmund

Burke wrote of "our manners, our civilization, and all the good things which are connected with manners, and with civilization," presumed by him to be in jeopardy in France. John Stuart Mill pondered the matter in an 1840 essay: "Take for instance the question how far mankind has gained by civilization. One observer is forcibly struck by the multiplication of physical comforts; the advancement and diffusion of knowledge; the decay of superstition; the facilities of mutual intercourse; the softening of manners; the decline of war and personal conflict; the progressive limitation of the tyranny of the strong over the weak; the great works accomplished throughout the globe by the co-operation of multitudes." Manners remained explicitly part of Mill's definition. The attainment of "physical comforts" and "the decay of superstition" also demanded the removal of sensory offense: a civilized hapticity required the comfort of, say, a soft bed, while the kind of practice a Briton like Mill might have associated with superstition—ingesting a strong-smelling substance to cure illness, perhaps—would have seemed an affront to sight, taste, and smell.[17]

In the United States, the nineteenth-century definition of civilization hewed close to that of the British. *Webster's American Dictionary of the English Language,* published in 1841, led its entry with "the act of civilizing, or the state of being civilized; the state of being refined in manners, from the grossness of savage life, and improved in arts and learning."[18] The 1900 edition defined civilization as "national culture" and "refinement," and included the quotation from Burke associating civilization with manners. Its definition of "civilize" began, "To reclaim from, or cause to come out of, a savage or barbarous state; to instruct in the rules and customs of civilization." A copy of this edition was sent to William Howard Taft, the first US Governor-General of the Philippines, in 1904.[19] Ethnologist W. J. McGee suggested that the difference between Anglo-Saxons and the "barbarous or semi-barbarous peoples of the world" had to do with whites' "sensitiveness to temperature, delicacy of touch and taste, [and] acuteness of vision and hearing."[20]

Civilization was defined against an uncivilized Other so as to reassure the Self of its own tenuously felt superiority. It was a process; transactional, not static. These features made it a concept well suited to the many purposes of empire at its genesis. Sir William Jones, who served as judge of the Supreme Court in Calcutta during the late eighteenth century and was the first Briton to learn Sanskrit, claimed that India had once been a great civilization, and that its history and language were therefore worth studying.[21] James Mill, a political economist who worked for the East India Company for seventeen years, disagreed with Jones. In his 1817 three-volume study *The History of British India,* Mill argued that India's civilization had never matched England's. "Our ancestors," he wrote, "however . . . rough, were sincere, but, under the glossing exterior of the Hindu lies a general disposition to deceit and perfidy." Muslims exhibited "the same insincerity and perfidy; the same indifference to the feeling of others, the prostitution and venality." Chapter 7 of Mill's first volume was titled "Manners." Its subheadings included "Proneness to Adulation, Perjury, Inhospitality, Cruelty and Ferocity, Timidity, Litigiousness, Proneness to Foul Language, Love of Repose, Avarice." Overall, Mill concluded, India was a "rude" nation, a natural target for the British civilizing mission. With the publication of *History*, Mill became the most important figure in the Anglicist school of Indology, which challenged Jones's more favorable "Orientalist" account of India's past. The book became required reading at Haileybury College, training ground for civil servants of the East India Company.[22]

Even those who adopted James Mill's corrosive view of Indian civilization refused to consider hopeless the cause of reforming Indian society, or some portion of it, someday. What historian John Darwin has called "liberal imperialism" emerged to counter the pessimists, especially those discouraged by Mill's insistence on India's backwardness. Despite the spiritual and moral drag of Hindu and Muslim superstition, it might be possible, and it would be desirable, to create a class of English-speaking Indians. John Stuart Mill, who (like his father) worked for the East India Company, was a liberal imperialist. He condemned "barbarous" Indian practices, among them female infanticide, *sati* (the immolation of widows), and "witchcraft," yet felt that with the proper institutions India could move ahead on the scale of civilization. He rejected the claim that Indians were inherently depraved, by reason of race or climate, and he felt that England might train an Indian "lettered class." In 1875 Oxford professor Henry Maine, who had served as legal adviser to the Viceroy in India, declared that India belonged to that "very family of mankind to which we belong." But institutions had "been arrested in India at an early stage of development," leaving the country "a barbarism" that nevertheless "contains a great part of our own civilisation, with its elements as yet inseparate and not yet unfolded."[23] Efforts persisted to bring civilization to India.

In the late nineteenth-century United States, civilization, as historian Gail Bederman notes, "was protean in its applications."[24] US officials invoked with fervor the imagined need to carry it to the Philippines, as if it were a gift. In January 1899, just after President William McKinley declared his intention to annex the Philippines through "benevolent assimilation," he told members of the First Philippines Commission, appointed by him to govern the islands, that "we accepted the Philippines from high duty in the interest of their inhabitants and for humanity and civilization."[25] The Commission agreed, in its initial report to the president: "The aim and object of the American Government, apart from the fulfillment of the solemn obligations it has assumed toward the family of nations by the acceptance of sovereignty over the Philippine Islands, is the well being, the prosperity, and the happiness of the Philippine people and their elevation and advancement to a position among the most civilized peoples of the world."[26] McKinley took this message to the Midwest during the fall of 1899, as he repeatedly invoked the desire of the United States to civilize its new possession. As he put it to one audience: "Our flag in the Philippines still waves there, and it waves not as the banner of imperialism, it waves not as the symbol of oppression, but it waves as it waves here and everywhere, the flag of freedom, of hope, of home, of civilization."[27] Little changed when Theodore Roosevelt became president following McKinley's assassination. In his annual message to Congress in December 1904, Roosevelt said that the islands were "at present . . . utterly incapable of existing in independence at all or of building up a civilization of their own. I firmly believe that we can help them to rise higher and higher in the scale of civilization and of capacity for self-government. . . . The justification for our stay in the Philippines must ultimately rest chiefly upon the good we are able to do in the islands."[28] There was disagreement among officials in Manila and Washington about how long it might take to civilize the Philippines, or just what that entailed. Some doubted that it was possible at all. But "civilization" was the word used repeatedly by those concerned with this American mission. Like Britons, the Americans believed themselves capable of refashioning Asians, and they would not countenance the possibility that they could not or should not do so.

The Elements of Civilization

By the early twentieth century the British and American concept of civilization contained a number of constituent elements, all of them related to the senses. One of these was religion. In imperial Great Britain and the United States, civilized people were Christians of a certain sort. The Church of England had explicitly rejected Catholicism in the sixteenth century, and Anglicans remained suspicious and fearful that Catholics might try to subvert their religious practices. The Islam and especially the Hinduism they encountered in India seemed even worse, though perhaps not so different from Catholicism, in their strangeness. Americans were overwhelmingly Protestant. Many had long suspected Catholics of seeking the eclipse of New World liberties through the extension of papal authority to the Americas. They linked Irish and Italian Catholic immigrants to criminality and depravity, and they fought wars with Catholic Mexico and with Spain, accused by the United States of having committed church-sanctioned atrocities in Cuba. Hindus and Catholics appeared to Britons and Catholics to Americans as foreign and dangerous, perhaps less because of the substance of their doctrines than of the vivid forms taken by their rituals. Hindu and Catholic practices seemed to threaten their senses and their bodies. Such Anglo-American fears underpinned the domestic sources of sensory offense taken in their colonies.

British visitors to India were routinely horrified by the religious manifestations they encountered there. They were suspicious of Sikh men, whose turbans appeared to conceal something sinister; of Parsis, who exposed their dead to carrion birds on Bombay's Towers of Silence; and of Muslims' alleged cruelty and fanaticism—the Self's unsettling Other.[29] Most disturbing were India's Hindus. In the seventeenth century, John Milton contrasted the "'liberty' and civil life and worship of his countrymen with the abjectness of peoples who were 'stupified [*sic*] by the wicked arts of priests' and 'merely worship as gods those demons they are unable to put to flight.'" Milton was describing Catholics, but as historian Lawrence James observes, "he could have easily been referring to Hindus as they were perceived by Britons" who later encountered them.[30] William Carey, an itinerant preacher who arrived in Calcutta in 1793, was appalled by what he witnessed there: "idols the very personification of sin . . . the lecher Krishna and his concubine Radha . . . No Bibles, no sabbath, no God but a log of wood, no saviour but the Ganges . . . no morality, for how should a people be moral whose gods are monsters of vice, whose priests are their ringleaders in crime . . . whose heaven is a brothel?"[31] The "lecher Krishna," "heaven is a brothel"—Carey, and many other Britons, deplored the alleged licentiousness of Hinduism. The nineteenth-century traveler Rosalie Roberts visited a Hindu temple in South India. She found the outside "wonderful," adorned with lights that made it look like "a fairyland." But the inside was "revolting. All the little niches had idols where there had been sacrifices and the blood was spilt there. There was the stench and the darkness, just the flickering light by the idols." Her senses affronted, she turned away in horror.[32]

As Britain confronted the implications of its formal control of India after 1858, a religious controversy arose at home that would come to intersect with its imperial concerns. It involved the rise of Ritualism in the Church of England. Ritualism represented for its adherents a corrective to the austerity of church practices over the previous centuries. The color and excitement of the Christian service had diminished, and the Ritualists hoped to restore them by energizing once more "the six points of ritual observance: the eastward position at Holy Communion, mixing water with wine in the chalice, the use of wafer bread, lighted candles on the altar, vestments, and incense." Ritualists defended the restoration of these practices as consistent with Anglicanism. Their opponents disagreed, claiming that Ritualism was Catholicism seeking to steal its way back into the core of British religious life. Parishioners complained about the re-emergence of ritual—"our light and beautiful highways are darkened and to our English sense rendered loathsome and terrible by these associations of the Inquisition," said one—and were unhappy in particular with the return of "incense much too profusely used, almost so as to render the procession at times invisible." Queen Victoria pronounced herself "shocked and grieved" that "the higher classes and so many of the young clergy [were] tainted with this leaning towards Rome!" The use of incense in Anglican churches was duly banned in 1868, and in 1874 Parliament passed the Public Worship Act, which forbade "any alteration in or addition to the fabric, ornaments, or furniture" of a church and deviations from the Book of Common Prayer. Ritualism nevertheless flourished through the end of the nineteenth century. In 1874, 136 churches in England and Wales had lighted candles and used vestments; eight years later, 581 used candles and 336 vestments. By the 1890s, the rise of Ritualism had created a crisis in the Church and led to the establishment of a Royal Commission on Ecclesiastical Discipline.[33]

The Ritualist Controversy coincided with the establishment of the Raj and thus increasing encounters by Britons with Hindu ritual. The "bells and smells" of Catholicism corresponded closely to the sensory practices of Hindus. Men called priests presided over both of these apostate faiths; both involved what to Protestants was idol worship, the frequent tolling of bells, the bodily proximity of worshippers to priests and to each other, and the heavy odor of incense. At the height of the controversy, Lord Arthur Charles Hervey charged that the ritualists "were as fanatical as the Indian mutineers," a comparison that many Anglicans would have found persuasive.[34]

The American Episcopal Bishop Charles Henry Brent arrived in the Philippines on August 24, 1902. Brent was to lead the newly established bishopric there; his mission was to proselytize for the true Christian faith and thus assist American officials with their civilizing work. Days after his arrival, he recorded in his diary: "This is sure[:] the people who come to these islands must do one of two things—be dragged down by the life here or elevate that life. If they are not missionary they will deteriorate morally—Evil communications corrupt good manners . . . or else good manners kill evil communications."[35] He was outwardly confident in his own mission, certain that there was no tension between secular and religious objectives, and convinced that his labors would have wide ambit. As he put it, "never before in the history of colonization has the avowed policy of the conquering country been so wholly unselfish. . . . We have set an ideal before our nation and before the civilized world that will tend to create a public conscience in every civilized nation which eventually will dominate the colonial policy of other civilizations. We have taken a course that will leave a deep impression on the life of man."[36] Brent traveled throughout the archipelago, often in the company of the US commissioners who governed the islands, trying first to assess the religious life of Filipinos, then trying to alter it as subtly yet surely as his position would allow. Brent believed he served two populations: the first Catholics, who had been converted to the faith under

Spanish rule; the second the Muslim and "pagan" inhabitants of the mountains and jungles, "savages" steeped in ignorance though not without redeeming characteristics. Toward the Catholics Brent felt ambivalence. In a 1904 assessment, he wrote: "Far be it from me to excuse, much less sympathize with, that encouragement of superstitious folly which Rome is guilty of. I am simply trying to say that though it hinders it does not nullify her work for Christ." Filipino Catholics had renounced paganism and believed in the divinity of Christ. Yet there was "grave moral laxity . . . under the shadow of the church and convents . . . in the Philippines." The Filipinos were by nature sensual and lazy, and the church had done nothing to discourage their licentious behavior. Instead, it pandered to their sensory excesses, which reflected its own. He despaired over the church-sanctioned system of *querida*, whereby men would take multiple lovers, and it was widely reported that Spanish priests had multiple mistresses too, and that they raped Filipino women and men as they felt the urge. Most of all, Catholicism encouraged Filipinos in their instinctive credulity. With the permission of the priests, "they will kiss the hand of a tinsel-decked scamp who having smeared himself with shoe-dressing announced himself as the 'Black Christ'; they will drink the foul bubblings of escaping sewage because someone has started the report that it was a miraculous well; they will listen with reverence to the myth of a wooden doll which, its priestly guardian affirms, takes periodical journeys of a supernatural character—and so one could easily go on." Along with the *querida* system, these popular sensory superstitions had unhappy consequences. Brent's reference to "foul bubblings" concerned the "miracle of Antipolo," in which people became convinced that a broken sewer pipe was the fount of a miraculous well with curative properties; instead, it contributed to the spread of cholera. The man calling himself the "Black Christ" tricked residents by deceiving them visually and demanded their loyalty by touch. In short, the church had betrayed its parishioners by condoning the violation of their bodies.[37]

Brent felt happiest upcountry, among ethnic groups different from the Spanish and Tagalog-speaking Catholics with whom Americans spent most of their time. In early 1903, he spread the gospel among the Igorots in Bontoc.[38] There were nearly two hundred thousand people in need of ministry, and as they were devoid of "the vices of civilization," the bishop had full scope to improve them as human beings. They had already made a start. Local militia members had "cut their hair" and donned "kahki [*sic*] clothing"; they were now "fine looking fellows." They were not ready to be baptized, but they asked Brent "to give them new names, like Christians," which would make it easier for the Americans to identify them aurally.[39] In June 1905 Brent sang the Eucharist and read scripture in Ilocano, then baptized dozens of evidently eager locals, altering at once their auditory and tactile environments.[40] Nearly twenty years later, Governor-General Leonard Wood, eulogizing President Warren Harding, said he was "confident" that the late president "felt that the two greatest blessings that have ever come to the Philippine Islands are, first, Christianity, which was brought by Spain, and with it came Western ideas of civilization, laws and methods of government. The second was the American flag."[41]

Ideas about civilization and the senses were also gendered. Envisioning civilization and imagining how it was meant to sound were considered masculine pursuits, requiring detachment, logic, and the ability to mobilize military and civil resources on its behalf. Women had different sensory roles to play. To them were reserved the still vital civilizing tasks linked to those senses regarded by late nineteenth-century Europeans and Americans as lesser—smell, touch, and taste—and then in the domestic sphere alone.[42] Men would make empires and plan how they should look and sound, in accordance with their definition of civilization. Women were charged with softening imperial subjects and their environments, teaching manners of the sitting room, the dining room, the kitchen, and the toilet. These tasks were in fact not always so easy to categorize and distinguish from each other, just as the senses worked in concert. And they were complicated and challenged by subjects who defied the clumsy binary thinking about gender that westerners brought from home.

The officials who launched empires were male. They made war in India and the Philippines in order to eliminate the alleged enemies of progress. Thereafter, the first requirement of governance was seeing—making legible—the state's subjects and their lands. Its second requirement was quieting noise and the babble of languages and educating subjects in the importance of well spoken, reasoned discourse, preferably in English. Women had a role to play in this task as teachers, though it was too much to expect them to impose discipline on unruly boys and men. There were roles for women in the home, in the realms of smell, touch, and taste, reputed to be keener senses in women. Detection of odors and interpretation of their meanings, the feel through delicate skin of the humid or smooth or harsh, the ability to cook and taste or manage a kitchen—in these ways women were to be particularly alert to the process of civilizing the empire. It would not be easy. In India, historian Margaret Macmillan has written, "the memsahibs struggled to keep Britain alive. . . . The struggle was absurd but there was a sort of heroism in it. They planted English flowers in their gardens and the heat withered them. They covered their furniture with chintz and the white ants chewed their way through. They got patterns for their clothes from Home but the native tailor somehow altered them subtly. They served English food even though half of it had to come out of tins. In a supreme gesture of defiance they reserved the hottest time of the day—between twelve and two—for receiving calls from gentlemen."[43] As for the Philippines, "American women in Manila largely set standards," according to writer Stanley Karnow. "Like the British *memsahibs* of India, they were determined to preserve their code of conduct in a foreign land." This proved difficult too, as it seemed to require them to avoid contact with Filipinos altogether, even those of high social class.[44] Empire's men worked outside the home. The offensive or dangerous odor of garbage or excrement required sanitary projects that only men could undertake. A rough road demanded male engineering; treating illness was left finally to the sight, hearing, and touch of male physicians. The job of imperial women was the olfactory, haptic, and gustatory refinement of subjects in domestic spaces.

There were two problems with the expectation that Anglo-American women would civilize the domestic and men the public spaces of empire. First, the tropical environment was thought to wear especially hard on western women, indoors or out. Discourse had it that white women were more sensitive to heat and other extremes of weather, more fearful of contact with the people and the animals found in Asia, and more inclined to have strong emotional reactions to the unpredictability and hazards of life generally in an Asian culture. The eighteenth-century author John Clark claimed that in the tropics, women's "lively bloom and ruddy complexions" were "soon converted into a languid paleness; they become supine and enervated, and suffer many circumstances, peculiar to the sex, from mere heat of climate and relaxation of the system," a view that endured well into the twentieth century.[45] American soldiers who had hoped their wives would join them in the Philippines nearly always changed their minds because of the perceived dangers of life in the islands.[46] Civilization could not be effected by women compromised by the harshness of life in the tropics, or by women who were because of it deterred from coming out at all. The second problem with the sensory division of labor in these empires was that Indian and Filipino subjects had different gender preferences and identities than did their occupiers. Women resisted the gaze and touch of a male doctor, especially if he was a foreigner. Indian and Filipino men did not behave with the same masculine affect that heterosexual white men demanded of themselves and others. British and American men frequently derogated the masculinity of Indian (particularly Hindu) and Filipino (mainly Tagalog) men. Hindus seemed to Britons soft, cowardly, and effeminate in their movements and behaviors.[47] In 1914 the cavalry subaltern Robert Baden-Powell wrote to his mother: "I like my native servants, but as a rule niggers seem to me cringing villains. As you ride or walk along the middle of the road every cart or carriage has to get out of your way, and every native as he passes you, gives a salute. . . . If you meet a man in the road and tell him to dust your boots, he does it."[48] Americans regarded the Filipinos with whom they worked as emotional rather than reasonable, inclined to crow in victory and sulk in loss, given to sudden anger and off-putting giddiness, and bound to others "less for their convictions than for their affections," as historian Theodore Friend observed.[49] These were hardly suitable subjects for self-rule.

Another element of the Anglo-American sensory definition of civilization concerned the maturity of cultures and peoples. Britons and Americans granted that India and the Philippines had long histories, even if (they felt) not very distinguished ones. On one hand, the buildings, infrastructure, and the land itself in these places were ancient, decrepit, rotted by age; on the other, the people who inhabited the two countries were fundamentally immature—small of stature, callow, gullible, and emotional. The lack of civilization in both countries had left their people underdeveloped, unable either to fashion or cope with modern societies. Indians and Filipinos, in short, resembled children and were thus unready to govern themselves.

They exhibited their supposed immaturity in a variety of ways. Like children, Asians lacked control of their sphincters, for how else could one explain the profusion of public excreta that disgusted and alarmed the Anglo-Americans? Indians and Filipinos seemed sanguine at the sight and smell of shit, much as children were, they were boisterous and loud, and the pulses and porridges they ate seemed to westerners better suited for toothless babies than civilized adults. Like children, Indians and Filipinos (claimed their rulers) lacked a sense of time, being always late for appointments and unable to stick to schedules. Indians and Filipinos were alleged to be naïve, petulant, poor with numbers and deficient in linear thinking overall, and quarrelsome among themselves and with their imperial masters. In India, the British allowed themselves to believe for a time that Indians would maintain for them the sort of fidelity that children gave their parents. They took satisfaction in being called by their subalterns "ma-baap," the Urdu term meaning "mother" or "parent."[50] The Great Rebellion of 1857–1858 thus seemed to Britons a betrayal of the most basic sort of trust, but it reinforced the idea that Indians were immature—indeed so much so that they were incapable of sustaining any sense of fidelity. The author of a manual for Britons bound for India advised her readers that servants "must be treated like children, kindly but very firmly." This was because "their brains are not properly developed and they cannot always see things in the same light as we do."[51] The same, the Americans thought, was true of Filipinos. Edith Moses's servants would not stay on task. "The Filipinos," she concluded, "are like children and love to do everything but the thing they are set to do."[52] Bishop Brent was taken aback by the abiding immaturity of Filipinos—"perennial children," he called them—and Governor Taft regarded "the child-like character of the people" as disqualifying them for self-rule anytime soon.[53]

The ascription of immaturity to subjects was an imperial construct. Clear authority and a firm grip were necessary to govern an Indian—"as incapable as a child of understanding what authority means," wrote Kipling—and Filipinos, "babies of the jungle," as the *New York Times* put it in 1899.[54] Civilization was for adults; to imagine that children were civilized was absurd. Tutelage was a necessary responsibility of civilized people attempting to guide and control the uncivilized.[55]

So too did self-declared civilized people in the late nineteenth century understand that the refinement of the senses was a necessary predicate for elevated class standing. Men and women of culture, of the better classes, respected their bodies and those of others. They were well dressed and smelled clean (which often meant the use of overpowering perfumes and colognes), spoke in well-modulated voices and avoided raucousness and noise, had smooth, light skins and wore refined garments, and ate carefully prepared foods in a mannerly way. The lower classes did none of these things, or did none of them well.[56] The higher orders avoided bodily trespass and thus sensory violation or the spread of disease. American public health nurse Ellen La Motte claimed that "the millionaire, the professional man, and the bank clerk' might . . . learn . . . what they needed to know to protect others from consumption," while "the day laborer, the shop girl, the drunken negro belong to a class which, *by reason of the very conditions which constitute it a class,* is unable to make use of what it learns."[57] "That was what we were taught—*the lower classes smell,*" wrote George Orwell.[58] By the nineteenth century, according to western elites, "disease, minimal amounts of dry grooming, and unwashed rags and underlinen meant that the bodies of the poorest smelled intensely, with strong animal odors, compared to the washed or scented population. The very poorest," writes author Virginia Smith, "were sometimes described by fearful people as 'savages,' 'brutes,' or 'animals'—traditional terms describing those beyond the boundaries of society, the untouchables, the impure."[59]

These were terms assigned to the lower classes by way of categories that were also racial, and conferred as well on imperial subjects by the representatives of empire. What described the poor in Britain and the United States also described the vast majority of Indians and Filipinos; here again, note the domestic then foreign application of sensory stereotyping. All had failed to achieve the sort of sensory refinement necessary for their inclusion among the ranks of the civilized. "So long it took me," recalled Iris Macfarlane, an Englishwoman in India, "to shake off my . . . assumptions that the lower classes and the coloured races didn't 'feel' things the same way, having simple nervous systems, like lobsters."[60] The language used by social reformers to describe the residents of urban slums in London and New York was the same as that used by those who encountered lower-class or -caste subjects in the colonies. It was exoticizing language, useful to those who spoke it as a way of classifying their subjects and making them legible, or of simplifying that which challenged or bewildered or frightened them. The British and the Americans regarded especially the poorest of their imperial charges, including beggars, for instance, as lesser men and women, and consigned them to the lowest places in the sensorium. They smelled bad. They looked alarming or repulsive, sounded loud and jarring, ate noxious food and drank foul beverages, and spread disease by contact. Like the poor of America and Europe, they were offensive in their apparent enthusiasm for spitting, belching, urinating, and defecating in public.

Savages, brutes, animals: here were terms of opprobrium, of class difference, of abiding ascriptions of Otherness. But their essence was racial. It was race, a word of staggering complexity and many dimensions, that Anglo-Americans deployed most often by 1900 to distinguish Selves from Others. Selves were racially fit, from good stock, rational, clean and decent, pure. Others were racially inferior, consigned, perhaps forever, to a status limited by their own inherent failings, their unhappy lineage, their depravities, their baseness. In the idea of race the concept of civilization and understanding of the five senses came together most powerfully in the late nineteenth and early twentieth centuries. People were regarded as uncivilized because of their supposed racial inferiority. Race-thinking emerged when there was a felt need to justify oppression and domination, and where vision could not reliably discern race. In British India this happened because Indians often exhibited (Britons admitted) more politesse than their own citizens, or were patently sophisticated and urbane, or came in a bewildering variety of colors, or were intimate with them in wholesome and affectionate ways, not infrequently producing offspring that defied once-stable racial categories imported from Britain. White Americans, who had encountered people of color at home before arriving in the Philippines, had been frequently confounded in their efforts to classify Others by race, taken in by mixed race people or those who "passed" as white.[61] And how to categorize Filipinos, some of whom looked like white Yankees, spoke elegant Spanish, and bathed with far greater frequency than the American soldiers who had come to civilize them? Race was supposed to be a science of classification, but it failed every test of predicting human behavior or even appearance. In the empires of Asia, the senses of the conqueror would be put to hard and immediate test in their effort to differentiate one race from another.[62]

Racial Others were those who offended the senses or threatened to violate the boundaries of the sensing body. They were regarded as filthy, diseased, and sexually aggressive, impinging on the permeable membranes of the Selves' sense organs and skins.[63] Anglo-Americans tried to construct racial boundaries between themselves and their imperial subjects. They did this in part with language. Whites referred constantly to Indians and Filipinos as "niggers." Britons and Americans separated themselves from those whom they ruled, reliant as they were on servants and functionaries but nevertheless hoping to see and hear as little of them as possible. In India, some public spaces were reserved for whites alone, and Britons avoided sitting near Indians on trains by segregating the cars, formally or through practice.[64] Kipling concluded his story "Beyond the Pale" with the moral that "a man should, whatever happens, keep to his own caste, race, and breed. Let the White go to the White and the Black go to the Black."[65] When a delegation of Filipino nationalists proposed to Secretary of State Elihu Root that the Philippines be made a state, Root dismissed them, declaring that "statehood for Filipinos would add another serious race problem to the one we have already. The Negroes are a cancer on our body politic, a source of constant difficulty, and we wish to avoid developing another such problem."[66] Bishop Brent rode into the Philippine highlands on a horse named Jim Crow; Philippine Governor-General Leonard Wood screened D. W. Griffiths's film *The Birth of a Nation,* which valorized the Ku Klux Klan, and found "nothing in it in any way objectionable."[67]

The bastion of a separate white racial identity in both British India and the American Philippines was the private club. Behind its walls, on its tennis courts and polo fields, in its restaurants and bars where the business of empire was transacted, only servants were permitted, and then only discreetly. It did not matter that Indian princes were far wealthier than the British who drank gin in the dark rooms, or that within the first decade of American rule in the Philippines there were Filipino legislators, commissioners, and medical doctors, none of whom were allowed inside the club as members. "Whiteness was all when it came to assessing worth" in India, recalled Iris Macfarlane.[68] Lady Chapman remembered that "clubs were strictly for white people," though she was certain that this was satisfactory to Indians ("Nobody seemed to wish to integrate").[69] While the policy eased to some extent after World War I, especially in remote posts, much could still go awry. An Indian doctor asked Kenneth Mason to put him up for membership at the club in Dera Doon. Mason invited the man to dinner, and all went well until the doctor suddenly cleared his throat and spat on the floor. Horrified, the Britons blackballed him.[70] Much of the narrative tension in George Orwell's *Burmese Days* results from the effort by the British civil servant Flory to convince his countrymen to admit the Indian doctor, Veraswami, to the club, the only social institution of consequence in their remote river town. The functionary Ellis won't hear of it: "My God, I should have thought in a case like this, when it's a question of keeping those black, stinking swine out of the only place where we can enjoy ourselves, you'd have the decency to back me up. Even if that pot-bellied, greasy little sod of a nigger doctor *is* your best pal. . . . Do what you like outside the Club. But, by God, it's a different matter when you talk of bringing niggers in here. I suppose you'd like little Veraswami for a Club member, eh? Chipping into our conversations and pawing everyone with his sweaty hands and breathing his filthy garlic breath in our faces."[71] Similar restrictions applied to club membership in the Philippines. Insistent on taking recreation with "their own kind," the Americans barred Filipinos from the Elks Club and the Army and Navy Club. Filipinos, observes Stanley Karnow, "could not play golf at the Manila Club or belong to the University Club, created by Taft for leading American civilians. Nor were they welcome at the Columbia Club, which Bishop Brent had founded as an American social center." Only in 1936, the year after he was elected president of the new Philippine commonwealth, was Manuel Quezon allowed "honorary membership" in the capital's Polo Club.[72]

Drawing on racial taxonomies developed by whites in Europe and North America over the previous century, Anglo-Americans posited the existence of a ladder of civilization. At its base was "savagery," a pre–social condition in which humans acted toward each other as individuals, primitive and violent; it was a state of existence, said Frank Murphy, the governor-general of the Philippines during the mid-1930s, that "leaves out the head." The next stage was "barbarism," in which society had started to form, though it retained such savage atavisms as sharp class distinctions and slavery. Civilization was meant to deliver men and women from barbarism.[73] Whether India and the Philippines were currently lodged in savagery or barbarism—Anglo-American views differed on this—they remained well short of civilization. In an 1875 lecture, British historian Henry Maine announced that Indian institutions had "been arrested . . . at an early stage of development," leaving the country "a barbarism." The British distinguished between the Aryans—light-skinned Europeans who, they said, had moved into India over centuries, carrying with them an old civilization, manifest in north India through the Sanskrit language, classical-looking Gandharan art, and even government—and the darker-skinned Dravidians, alleged to be racially inferior indigenes who lived south of the Ganges, and who by "intermingling" with the Aryans had cost the latter "their purity of race." The result overall was India's "downward trajectory" on the ladder of civilization, particularly evident in its vulgar and "barbarous" Hindu architecture.[74] The Americans posited a similar, binary distinction among Filipinos: on the one hand the Spanish-educated Tagalogs found mainly in cities and towns; on the other the rough people of the hills and forests who hovered between savagery and barbarism, some yearning to be Christians, others still hunting heads.[75] Neither group was yet civilized, and all Filipinos were said to bear features characteristic of their "race." They were "slow, oh my how slow, and lazy, and one sometimes wants to get out with a raw hide and encourage them to work a little more. Their ways are not ours and their thoughts are not ours, and perhaps never will be," wrote Frank Laubach to his mother. "We have not been able to find a servant that is not either lazy or thievish or else eternally slow and dumb."[76] William Howard Taft reflected frequently on the racial character of Filipinos. "These people are a peculiar race," he wrote to Justice John Harlan in June 1900. "They are polite, appear light hearted, but are not industrious. They may . . . work for three or four days in the desultory manner in which they work in this country, and then more than half of them will quit with the advanced wage in their pockets. . . . They . . . are the most gullible people in the world. . . . The great mass of them are superstitious and ignorant. . . . The idea that these people can govern themselves is . . . ill founded. . . . They are cruel to animals and cruel to their fellows when occasion arises. They need the training of fifty or a hundred years before they shall even realize what Anglo Saxon liberty is."[77]

"They are cruel to animals" was a frequent charge of Britons and Americans, and peculiar in that the Anglo-Americans commented often on their subjects' proximity and even resemblance to animals. According to the British, India was a land of elephants, tigers, buffalo, cows wandering through city streets, sinister-looking pariah dogs, monkeys, insects, and snakes. Indians whipped the horses and oxen that pulled their carts, and despite professing their worship of cows, Hindus neglected them shamefully. Britons claimed that Indians looked like animals, among them the beggar children who clung to the windows of a departing train, "screeching and looking at us with great big spaniel's eyes until you had to tap their knuckles, so that they would drop off all along the platform like little flies."[78] Aspects of the Indian personality were said to resemble animals. Like insects, Indians were irritating. They were as treacherous as snakes, dangerous as crocodiles or tigers, mischievous as monkeys, or as passive toward their fate as bullocks or elephants. The same was true of American perceptions of Filipinos. "Everybody that comes out here thinks for a while we ought to treat these people like human beings, but they soon get over that," Winifred Denison wrote to his grandmother in 1914.[79] Edith Moses likened her servants to monkeys or baboons, "for the probability is," she instructed a prospective visitor, "that a half-naked, dark-skinned creature is rushing up and down the hall on all fours, with big burlap socks under his hands and feet."[80] Nicholas Roosevelt wrote an extended meditation comparing Filipinos to carabao, the buffalo prized by farmers and used for transport throughout the archipelago. Like the carabao, Roosevelt asserted, the people of the Philippines were inclined to be placid and patient: "Nothing disturbs the slow serenity of the carabao. No power on earth can hurry him."[81] The pigs that ranged freely throughout the islands disgusted Americans. Pigs were dirty, ugly, and smelly, and carried diseases including trichinosis and hog cholera. By the nineteenth century the pig was widely associated "with offenses against good manners."[82]

Britons and Americans frequently commented on the prominence of Indian and Filipino sense organs, physical manifestations of their bearers' supposed racial inferiority. With civilization came refinement of the senses and of eyes, ears, noses, skins, lips, and tongues. That those who were not yet civilized had what whites regarded as protuberant eyes, pendulous ears, large, flat noses, dark, coarse-seeming skins, and thick lips came as little surprise, though of considerable interest, to Anglo-Americans. The apparent preoccupation with the "lower" senses exhibited by lesser peoples explained their distorted features.

The nineteenth-century naturalist Lorenz Oken ranked people on a ladder of the senses: at the bottom was the African "skin-man," then came the Australian "tongue-man," Native American "nose-man," Asian "ear-man," and, at the top, the European "eye-man," though in practice these associations were not so rigid—that is, westerners regarded all people of color as having acute "lower" and dulled "higher" senses.[83] The underdevelopment of their higher senses also purportedly explained the extraordinary and more primitive abilities of Others. Africans were said to be able to withstand the hottest sun because of their opaque and toughened skins. Indians had keen senses of smell and insisted, said the British, on sniffing others constantly, like animals. Filipinos, according to the Americans, had a good sense of touch, being dexterous with musical instruments, for example. But their food was often inedible, possibly because they could not taste it properly with their bulging lips and poorly formed mouths. Following the capture of the Filipino independence leader Emilio Aguinaldo in March 1901, the *New York Evening Journal* compared his facial features to those of the American General Frederick Funston, who had caught him. Funston had a "strong chin," while Aguinaldo's "lips are red and thick. The lower lip hangs down heavily. The upper lip turns up coarsely. His brutality is plainly shown."[84]

Each of the five senses—how it was exhibited, how it was deployed—was thus assigned a place on the scale of civilization and a racial identity. Sensory organs and features of Others gave evidence of their racial inferiority, deeply ingrained, fully embodied, and likely to be enduring. Dark skin indicated dirt, danger, coarseness, a darkness within. In the city of Nagpur and after traveling in "all the wild and primitive places" of the countryside, Carol Hyde found "a few white faces . . . such a treat after all the dark and dirty ones!"[85] Erica Farquharson watched her nursemaid (*ayah*) try to get Farquharson's baby to accept her, but the child screamed " 'dirty, dirty,' when Ayah's small brown paws were stretched forth to wash or dress."[86] In the Philippines, Americans came to regard all Filipinos as likely carriers of disease, transmittable to whites through the slightest contact.[87] The colonized countries stank of excrement and death, but also of the "ethnic" or "racial" smell of men and women of color, who were alleged to have a "hircine" (goatish) odor that no amount of washing could remove, that no cologne or coconut oil could cover up.[88] Anglo-Americans were physically uncomfortable in India and the Philippines, where they feared contact with the "oily, black bodies" of the "natives," suffered in the moist heat, and marveled at the proximity of dark skin to harsh fabrics that would have irritated the refined, smooth skins of whites.[89] "Native" touch supposedly polluted food, which was in its essence bad for whites in any case: the "molten curries and florid oriental compositions" of India, the "indigestible" rice cakes, grasshoppers, and dogs eaten by Filipinos—and all in the most gruesome way, with fingers and the sounds of slurping and crunching.[90] "Creatures of the inferior races eat and drink," according to *Mrs.*

Beeton's Book of Household Management, an 1861 manual popular with Britons in India. "Man only dines."[91]

Not just the people of Asia but the environment itself was racialized by the imperialists. Nature in the tropics was especially powerful, and over time it damaged those who lived in it. Few Anglo-Americans doubted that there were genetic reasons for the alterity of Asian Others. There were also environmental ones, which meant that whites, too, would gradually be debilitated by their exposure to nature. The degradation of races that had always lived in the tropics was, whites insisted, on display for all to see. Now the danger was the deterioration of those who had come to civilize Indians and Filipinos.[92] In a series of articles published in 1898 as *Control of the Tropics*, the British sociologist Benjamin Kidd warned: "In climatic conditions which are a burden to him; in the midst of races in a different and lower stage of development; divorced from the influences which have produced him . . . the white man does not in the end, in such circumstances, tend so much to raise the level of the races amongst whom he has made his unnatural home, as he tends himself to sink slowly to the level around him." In "the relationships of the Western peoples to the inferior races" lay the future of "our civilization."[93] In India, Andrew Balfour worried that "the skin of the European long resident in the tropics undoubtedly darkens . . . his descendants tend, though not invariably, to have dark skins," and Sir Richard Havelock Charles, professor of anatomy at Lahore Medical College, insisted that the Indian sun caused whites to develop " 'a congeries of mental and sensory disturbances' and morally to degenerate."[94] Britons in India were susceptible to the pernicious effects of "Burmah-head" or "Punjab-head"; Americans in the Philippines were warned against "Philippinitis," a condition, according to a 1908 travel guide, "of mental and physical torpor, with a lack of interest in one's surroundings, ambition wanting, a general disinclination to mental or physical exertion, forgetfulness, and irritability."[95] "Certain it is," wrote Bishop Brent, "that the Orient is no fit place for persons, especially young men, who have not moral stamina."[96] American soldier Charles Routt hoped to stay on in the Philippines after he was mustered out, but noted, "the trouble is a man becomes like an Oriental himself after a time in this climate."[97] Thirty-five years later, writer William Anderson still worried that whites were coming undone in the Philippines. "Let it be said emphatically that the tropics are an unsuitable place for the white man," he wrote. The sun damaged his skin. "The general tendency of the white man in the Philippines is to deteriorate mentally, morally, and physically." White men turned to alcohol or "other stimulants. . . . With the lack of moral restraint, many a man has gone wrong in the tropics who otherwise would have been a good and useful citizen had he remained in the United States."[98] Fear of physical and moral degradation, combined with hope that the process could be halted or reversed with the appropriate care, helps to explain the Anglo-American fetish with soap, to be imported to the tropics and used by the "natives" and themselves. Soap had mystical qualities of purification; it could scrub clean and white the maculate dark skins of the empire's Asian subjects, if only metaphorically. Advertisements for Pears' Soap claimed that it could be a "potent factor in brightening the dark corners of the earth as civilization advances." One ad depicted a black man on a beach, "examining a bar of soap he has picked from a crate washed ashore from a shipwreck. The ad announces nothing less than the 'Birth of Civilization.'"[99]

The Senses and the Emotions

Anglo-Americans thought there was another difference between themselves and Asians: westerners were rational, Asians emotional. This difference ran as deep as race. It was connected to gender (women and the effeminate were emotional), maturity (babies and children had not yet learned to reason), and significantly to the five senses. "The life of the senses in intimately linked to the life of the emotions," anthropologist David Howes has written.[100] To each sensory stimulus there is an emotional response, or several responses. Encounters with the unfamiliar often inspire the most powerful sensory and thus emotional reactions; the perceived strangeness of the Other is registered in the strength of the body's response to it. Senses inspire emotions, create impressions of Others, and then prompt behaviors toward them. British and American men prided themselves on their rationality, intellect, reserve, and coolness under fire. These faculties, they claimed, were needed when governing men and women who appeared to live according to their instincts, heeding their hearts not their heads. "At best we are an alien, and worse than that an unbending and unsympathetic race," wrote a British official in India during the 1870s. "The race we are called upon to rule is essentially an impulsive and a feeling one . . . we never thaw to them and they never open to us."[101] An American visitor to Manila in 1901 concluded that the Filipinos "are a volatile people, easily led, easily swayed by passing emotions and influences, and lacking that true stability of character which lies at the base of popular government."[102] Misunderstanding this fact of life could be dangerous, given the suddenness with which emotional Indians or Filipinos might erupt in violence.

The greatest apparent threat to whites from Asian bodies or the tropical environment was violation of the boundaries of the body. Offense against corporeal taboos, trespass of body membranes, unsolicited penetration of the skin or through the orifices—all triggered in whites a powerful emotional response, for all threatened to contaminate or endanger the body with the presence of the Other. Such violations elicited fear, anger, revulsion, and frequently disgust.[103] What disgusted westerners in 1900? The sight of pustules on a body or the digital abridgments of lepers, sharp, fecal odors, the touch of "ugly people," food that was slimy or greasy or rancid, drink that should not have been warm but was, the sound of spitting and hocking and the sight of snot or red spittle on the ground, distortions or excrescences of the body and of the sense organs especially—tattoos, piercings, swellings, rashes, the presence of blood or pus or mucous—all uncivilized, all seemingly common among class and racial Others, all apprehended in sickening abundance in India and the Philippines. American medical missionary Frederick Meyer, writing from a hospital in Capiz, made confrontation with disgust an emblem of his faith: "In spite of the reeking stench of some of the neglected cases, the gruesome cuts with oozing brains, the eight-inch worms coming from the mouth, nose, or even through appendiceal perforation, the thirty maggots lodged with dogged determination in the nasopharynx of a poor comatose fellow, things distasteful to the eyes, ears, nose and throat, the hospital force feels it is accomplishing a real service to the community in the name of Christ."[104]

Imperialists, Anxious and Exhilarated

The conviction that their mission to civilize Others was just gave Britons and Americans confidence in their imperial ventures. But the constant threat of violation and contamination, the presence of their bodies in hazardous, tropical places, also led to intense anxiety. And it was not just that they feared contamination. The "assault" on all the senses could also be exhilarating. With the dangers of empire came also powerful temptations, a desire to know the Other in the most intimate ways. The frisson of horror must contain not just fear but excitement, the illicit pleasure born of the possible embrace of the forbidden. The instinct of the British following the Great Rebellion, and the Americans practically on arrival in the Philippines, was to isolate themselves from their subjects. By 1858, "gone were the days when the British in India would slip into native clothes, smoke a hookah and take a native mistress," notes scholar Indira Ghose.[105] Now they must so far as possible remove themselves from the "natives," a strategy "built upon distancing and denial."[106] Contact with Indians and Filipinos threatened contagion, for microbes were said to lurk in dark bodies unseen and were thus especially dangerous. The Americans blamed an eruption of cholera among their soldiers in April 1902 on their "indiscriminate mixing with the [Filipino] people."[107] "We astonish the natives when we arrive in a pueblo by bringing our food, bedding, and little alcohol stoves," recorded Edith Moses. "On account of the cholera we prepare our own dinners and refuse the excited invitations of the presidentes [mayors], who have expected to entertain us."[108]

And yet perfect isolation was never fully possible. Virtually all of the British and many Americans needed servants, including those who bore them bodily up hills and across rivers, helped them dress, removed their wastes, and, in India, suckled their infants. The civilizing mission demanded that Anglo-Americans initiate physical contact with their subjects: not all vaccinations could be done by Indians or Filipinos; lepers taken to hospitals (in India) or to Culion colony (in the Philippines) required steadying by western hands; the Christian baptism of "savages" was a tactile act. Discipline meant slapping, punching, and beating "natives," and despite suspicions about their loyalty Indian and Filipino soldiers and police officers remained vital for maintaining public order. Then there were the seductions of empire. Officials worried about their soldiers or subordinates "going native." This might mean something fairly innocuous, such as dressing like a Filipino or eating Indian food. The great fear of British and American officials was sexual contact between their nationals and the local people. This occurred constantly, to the embarrassment of the authorities, who nevertheless insisted that men would be men, and that regulation of Asian bodies was the best approach to the problem. The Indian Contagious Diseases Act of 1868 required the registration, medical inspection, and, if deemed necessary, isolation and treatment of prostitutes in "lock hospitals" and placed certain areas off limits to them. Similar policies were undertaken in the Philippines where, as Bishop Brent wrote, American "young men . . . are immediately exposed to extraordinary temptations."[109]

The pursuit of civilization nevertheless went forward. It could succeed only if some portion of the populations of India and the Philippines were prepared to accept it. This required that certain Indians and Filipinos must be less racially debased than others. Of this possibility the British were at the turn of the century less sure than the Americans. Many leading Indian intellectuals, politicians, and artists were Bengalis, or so thought the British governors in Calcutta who were most inclined to encounter them, and however sophisticated they seemed, Bengalis seemed to the British poorly suited for self-rule. Bengali men were alleged to be effeminate, and therefore weak, cowardly, and cunning rather than straightforward and truthful. The Bengali "lives in a constant vapor bath," declared Thomas Macauley. "His pursuits are sedentary, his limbs delicate, his movements languid. . . . Englishmen who know Bengal, and the extraordinary effeminacy of its people, find it difficult to treat seriously many of the political declamations in which English-speaking Bengalis are often fond of indulging."[110] The streets of Calcutta reeked of garbage and excrement; minor officials, called *babus* (with contempt by the British) were said to chatter pointlessly and in what the British called *chi-chi* English, offending civilized ears; and even the best Bengalis wore strange clothes, ate peculiar foods, and spat on floors. Yet some British officials asserted that Indians of the highest social station and intellectual achievement might exhibit characteristics of advancement or the potential for it. Many spoke English, and a number had been to British universities. The best men of the "martial races"—Muslims and Sikhs—did not share Bengalis' cravenness. High-caste Hindu Brahmins were at least as class conscious as their British counterparts, and British liberals admitted that the better sort of Indian often had good manners and knew how to behave in polite society. In the end, Macauley remained willing to consider civilizing the best of them. He thought the British could create a class of Indian "interpreters between us and the millions whom we govern," a class "Indian in blood and colour, but English in taste, in opinions, in morals, and in intellect."[111] When Edwin Montagu became viceroy in 1912, he urged that Indians be recruited to "every branch of the administration" with a view to "the gradual development of self-governing institutions."[112] He had in mind the best sorts.

So too did the Americans envision the Philippines as a bifurcated society, in which a minority of men might, with time and training, learn to govern the incorrigible masses. The first Philippine Commission distinguished between what it called the "barbaric" tribes, including "Negritos" and "Indonesians," and the "Indios Filpinos," whom it described as "civilized and Christianized" because of their previous contact with the Spaniards and other "foreigners."[113] Philippines Education Commissioner David Barrows put it somewhat differently in testimony before the Senate Insular Affairs Committee in early 1902. There were in the archipelago, he said, "two generally large elements, one of which is commonly known as the 'gente ilustrada,' which is the cultivated class, and the other is the 'gente baja,' or the subordinate class." The former class was "very small," perhaps "a dozen families." Its members were "ambitious," "hospitable," and "charming," comparable to the similar class in Japan.[114] They were not quite ready to strike out on their own. "Our only hope of success in dealing with the Filipinos is the development of a large conservative element among the educated people, who by political training and experience shall learn self-restraint, and the creation of a public opinion among the present ignorant mass whom nothing can reach but a wide system of popular education," wrote Taft to a friend in early 1904. "Without this conservative element and this popular opinion, useful self-government among the Filipinos is impossible."[115] In her travels through the islands with her husband and other commissioners, Edith Moses met with the best men in town after town. "The young Filipinos we meet in society are very polite, and desire to be thought men of the world," she wrote. "They are the rich and prominent citizens, but at the public meetings of the Commission there are many natives"—presumably not the rich and prominent—"who wear their shirts outside their trousers." At Baguio in April 1902, she met the town's *presidente*. One of the burdens of his job was the need to wear for ceremonies a white suit, hat, and shoes, "the insignia of his office" designed to impress with their appearance.

When the man's term ended he bequeathed his official clothing to the next incumbent and "joyfully return[ed] to a 'gee string'; on public occasions, however, he may don a shirt."[116] There was agreement that the "gente baja," despite the romance of them, were unready for self-government. Eli Lundy Huggins wrote to his sisters when he "saw for the first time two wild pagan mountaineers, Igorrotes. They were naked except for loincloth, and profusely tattooed, bodies and faces, in blue. They evidently are of a different race from the converted, catholic natives of the coast. They have more aquiline features, and are emotionless and inscrutable in their expressions and appearance, whereas the catholic natives are suave and ingratiating in their expression and manners."[117] Charles Denby of the Philippine Commission asked Harold Ashton, who had lived in the islands for years, whether he thought the Filipinos had the ability to govern themselves. "Let him have his carabao in peace; don't tax him directly, and he will sit in the sun and not bother his head about the right of taxation among other things. . . . He wants to be left alone," Ashton replied. Denby repeated the question: "What is your opinion as to his capacity for self-government?" Ashton responded, "he has absolutely none," though he added that "I am speaking of the rank and file, not of the people you see going about in patent leather boots."[118] For those, perhaps, there was hope of redemption.

Indians, Filipinos, the Senses, and Civilization

Indians and Filipinos were hardly passive in the face of their subjugation. They resisted in various ways the definitions of civilization and the racial categories that the Anglo-Americans sought to assign them. They did so by articulating their own versions of what it meant for a society and a people to be civilized and by rejecting efforts to denigrate them for their treatment of the senses, by which westerners meant to gauge their decency, their refinement, and thus their fitness for self-government. To some extent, Indians and Filipinos tried first to establish that the British and Americans, even by their own standards, fell far short of civilized behavior, and that they themselves were cleaner, more mannerly, and more refined than their putative guides and insistent tormentors. But they also developed their own versions of what it meant to be civilized. Both versions were fully implicated in nationalism. In India, the idea of civilization was meant to distinguish that nation from its imperial ruler: it was to be an expression of tradition, community, and culture, not, as Indians argued was the case with Britain, merely a cover for the extension of brute power. It resided as well in a longstanding determination among devout Hindus to establish a rigid boundary between the pure and the polluted, especially with regard to the preparation and consumption of food. In the Philippines, nationalists recognized that the surer path to independence was to develop a discourse of civilization that derived much of its substance from a Spanish colonial past and the vanity of Americans who proclaimed their desire to civilize and democratize their subjects. Both Indians and Filipinos saw fit to mimic, so far as possible, Anglo-American practices of the body, even while retaining those they considered desirable and vital to their identities and promoting, with some success, hybridized versions of these practices that westerners came to adopt.

Indians were keenly conscious that the British were judging them by their habits and manners, and that insofar as their future autonomy required persuading Britons that their everyday practices of deportment and hygiene were sufficiently refined, they tried to meet the expectations of the imperialists. They did this on their own terms and without granting that the British were hygienically superior to them, yet with manifest anxiety that their efforts would be met with scorn.[119] The Persian code of politeness, embodied in the concept of *tahzib ul akhlaq* (the polishing of manners), was championed by Indian intellectuals in the late nineteenth century, and while it emphasized personal responsibility for refinement it was otherwise consistent with the broadly social aims of Britain's civilizing mission.[120] In the late nineteenth century, a number of Indian reformist men wrote advice manuals for women, prescribing behaviors designed to show the British that Indians too were civilized. Analyzing a number of these, historian Judith Walsh concludes that they prompted family debates over proper behavior, "as people suddenly [found] themselves faced with the need to justify yet one more aspect of indigenous daily practice—the use of hands rather than silverware for eating, or the use of a *neem* twig rather than European tooth powder for cleaning one's teeth. These might be items of daily habit or practice whose existence the debaters had previously considered entirely unproblematic, of which they might not even have been consciously aware, yet whose place within the daily scheme of things they suddenly [found] necessary to consider and defend."[121]

One of these manuals, written by Satyacaraṇ Mithra, included a series of instructions given by a husband to his wife concerning hygienic practices. He urged her to rise early, urinate and move her bowels, then wash her face and "clean your teeth with coal powder. Or if you use a *neem* twig or a twig from an *asheora* tree, that would be even better"—though in neither case should she follow the British habit of using tooth powder. A European woman would next start knitting, but it was better to clean the house, for that was good exercise. Next came a massage with mustard seed oil, which would prevent "scabbies and ringworm," scaly skin, and "a bad odor." Here the wife interjects: "I've finally understood something. That's exactly why I used to get such a strong, goatish smell from the European lady's body! Husband: Where? Wife: One day when I was the studying at the Bethune School, a European woman came to test us. There was a nasty odor from her body." All the more reason that bathing must be done daily, in a river or a pond with ample sand for scrubbing and "no rotten things in its water." Then came flower picking, for "enjoying the lovely scented air of the flower garden in the early morning purifies the mind and improves the health of the body." To the kitchen: "You should eat all the things which should be eaten to improve your health. Don't prepare the same kind of vegetable dish every day—it's better to vary it from time to time. You should not eat quickly. You should chew your food slowly and swallow." Finally, "after cooking and eating, you should come to your husband piously and in a cheerful state of mind. It is each wife's duty to zealously endeavor to infuse pure and holy feelings into her husband's mind."[122] B. N. Lahari, who began training to become a senior police officer in 1921, thought that he was warmly received by his British colleagues "because he did not chew betel or play Indian gramophone records"—he did not offend British senses—"and because of his willingness to engage in mess horseplay and fight back."[123] Advice manuals urged Indians among the British to dress respectably, keep visits short and apologize for their duration in any case, avoid overwhelming newcomers with insistent offers of help, and to offer visitors cigarettes or cigars rather than *pan,* betel and lime paste wrapped in a leaf.[124] Syed F. A. El Edroos noted that at parties, Indian hosts had traditionally sprinkled rose water on their guests. "However, as this makes the clothes wet Indians of the new school or those wearing European dress take it either on their handkerchiefs or on their bouquet." Next came the *itra* (scent), either poured on the hand or rubbed on clothing. "But as the smell of the Indian scent is too strong for European ladies and gentlemen it is applied to the bouquet only, which can after leave-taking be easily put aside." If an Indian managed to get into a British club, any number of behaviors were prohibited: there was to be no expectorating or noisy throat-clearing, suppression of "those ebullitions which are considered amongst his own people to indicate that he has fed well," no hiccupping, sniffing, snuffling, humming, loud laughing, or yawning, nose-blowing only with a handkerchief, avoidance of "all allusions to ailments, especially in the presence of ladies," and no "fingering the nose or laying hold of the ears during conversation."[125]

While some Indians tried to imitate the British in order to please them, others were critical of British habits. "The Indians thought we were very dirty because we sat in the bath and washed ourselves in the water in the bath, whereas they always washed in running water," recalled Evelyn Dagmar Bogle.[126] Emma Roberts discovered that Indian newspapers, written in Persian and resembling British tabloids, often lampooned British behavior. She included in her memoir one of their descriptions of a British dinner party: "The *gentlemen of exalted dignity* had a great feast last night, to which all the military chiefs and lieutenants were invited. There was a little hog on the table, before Mr—, who cut it in small pieces, and sent some to each of the party; even the women ate of it. In their language, a pig is called *ham*. Having stuffed themselves with the unclean food, and many sorts of flesh, taking plenty of wine, they made for some time a great noise, which doubtless arose from drunkenness. . . . After dinner, they danced in their licentious manner, pulling about each other's wives."[127] Striking here is the catalog of British sensory violations, with the bright light of contempt turned by the ruled on the ruler. It is worth recalling Gandhi's (perhaps apocryphal) response to the question, "Mr. Gandhi, what do you think of western civilization?" "I think," he said, "that it would be a good idea."[128]

Gandhi thought long and hard about civilization, as did his compatriot and rival Rabindranath Tagore. Both concluded that Indian civilization was by all measures very different from western civilization. For Gandhi, civilization resided in India's past. It had nothing to do with religion, or at least a particular religion, for Muslims had contributed to it as surely as Hindus had. What passed for civilization in Europe was materialism and technology—soulless things. It was in fact better understood as intellectual and spiritual. Greece, he argued, was a greater civilization than Rome, though the latter had conquered the former. He recalled an incident from his childhood, when his father, a government official, was summoned to a *durbar* during a visit by the governor. His father felt compelled to wear stockings and boots, rather than the soft leather slippers he usually wore. "If I was a painter," Gandhi recalled, "I could paint my father's disgust and torture on his face as he was putting his legs into his stockings and his feet into ill-fitting and uncomfortable boots. He had to do this!" Such were the demands of the "civilized" conqueror, and such was the unhappy symbolism of their crass mission.[129]

Tagore's understanding of both western and Indian civilizations was more sharply drawn than Gandhi's. Whereas the Europeans and Americans associated civilization with the state and thus power, Indian civilization had no state to which to attach itself, and thus resided in culture or society. Moreover, western civilization was meant to exclude, "to expel and to demolish all others for self-preservation," or to "homogenize" white societies by expunging other races from them. By contrast, Indian culture had always been "syncretic," absorbing into itself the contributions of every member of society, welcoming diversity. Here was a more humane way to imagine civilization, and, not incidentally, a polity. The basis for nationhood in India was not the history of a state or the power to exclude or punish, but instead the persistence of cultural achievement and social tolerance. The unity of an Indian state would ultimately derive from this.[130]

Whatever small regard Americans had for Filipinos, the *gente ilustrada,* or the *ilustrados,* had from the first sought to emulate European habits and adopt European modes of civilized behavior. They protested against American hypocrisy, the professions of liberty and democracy made by soldiers and officials who denied these to Filipinos. They followed the example of José Rizal, martyred in late 1896 by Spanish authorities at the behest of Catholic friars in the archipelago, whose perfidies he had exposed in his 1887 novel *Noli Me Tangere* (*Touch Me Not*). Rizal had been educated in Spain and had witnessed there a flowering of new ideas and spirited political debates such as were prohibited in Spain's Philippine colony. He had the temerity to ask why this was so. Rizal spoke several European languages, had an American common-law wife, was a naturalist and a physician, and wore to his execution a European-style black suit, white shirt, and bowler hat. His death sparked outrage, and men far more radical than he emerged in Philippine politics; against them the Americans would do military and ideological battle after 1898. But Rizal remained for many educated Filipinos, including those with a Spanish parent and called *mestizos*, a model of progress, dignity, and self-restraint. The Americans regarded him sympathetically, as a victim of a sinister Catholicism familiar to them at home. Theodore Roosevelt proclaimed Rizal the Philippines' "greatest genius and most revered patriot," and promised to "carry out exactly what he steadfastly advocated."[131]

This did not mean that Americans found Filipinos civilized. They thought that even the *ilustrados* could be uncouth and far from ready for self-rule. Filipinos staked their claim to self-government by using American words and deeds to demonstrate that neither people had a monopoly on decency and propriety. Americans, they insisted, were violent, racist, licentious, and crude. Above all, they were hypocrites. In February 1899, days after hostilities broke out between Filipinos and Americans outside Manila, a supplement to the paper *Heraldo Filipino* laid charges against the interlopers:

> You ought to know by this time that these people can teach us nothing good. What we can learn from them is all evil. . . . They are worse than the wild people who live in the woods, they have not the slightest idea of looking at things from the point of view of a man of honour nor have they the slightest respect for reason, for this does not control their actions in the least. Without the slightest attention to civility they rush into houses and if they find the people eating, without saying a word, they take what they want from the table, put it into their mouths and go as they came. . . . Their habits and manners are a disgrace to the country where they were born. In no history have such customs and manners been described even in that of the most ignorant people. They search women who pass, feeling all over their bodies, taking from them money and whatever else they carry and if they come on them in a lonely place they strip them naked after violating them and do not leave a rag on them. Are these those honest men of whom we have heard? Are these the people who were going to teach us good habits? Are these the people who were going to guide us? The race which does these

> things is the most hated one in the world, it is the race which commits most cruelties, it is the race which does not treat its mother with respect; in this race there is not the slightest idea of personal dignity, it is a race which does not know what honour is, which does not possess the slightest vestige of regard for good manners.[132]

Three years later, with the war winding down but not yet over, Lorenzo, Manuel, and Mariano Lopez, brothers of Sixto Lopez, a rebel general who had surrendered (and been deported), were arrested by the Americans in Batangas and imprisoned for five months. The Lopezes were a good family, well off and English-speaking. Manuel wrote to their sister, Clemencia, from prison, outraged that an American lieutenant had forced the brothers to remove their hats in his presence, and incensed that the officer had called him "a great insurrecto!" Manuel considered this an "affront to me" by "an official who is wholly without breeding." The Lopezes were not allowed to have "food brought in" by their family, but "were obliged to eat wretched food" like the other prisoners. They were transported to the island of Malagi, first on a steamer in which they were placed in the hold like "animals," then transferred to a different steamer with more space and portholes through which to breathe—but where even the best accommodation "was the place provided for the transportation of horses!"[133] Their outrage was understandable. It was that of men of "breeding" and class who were insulted that the self-proclaimed agents of democracy and decency, though mere soldiers, had treated them as if their race mattered more—as if they were ordinary Filipinos.

The *ilustrados* tried at all times to reassure the Americans that they had more in common with their rulers than with the *gente baja* of their own country. It was true, they said, that the Filipino masses lacked refinement, but the Americans could trust them to discipline their less refined countrymen and women, to train the masses in respect for the senses and the ways of civilization such that they and their occupiers shared. The Americans tended at first to regard such professions of solidarity with amusement, ignoring as they did the racial divide that they inscribed on their own relations with all Filipinos. That was the tone of Colonel Arthur Ferguson's letter to Governor-General Taft in early 1902. "We are favored," he wrote, "with a long and characteristic document from Paterno"—Pedro Alejandro Paterno, a *mestizo* lawyer who had sought to mediate between US and insurgent forces—"relating to a scene he had witnessed in the vicinity of Manila, which brought the blush of shame to his cheek and gave his moral being a severe jar." Paterno had happened upon a cockfight, long a favorite pastime of ordinary Filipinos, but an activity looked upon with dismay by the Americans, and thus by Paterno. He found there "a motley gathering of men, women, and children engaged in nefarious games of chance in which they indulged during the intervals between the cockfights. This scene was so abhorrent to his nature that he paints it in all its grewsome [*sic*] colors, and calls upon the Governor to lose no time in commissioning some 'delegates' to visit the spot, ascertain for themselves the true facts, and then take the most strenuous measures against a continuance of such debasing practices as cock-fighting on week-days"; evidently weekend cockfights remained acceptable.[134] The "blush of shame" Paterno felt came quickly to a man trying desperately to establish that his people were as civilized as those who now governed them. The Americans were not yet convinced.

Ten years later, an editor of *La Vanguardia* came closer than Paterno to the hard truth. The writer had seen on a Manila street an American; he didn't know who he was but the man had looked at him with "the imperious haughtiness" of a "man of a superior race." He had a "humiliating gaze" aimed at those around him. If a Filipino got in his way or accidentally brushed him as he walked past, the American pushed him aside. After all, "what treatment can a semi-savage, who eats rice with his fingers and talks a language which is not a language but string of ill-sounding monosyllables which vex one's ears, expect? Why should one show any consideration for persons who belong to the lowest social scale, who have a flat nose, thick lips and simian aspect, with tattooing and breach-clouts, who eat raw meat, the last representatives of an inferior and primitive caste destined to disappear before the impulse of civilization?"[135] Such was the contempt Americans displayed for their allegedly inferior subjects. To many Filipinos, efforts to demonstrate that they were civilized must have seemed hopeless.

In such ways did Britons and Indians, Americans and Filipinos, regard each other. Determined to bring their version of civilization to the benighted people of Asia's tropics, the Anglo-Americans confronted men and women they considered to be savages or primitives who failed to respect the senses and who threatened by their presence the boundaries of the westerners' bodies. Violations of sight, sound, smell, touch, and taste represented to the westerners a lack of refinement and decency. They construed difference in several ways, but most of all as racial ones. They recoiled in fear and sought to distance themselves from those whose habits reflected their crudeness and terrified them so. Yet they could not fully isolate their bodies, for their mission was correction, sanitation, hygiene, and liberation, all of which required sensory contact with those they confronted in their empires. They needed help from their subjects too, which required exposure to them. And there were attractions and temptations of the Other, including relatively innocent ones such as food and adventure and, not innocently, sexual exploitation. Indians and Filipinos had their own understandings of what civilization meant, and who in fact was guilty of sensory transgression and fundamental misbehavior. Their goal, increasingly, was to get the foreigners out.

Elites in India and the Philippines would do what they must to achieve liberation and establish independent nations, acquiescing if need be to Anglo-American demands that they alter their habits, but just as often insisting that the sort of sensory practices, the "civilized" behaviors which their occupiers demanded, were in truth not very civilized at all.

2

Fighting

War and Empire's Onset

> War is hell on [the senses]; the violence of it engraves sensory memory in ways other experiences cannot approach, memory so powerful it can be relived, over and over again. Indeed, as far as the senses are concerned, all war is total war, pushing them to their limits and beyond, dulling and then overwhelming and then dulling them again. Distinctions become muddled, nerves fray, and the sense of self shatters.
>
> —Mark M. Smith, *The Smell of Battle, the Taste of Siege* (2015)

Empires begin in violence. British India and the American Philippines are examples of this axiom. Britons came first to India long before the United States had imperial aspirations—indeed, long before there was a United States: British traders arrived in Gujarat in 1608, a year after the founding of Jamestown, the first viable English colony in North America. Throughout the seventeenth and eighteenth centuries America and India were comparable to each other in their status as subordinates of Britain, but crucially the North American colonies were holdings of the British crown and subject to regulation by government, while India was the domain of the East India Company, a crown-chartered private stock organization formed by aristocrats and merchants intent on dominating the trade of South and East Asia. While the British settled into their first factory in India, granted them by the Mughal emperor, Jamestown settlers struggled to survive against the resistance of the Powhatan people, whose permission to settle nearby the English had neither solicited nor obtained. The company began building a stronger presence in southeast India, at Madras, in 1639, the year before the bloody North American Beaver Wars pitted Iroquois against Algonquian, each sponsored by European rivals. These rivalries affected India too, and they prompted the company to protect its economic position by recruiting a larger military force of mercenaries and adventure-seekers to counterbalance particularly the French. In 1757, as the French and British fought for supremacy in North America, an East India Company force under the command of Robert Clive won a decisive battle against the army of Bengal and its ruler, or *nawab*, Clive having first bribed most of the *nawab's* officers to lay down arms or turn them against their prince. The company now ruled the wealthiest province in India. The American Revolution was nearly two decades off.

There followed a century of uncertainty concerning the extent of British power in India. The government concluded that it could not countenance the collapse of the East India Company, too lucrative to be allowed to fail, and so superintended its budgets and its foreign and military policies. The company had an inconstant relationship with Indian authorities. Over some—the leaders of the princely states of Hyderabad and Mysore and vast Rajputana, for example—the British had little sway. For a time, the company paid tribute to the Mughal emperor in Delhi. In 1830, the Chief Justice of Bengal asserted that there was "no definite opinion, either as to the true character . . . of the sovereignty of the crown, nor of the dependence of the laws on Parliament, nor as to the rights either of political power or of property of the East India Company, nor even of the relations in which the many millions of natives stand to the political authorities by which they are entirely governed."[1] The company's army nevertheless grew. It meant to keep order inside British possessions and to extend them, at the expense of European rivals and Indian aspirants to autonomy. The company banned *sati*, pursued the notorious *thugs*, and made English the language of instruction in Indian schools. Whatever the supposed racial limitations of their subjects and the company's lack of official status, the British believed that reform of Indian society was not only possible but also imperative. By 1857, many in Britain believed that such efforts had begun to succeed.

The Crown, meanwhile, had no success retaining its North American colonies. The British were distracted by political upheaval at home through the seventeenth century, still at odds with the French, and unable to keep their American subjects from antagonizing the Native Americans or challenging British political and economic authority. In the aftermath of the Seven Years War (1756–1763), in which they had defeated the French and their indigenous allies largely on behalf of the colonists, they announced a series of measures designed to tighten their control of colonial legislatures and the freewheeling trade practices that had long subverted all attempts to rein them in. Some Americans rebelled, and when the king, George III, tried to suppress them, they declared independence. The United States, established in 1783, would remain for some years little more than an aggregation of states faithful to a legacy of persistent localism, but over time, through a combination of abundant land, shrewd leaders, ruthlessness in its treatment of black labor and native peoples, and no little luck in its diplomatic timing, it would become an economic power and feared in its hemisphere. The United States absorbed territory across North America to the Pacific. It fought a war with Mexico and annexed its northern lands. The Civil War determined finally that slavery in the country would be expunged. Postwar immigration fed a growing labor force; concentrations of capital gave rise to a vigorous industry, and by the centennial year 1876 the value of US exports had outdistanced that of its imports. As the end of the nineteenth century neared, the nation had ever greater interests in affairs beyond its shores and a fresh capacity to pursue them. Then, in 1895, Cubans rebelled against their Spanish rulers.

These brief narratives have brought two nations to the verge of formal empire, in India and the Philippines respectively. India would not be Britain's first overseas imperial possession; by 1857, the British had long held colonies in the Americas, Africa, and Asia. The United States, only recently a colony itself, had through the nineteenth century expanded on land, and whatever its interests in projecting its power across water, it had by the 1890s been content mainly to increase its trade with other nations, neglecting to create a military force that would have been necessary for pursuit of a more formal empire. Yet the fact that the British assumption of power in India and the American absorption of the Philippines were separated by forty years does not make them analytically incommensurable. Both were examples of "liberal imperialism," undertaken by nations intent on bettering the condition of their subjects and certain that the imposition of their institutions would do so. Influenced heavily by political, intellectual, and particularly scientific debates at home, the decisions were represented by the Anglo-Americans as acts of rescue: in India from "natives" who were pathologically determined to murder Europeans; in the Philippines, first, from Spaniards whose despotism had left the islands in destitution and ignorance, then from a small minority of Filipinos who misrepresented benign American intentions in order to pursue their unrealistic goals of independence—though ultimately, in both cases, empire required the establishment of alliances with local elites. Each power watched the other shape its colony, and on the whole each approved of what it saw and regarded it as ratification of its own choices. "The more the American lives in the Philippines and comes to understand the Orient the better he comprehends, and the more he is drawn to sympathize with, the work which Great Britain has done, and is doing, in the world," editorialized the *London Times*.[2] Robert Clive was an "embarrassment" to mid-nineteenth-century British policymakers, men such as James Mill and Thomas Macaulay "for whom the Raj," writes Lawrence James, "was one of the highest attainments of Christian civilisation."[3] The American architects of empire in the Philippines—William Howard Taft, Elihu Root, and Theodore Roosevelt, among others—had the same sense of mission in mind.

But first there would be war. And in these wars for empire, as in all wars, every sense would be excruciatingly heightened.

In war, soldiers strain to see the enemy as their self-preservation depends on it, and where the enemy is stealthy or elusive laying eyes on him requires remarkable concentration of vision. It is imperative to hear the enemy when vision is occluded—at night, or by artillery smoke—and men must respond promptly and correctly to the battle commands or bugle calls of their own side. The odors of war are acrid, among them unbathed bodies, smoke and fire, human wastes, blood, and rotting corpses. Soldiers feel battle acutely: their uniforms, heavy with dirt, scratch their skins; their boots pinch; bullets or shrapnel sting or come too close for comfort. War has its own tastes, as food and drink become the soldier's fantasy and his keenest desire; he suffers privation and frequently recoils from the rations provided him.[4]

The Great Rebellion had a variety of causes. One important one was the British removal from power of Indian princes, or the company's absorption of princely states for which there was no male heir. Wajid Ali Shah of Oudh, whose state contained the city of Lucknow, was exiled to Calcutta, while Nana Saheb, a leading Maratha prince, was reduced to a pension and a rump court in Bithur. In 1853, the British seized control of Jhansi. These assaults on the old order, justified by company authorities in the name of good government and economic justice, were resented not just by the deposed princes but by many of the ordinary Indians over whom they had ruled. The takeovers fed longstanding fears that the British were trying to impose their values on Indians, in particular that British evangelicals sought the demise of Indian religions in favor of Christianity. Hindu soldiers, or sepoys, remembered their humiliating participation under British command in the Afghan expedition of the late 1830s, during which they had been prevented from taking customary daily baths, given repellent sheepskins to wear against the cold, and forced to accept their food from Muslim cooks, thereby "losing their caste" and becoming "much dissatisfied and disgusted."[5] New military policies had increased the recruitment of lower-caste sepoys, alarming their self-proclaimed social betters, and there were rumors that Indian soldiers would be sent overseas, to which high-caste Hindus, whose beliefs forbade crossing oceans, objected. From Delhi, Mohan Lal explained to a British correspondent why wealthy Indians supported the rebellion. Despite their having done better than they would have under "any native Government," Lal observed "that nothing but the distant and the contemptible manner with which they are treated by the generality of English gentlemen wounds their heart and compels them to forget the blessings of British rule."[6] Lal was a Hindu; the Muslim S. A. Khan echoed his view. There was a time, he wrote, when company officials had treated their Indian subjects with kindness, had "carried their hearts in their hands." No more. British "pride and arrogance" had caused authorities "to esteem the Hindustanee as nothing in their eyes," and had made Indians in turn "look upon" the British "with dread," such that "even natives of the highest rank never come into the presence of officials, but with an inward fear and trembling."[7]

In this testimony from aggrieved Indians resides the first hint that insults to the body, more precisely affronts to the senses, played an important role in igniting the Great Rebellion. Indians resented the "contemptible manner" and the "pride and arrogance" they saw in the eyes of the British, whose cold gaze they suffered whenever they sought an audience, and whose sharply raised voices gave them orders that seemed to reflect such hubris. Hindus borne to Afghanistan recoiled from having to take bread from Muslims at British insistence and shuddered at the touch of an animal's skin against their own. The standard military uniforms, made of "thick unyielding European cloth," were nearly as bad. "I found it very disagreeable wearing the red coat," Bengal infantryman Sita Ram Pande recalled. "It was open in front, but was very tight under the arms. The shako"—a cylindrical felt hat with a visor—"was very heavy and hurt my head . . . I always found it a great relief when I could wear my own loose dress."[8] In early 1857, as British suspicions grew that something was afoot, officers increasingly confined or punished Indian soldiers, placing the harsh rasp of manacles on the hands and feet of plotters and loyalists alike.[9]

Most of all, the sense of taste, or the placement of apparently unclean substances in the mouth, triggered the rebellion. During the early months of 1857, reports began to surface of the mysterious transport of chapattis—flattened wheat cakes that are the standard bread of North India—from village to village, carried by *chowkidars* (watchmen) or, in at least one case, a dog. One morning in March, Mark Thornhill, Magistrate of Muttra, found four of the cakes on his desk. His inquiries revealed that his *chowkidar* had accepted them from a man, "with instructions to make four like them and to take these to the watchman of the next village who was to be told to do the same."[10] Seeking the meaning of "the chapatti movement," the British discovered that according to local myth, the dog was the Maratha god of the sword, so that chapattis brought by canine were perhaps an incitement to violence.[11] Or the spread of the cakes might be a sinister invitation to the plotters to share food; the *thugs* were said to have eaten sugar together to affirm their solidarity.[12] "Government was quite nonplussed," recalled Ruth Coopland. "Some thought it was a ceremony to avert cholera, which had been frightfully prevalent in the North-West Provinces the year before; others said it was of superstitious origin; and *some* hinted at treason."[13] In the sepoys' view, the chapattis were a plot by the government to force them to eat in common food that had been polluted by the touch of a lesser caste or an alien religion.[14] With the chapatti movement came ominous reports of food secretly poisoned by the British or by Indian merchants at their behest. In the same month that Thornhill discovered chapattis on his desk, shoppers at the market in Cawnpore found the staple flour known as *atta* for sale at a dramatically reduced price. A rumor spread that the *atta* had been adulterated with the powdered bones of cows (abhorrent to Hindus) and pigs (inedible by Muslims). Clarified butter (*ghee*), another staple of Indian kitchens, was alleged to have been mixed with animal fat, and when salt appeared in Rajasthan stained red by the ochre previously carried in the burlap bags that held it, locals feared it had been drenched in cow's blood. At the Barrackpore barracks of the 43rd Bengal Native Infantry, fifteen miles north of Calcutta, Major-General J. B. Hearsey received an anonymous petition from his sepoys. "The Lord Sahib has given orders . . . to all commanding officers to destroy the religion of the country," it read. "We know this. . . . The officers of the Salt Department mix up bones with the salt. The officer in charge of the ghee mixes up fat with it; this is well known. These are two matters. The third is this: that the Sahib in charge of the sugar burns up bones and mixes them in syrup the sugar is made of; this is well known—all knows it."[15]

These fears anticipated and ultimately reinforced the most visceral trigger of the Great Rebellion. Along with proliferating chapattis, spoiled flour, and tainted salt, sepoys believed that recently issued cartridges for their Enfield rifles had been lubricated with pig or cow fat. Soldiers loaded the cartridge by biting off its top. Biting rather than tearing the cartridge was often necessary because the grease thickened the paper and made it slippery, but even if the cartridge could be torn by hand, tactile exposure to a pollutant was nearly as bad as its placement in the mouth.[16]

Rumors of the animal lubricant circulated through bazaars and barracks in early 1857. At Barrackpore, sepoys showed their outrage by burning buildings. General Hearsey launched an inquiry, during which he tried to reassure the men that only mutton fat and wax had been used on the cartridges. A British officer questioned one of the dissidents: "What reason have you to suppose that there is anything in the paper which would injure your caste? Answer: Because it is a new description of paper with which the cartridges are made up and which I have not seen before. Question: Have you seen or heard from anyone that the paper is composed of anything which is objectionable to your caste? Answer: I heard a report that there was some fat in the paper. It was a bazaar report . . . My suspicion of the paper proceeds from its being stiff and like cloth in the mode of tearing it. It seems to us different from the old paper."[17] The British had by this time privately acknowledged having made a mistake: there was almost certainly cow and pig fat in the lubricant of cartridges that had been sent to depots near Calcutta. They tried to prevent any of the affected ammunition from reaching the sepoys and promised them that the lubricants were now innocent or that they could apply their own. But it was too late. On the afternoon of February 26, soldiers of the 19th Bengal Infantry Regiment at Behrampur, 110 miles north of Calcutta, refused to accept their cartridges for firing practice. These sepoys mutinied that night.

The British tried to contain the flames with a mix of suasion and forcefulness; in the Punjab, the Judicial Commissioner Robert Montgomery disarmed his regiments and thus prevented them from rising.[18] Elsewhere, though, the troops would not be calmed. British authority collapsed throughout north central India, garrison by garrison, city by city. Cawnpore erupted May 4–5, Meerut on May 10, and Delhi, home of the last Mughal Bahadur Shah, who joined the rebels, was besieged the next day. Oudh became the epicenter of the rebellion: Lucknow was invested by the mutineers on June 30, and a British relief force was turned away over the summer.

British authorities were incredulous that their sepoys would turn against them. They had difficulty understanding how their former allies could resist or conduct sieges so effectively, though in the end they chalked this up to the superiority of their British training. Most of all, they could not fathom that unsubstantiated rumors about rifle cartridges could be serious enough to inspire such violence. Yet grievances concerning abuse of the senses, a violation of the body, were far from trivial to Indians who claimed to suffer them. Again and again sepoys insisted that suspicious chapattis, reddened salt, and above all cartridges greased with animal fat were polluting, and therefore clear betrayals of trust by their masters. An official writing to Robert Montgomery about the situation in Delhi reported: "I have been told by sepoys that they had 3 complaints. First the messing system in the jails 2nd the cartridge and 3rd the bones ground up in their otah [*atta*]"—but he could not help adding "the annexation of Oude [Oudh] is I firmly believe the root of this outbreak."[19] He underestimated the intensity of feeling surrounding the cartridge issue. When sepoys, Muslim or Hindu, at the posts that mutinied in 1857 said they were angry that their cartridges had been lubricated with substances that would violate their religious beliefs, their words ought to have been taken at face value.[20]

The British would say, during or in the aftermath of the rebellion, that they had seen it coming—or rather, that they had felt it coming with all their senses. The portents were unnatural: strange storms or winds, fierce heat, cosmic disruptions that foretold terrible events. On May 5, 1857, Lieutenant Edward Martineau wrote from Fategarh that the state of the army was "as bad as can be." "We make a grave mistake," he continued, "in supposing that because we dress, arm and drill Hindustani soldiers as Europeans, they become one bit European in their feelings and ideas. I see them on parade for say two hours daily, but what do I know of them for the other 22? What do they talk about in their lines [and] what do they plot?" Then: "I can detect the near approach of the storm, I can hear the moaning hurricane, but I can't say how, when, or where it will break forth."[21] The northern heat that spring was "scorching," remembered artillery officer Vivian Majendie. The men were "tormented by flies . . . or prickly heat. . . . How shall I ever forget these long hot mornings when one's only amusement—if amusement it can be called—was watching the thermometer gradually working its way up to 114° or 116° or even 125°, or gazing listlessly out at the quiet camp, where not a human being, except a sun-dried nigger perhaps, was to be seen, and over which swept the terrible furnace-wind of Hindustan with its clouds of parched dust pungent as dry snuff?"[22] In Gwalior, Ruth Coopland was awed by a dust storm "filling the air to a great height with fine dust, rendering it almost dark, and casting a lurid light over everything."[23] After the powerful storms "the air would resound with the croaking of frogs; masses of insects flitted about." India in early 1857 seemed to the British a sensory nightmare, "'a detestable country.' Its people were 'savages'; its food inedible; its climate horrible; the whole 'damned place' seemed full of revolting insects that ate huge holes in new, expensive uniforms, of soggy peaches that tasted like turnips and cantankerous camels that smelled like drains."[24]

In late 1856, Elizabeth Sneyd began having aural premonitions of terrors to come. One night, she and her youngest daughter "were suddenly awakened by a most unearthly, dreadful sound of a multitude, as it were, of human voices blended together as one, uttering a most fearfully loud and awful groan of intense agony and distress as it were, which seemed to issue from the floor of our room . . . and we both jumped up exclaiming 'Oh! What was that dreadful sound?' I got up to examine the room, open the doors, *and* looked about the verandah, in front and outside the house into the compound to see if there were any natives or wild beasts congregated there; but nothing was to be seen of any kind about that bright, calm, clear moonlight night." She had another frightening episode in early 1857, at Shahjehanpur, with her husband Henry away: she heard the "sound of low voices and trampling of feet in the verandah." There she found a number of armed sepoys, who claimed they were looking for "badmashes." Weeks later, when she arrived in Cawnpore, her hotel room was dirty, and the sepoys failed to "salute" her as they usually did; instead, they did "nothing but point and laugh at me amongst themselves, while talking a great deal together in an undertone, keeping seated on the ground the whole time. My mind misgave me—it appeared very ominous of evil." When she requested a meal, she was given leftovers from "the natives' dinner," which she refused to touch.[25] Amy Haines and her family were in Lucknow in the months before the rising. It was a city of "odd sights that used to distract me out of my senses." The family thought the people "indecent" and "abusive"; "nobody boasting any modesty dare venture out, without their sight and ear being insulted with obscene language and indecorous manner." Graphic paintings in the streets appalled her, and the brightly colored Indian clothing could not, she claimed, conceal the filthiness of the residents. Her father decided that the family must leave, "for he said that in the insolence of the natives he saw the shadow of coming events."[26]

In the weeks before the rebellion, the British noticed changes in the gestures of sepoys and other Indians, or thought they did, including the apparent refusal to salute Elizabeth Sneyd, and a shift in the "demeanor" of the Sutherland family's servants in Lucknow.[27] At Mainpuri in mid-May, just before unrest began there, the British arrested a soldier on guard-duty who shot at a crow. "Thereafter the sepoys . . . 'assumed a threatening and defiant demeanour and to every keen observer their angry looks showed too plainly the approach of a gathering storm.'" Elsewhere, a "European woman in the bazaar was 'impudently stared at by a respectable looking native who came close up to her *jampan* [carrying chair] and then twisted his moustache in her face.'" These seemed expressions of insubordination. Equally troubling to the British were deceptive or treacherous gestures. On the verge of the outbreak, magistrate William Edwards was nearly guided by a seemingly loyal sepoy into a dangerous part of town. "The man's earnest and respectful manner quite deceived me," Edwards recalled.[28] After the mutiny in Ferozepore, some two-fifths of the soldiers of the 57th Infantry remained in their quarters. They seemed, wrote their general, "quiet and tractable," but they "have an appearance that I do not like."[29]

Following the first risings, the waves of the Great Rebellion broke in the spring and summer of 1857, intensifying the assault on the senses the British had long experienced in India. They were badly prepared for the conflict. Company armies consisted of some four thousand European and three hundred thousand Indian troops, and while many of the sepoys remained loyal or sat out the rebellion the odds did not favor the British. Immediately the officers called for reinforcements from Britain and other parts of the empire. The newly arrived soldiers were unused to conditions in India, and they found the sights, noise, heat, dust, odors and food far different from what they had known elsewhere and far more difficult to manage.

Problems of vision were vexing and various. British officers remarked on the seemingly innocent look of their sepoys just before the mutiny began. Their "demeanors" sometimes became more sullen or angry, but not always. Telling friend from foe is a common problem in war. It was especially hard during the rebellion, because the British depended on Indians to keep them informed, protect their families, and fight alongside them against the rebels, even though no uniform distinguished them from their enemies. In the Punjab, Henry Lawrence found that "so contradictory and anomalous were appearances" that he nearly mistook for loyal the 45th NI (Native Infantry)—"adepts in duplicity"—while regarding with suspicion the ultimately passive 57th.[30] Oversight required constant, exhausting vigilance; the judgment of the eye was undependable, as the British well knew.[31] When the sepoys did strike, it seemed to Britons an outrageous betrayal. Emma Sophia Ewart, whose husband John was a lieutenant colonel, wrote her sister Fanny in May of her "miserable reflection that all this ghastly show is caused not by open forces, but by the treachery of those we have fed and pampered and honored and trusted in for so many years."[32] The Ewarts would be killed days later. Alarmed by developments, the Legislative Council of India, with the assent of the Governor General, passed a law giving the police or other authorities the right to arrest any Indian "upon reasonable suspicion that he is a Mutineer or Deserter and amenable" to the rebels' cause. This was hardly sufficient to end the uprising, but it eroded any presumption that a "native" might somehow look innocent.[33] John Kaye described a hypothetical "British Magistrate, returning from his evening ride, [who] was . . . met on the road near the Bazaar by a venerable Native on an ambling pony—a Native respectable of aspect, with white beard and whiter garments, who salaamed to the English gentleman as he passed, and went on his way freighted with intelligence refreshing to the souls of those to whom it was to be communicated. . . . This was but one of many costumes worn by the messenger of evil . . . there was nothing outwardly to distinguish him."[34] Robert Montgomery's report just after the rebellion cautioned readers about its conclusions. "Such are the main facts of the *outward* conduct of the people during this period of trial," he wrote. "What their *inward sentiments may have been,* and whether their loyalty could be depended upon, *beyond a certain point,* is a different question." In the end, Montgomery decided, "it is hard to read the hearts of the Punjab people; and it were vain from outwardly favourable symptoms to assume the existence of loyalty, which perhaps may never be felt by an Asiatic race towards European rulers."[35]

Once their enemies had decided to rebel, the British claimed, they abandoned all pretense of innocence and allowed their hatred and anger to show. Attempting to escape by steamer down the Ganges for Calcutta, Elizabeth Sneyd watched from her carriage as sepoys brandished their ramrods "whilst making horrid faces and sneering and shaking their heads at me in the most insolent and contemptuous manner possible." She responded with a visual code of her own: "I kept perfectly still without saying a word, as I looked calmly and steadily at the vile wretches."[36] Taken captive at Gwalior, Ruth Coopland recalled her terror: "No words can describe the hellish looks of these human fiends, or picture their horrid appearance. . . . Hundreds of sepoys now came to stare at us," making British women the objects of their gaze.[37] When battles ended, British soldiers thought they knew how to distinguish living rebels from loyalists—the former looked guilty. "We have met upwards of 100 [sepoys] going to Allahabad and various places with their papers all correct," wrote Captain Chardin Johnson in his diary, "but who have been in Oudh and Cawnpore during all the outrages committed there, some too with blood-stained arms, all of them mutineers of more or less hideous character."[38] Even in death, the sepoys' hatred for the British was clear. Robert Young joined the siege of Delhi in the summer of 1857. When the city fell to the British in September, Young entered the hospital. There he saw sepoys "scowling in death their eyes wide open, glaring as it were with hatred; they were in every possible attitude, often of attack, just as they died." Young found it "sickening to behold them, and the stench was unbearable." The bodies were hauled by elephant to the river and thrown in.[39]

Yet the British were frequently denied the sight of the enemy. The battlefield was masked by dust or smoke or the darkness of India the soldiers swore was deeper than any they had known. In the "blinding" blowing sand, troops and horses blundered into each other.[40] Indians under siege sheltered behind battlements, firing at their besiegers with cannon and musket when the opportunity presented itself. "These rascals are giving us an immense deal of trouble," complained a British officer before the gates of Delhi in June. "They all sneak behind walls—if we could only fairly see them I think we should easily exterminate them."[41] The rebellion by its nature frustrated the eye; it was a conflict in which the fighting produced "mental hallucination" and "optical illusion," as one officer put it.[42] The circumstances of the rising moved the British to try to fool the eyes of the sepoys. In May 1857, with Europeans under siege in Delhi, field surgeon S. H. Batson volunteered to take a message to Meerut to requesting help. He dyed his face, hands, and feet brown and dressed as an Indian holy man ("faqueer"). He was discovered by villagers, who noticed his blue eyes, but his familiarity with Indian languages, religions, and "manners" saved his life. A sympathetic real "faqueer" gave him proper clothes and "necklaces of beads" and instructed him to say he was from Kashmir, where people had blue eyes. In the end there was nothing Batson could do to help the British in Delhi, but he had escaped by tricking optically his potential captors.[43] Amy Haines saved her life by masquerading as Muslim. She remembered that "my oriental dress had so altered me that I excited little suspicion when necessitated to go from one place to another. So well did I personate the Mahomedan women that could my own dear parents have seen me, I am sure they would have wondered at the alterations in their child."[44]

After the Crown had taken charge in India and the military controlled the cities in 1858, it was the vision of carnage perpetrated by the rebels that caused the British to demand revenge. A massacre at Cawnpore, reported widely by the British press in gory and embellished detail, particularly inflamed sensibilities. In June, a vastly outnumbered party of Europeans had been promised safe passage out of the city by Nana Sahib. But as they were boarding boats for Allahabad, the Europeans were attacked by sepoys. Most of the men were killed; women and children were taken captive and placed under guard in Cawnpore. On the night of July 15–16, with British forces about to enter the city, butchers—many of the sepoys refused the order to do it—slaughtered nearly two hundred Europeans, hacking off limbs and throwing bodies down a well. When the British troops arrived on the 17th, they were sickened and enraged. There was blood on the floor and walls and stark visual reminders of the lives of those who had been killed: locks of hair, bits of jewelry, and children's shoes. Colonel James Neill, left in charge of the Cawnpore garrison, ordered the accused leaders of the insurrection to clean up the site, wiping or licking up the blood and being forced to eat pork (Muslims) or beef (Hindus) before they were hanged.[45] When Chardin Johnson visited the city nearly three months later, he found a memorial to Indian perfidy and British courage. The house was still "covered with blood stains on the walls and floor. In the compound outside I saw masses of hair clotted with blood and pieces of dresses etc." He found inscriptions scratched into the walls, allegedly carved by the victims, "describing the horrors they underwent and calling upon their countrymen to avenge" them, though Johnson conceded that many of the inscriptions had likely been made since the killing. Still, "it was a sad sad sight, and many of us could scarcely help crying."[46] Their own version of liberation had routinely involved the summary hanging or "blowing from guns" of suspected rebels, as Indians well knew. The sight of mass murder in Cawnpore was evidence, said the British, of Indian barbarity, and the only fit response to it was one in kind.

Soundscapes too are changed by war. Premonitions of war are borne by whisper and rumor, while war itself brings the thunder of marching, the whistle of bullets, the roar of cannonballs, the sounds of soldiers yelling in triumph or

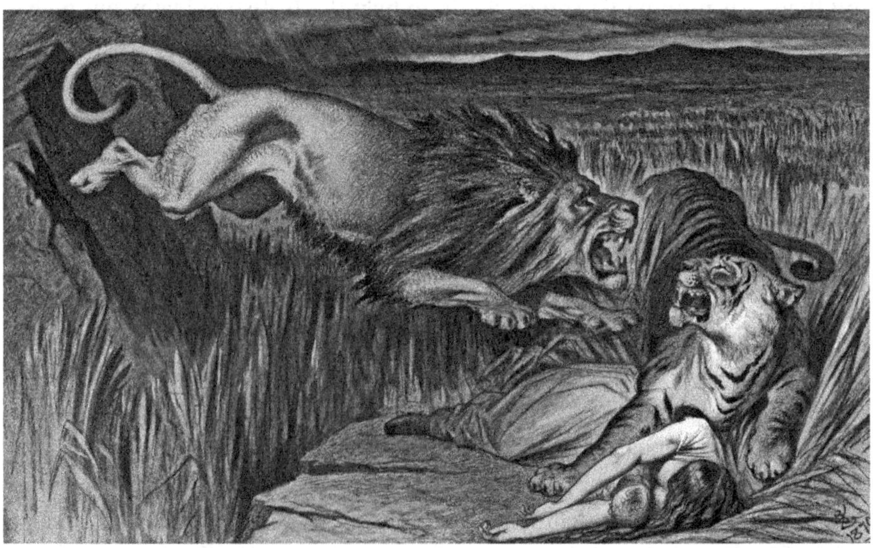

Figure 2.1 The British Lion's Revenge. Drawn by Sir John Tenniel, this cartoon appeared in *Punch*, August 22, 1857. A British woman and child—civilization and whiteness—lie beneath the Indian tiger. The image was well designed to inflame British public opinion. Courtesy of Library of Congress, Prints and Photographs Division.

fear or pain. Noise is sovereign during combat. More subtly, language differences exacerbate confusion between allies and enemies alike. A tone of voice, a hint of sarcasm, a change in the pitch of speech—all of these can signal a shift in feelings of loyalty between officers and soldiers. Sound is vital for intelligence and as a way to alert civilians and troops about what is happening despite the visual occlusions of war. Quiet can be a relief, or it can be ominous. Armies think it vital to silence their enemies, initially by disrupting their means of communicating, finally by eliminating their resistance completely; when the guns fall silent, it is essential that those of one's opponent have done so first.

Few British officers could understand the language of their Indian soldiers, and most sepoys knew only terse orders in English. The rebellion made the language barriers seem worse, limiting vital communication on all sides. The discomforts of being in the military were to some extent aural. After their noonday meal, "men and officers stumbled back to their tents . . . to lie sweating sleeplessly in the heat, disturbed by the howls of pariah dogs, the yelling of jackals, the gurgling groans of camels the beating of native drums, the squeals and kicking of horses, and the droning chanting of Indian servants who in spite of all edicts on the subject could not be prevented from singing."[47] In the midst of the rebellion, the *Times of London* ran a story about a court of law in Calcutta. It was difficult, an observer admitted, to get anything done there. "The din, the hubbub, the discordance of the many voices, Bengali, English, and Hindostani, is truly astounding," he wrote. "On the one side are heard the gentle tones of a mild Hindoo, pouring in soft suppliance his griefs, with accompanying promises, into the ear of some native Amlah [a court official]. On the other side, the ear is assailed by the harshest languages, often the most virulent abuse, bandied between two witnesses, or lookers on, apparently in the last stage of a violent altercation; and to this is added the unnecessary vociferations of some dozen policemen, who rush, gesticulating violently, to the spot to increase the confusion."[48] The inability to understand Hindi especially had consequences on the battlefield.[49] British officers and civilians heard a new "insolence" in the voices of their soldiers or servants.[50] There were certain words British officers used that their sepoys understood. A British civilian in India recalled that "the sepoy is . . . addressed as 'suar' or pig, an epithet most approbrious [*sic*] to a respectable native especially the Mussulman, and which cuts him to the quick. The old [officers] are less guilty. . . . But the younger men seem to regard it as an excellent joke, as an evidence of spirit and a praiseworthy sense of superiority over the sepoy to treat him as an inferior animal."[51]

Once the rebellion started, the British tried to secure their own lines of communication and to prevent the sepoys from communicating among themselves. They could not always control roads, rivers, and telegraph lines. When the telegraph in Lahore went down, men in the cantonment found the abrupt "silence . . . oppressive."[52] Cawnpore was in every way cut off.[53] In Googaira, British troops seized "the drums with which the rebels used to sound the assembly, and collect their forces in the wilderness."[54] The newspapers were strictly censored. A new law required a government license to operate a printing press; another "prohibited the publication or circulation" of "any particular newspaper, book, or other printed paper" deemed subversive by the authorities.[55] Editors were banished or imprisoned for publishing "treasonable matter," or put under surveillance.[56] And the British tried to intercept and open every letter addressed to a sepoy.[57] As Robert Montgomery observed, "no man's tongue was his own property."[58]

War came "like a thunder-clap," bringing its soul-wrenching din. In the Punjab, Henry Lawrence's pre-emptive crackdown on the sepoys was announced with the "ringing rattle" of artillery loading and the "tramp" of loyal soldiers moving into place at their front. The sepoys were struck "dumb before the newly-aroused volition of the Anglo-Saxons."[59] The British rang church bells or fired off shots to warn of the enemy's approach.[60] In Delhi, the rebellion was heralded by the explosion of the magazine.[61] To captives, the sounds made by the sepoys were terrifying: "their wild shouts of laughter mingled with the crackling of the flames. . . . We heard them disputing, and the clang of their guns sounded as though they were reloading them" (Ruth Coopland, at Gwalior), and "the entreaties of the wounded to be helped out of the flames . . . was more than one could bear; and their cries and dying groans heart-rending" (Amy Haines, Cawnpore).[62] From Lucknow, in the summer of 1857, Brigadier John Inglis took charge of the garrison trying to hold the Residency portion of the city against the rebels. "Few troops have ever undergone greater hardships, exposed as they were to a never-ceasing Musketry fire and Cannonade," he wrote to the Military Department in Calcutta. Between actual attacks, Inglis's men were subjected to "the hardly less harassing false alarms which the Enemy have been constantly raising." The rebels opened fire, "sounded the advance, and shouted for several hours together, though not a man could be seen, with view, of course, of harassing our small and exhausted Force, in which object they succeeded." The enemy crept so close at times that they could converse with the Indians who had remained loyal and tried to persuade or threaten them to desert.[63] The British were the besiegers at Delhi that summer. As the British attack began, wrote G. E. Baynes, they were met by "a tremendous musketry fire" and "the enemy yelling and shouting at us" from the city walls.[64] Robert Young was there too, having heard through the siege "the din of the bullets . . . enough make the bravest new hand at times quail, especially when the round shot came singing along." The assault began with "the roll of musketry," which grew "louder and louder" and was accompanied by the "booming of the heavy guns."[65] The noise was fearsome.

As each battle ended, the noise of combat was replaced by the sounds of victory, including the music of bands. Chardin Johnson heard "a capital selection from the Travatore, including 'Ah che la morte,' which called to mind other times and scenes."[66] One officer came across a pile of broken furniture, which included several wrecked pianos. A group of Gurkhas, who had fought alongside the British, were pulling their swords over the instruments' wire strings "as they danced like demons to their own horrible discords"—a celebration of victory, or perhaps a show of contempt for losers and victors alike.[67] The British also recorded pleas for mercy from sepoys whose "treachery" could not be proved. "Is it justice," asked one rajah, "to turn a deaf ear when the king has sent his very women to plead at the foot of your throne?"[68] British ears remained for the most part deaf in this regard. Nor did the British record the groans of wounded prisoners, the squeak of the hangman's rope, or the blasts of cannon that blew apart hundreds of the vanquished sepoys.

The sense of smell was assailed by the fighting. The storms that people saw and heard and felt as the rebellion approached also carried a distinctive odor—until, that is, the dust they carried entered nostrils and dulled olfactory nerves. In their attempts to hide from the enemy, British civilians and soldiers often took refuge in noisome outhouses and latrines.[69] Correspondents who came to India to cover the uprising found the terrible heat of the place accentuated smells best understood by those in London who might, wrote one, "stand over the grating of a Strand cook shop in the dog-days" of summer—though even then they would have but a "poor idea of the nastiness of the blast."[70] In Cawnpore, the odor of the barracks in which the British sheltered soon drove them to open trenches; in Lucknow the sweepers fled, and the latrines "were soon filled to overflowing."[71] Elizabeth Sneyd was fortunate to escape downriver from Cawnpore, but she suffered from "the intolerable smell arising from a quantity of half dried bullock hides and other merchandize being taken to Calcutta" on the boat.[72] The reek of blood and rot and of the dead, animal and human, was everywhere. "We occupied the post," recalled Francis Maude and John Sherer of their time at Lucknow, "and as I lay there, on the second night, the effluvium from the festering heap of bodies . . . was so overpowering that I was totally unable to sleep."[73] During the siege of Delhi, an officer wrote to the *Glasgow Herald* that the sepoys defending the city "have their dead and wounded altogether, and the stench is frightful, even outside" the battlements.[74] Robert Young, on picket duty, was forced "to ride through hundreds of dead and putrid camels, the stench from which was abominable, and almost stifled me in spite of cigars, eau-de-cologne, &c."[75] "It is time we were off," Chardin Johnson wrote in his journal at Delhi in November. "The smells, dead Pandies [Indians] and whatnot, are becoming unbearable."[76] Overcrowded military hospitals lacked ventilation, and in at least one case the outdoor latrines lay "close to one of the wards and the kitchen, where great annoyance is experienced from the smell."[77] The British also reported on alleged Indian abuses of the nose and Indians' contempt for British smelling practices. The leaders of the rebellion were said to cut off the noses of Indian "traitors," and an Indian cavalryman, who saved the life of the Englishwoman Amy Haines, nevertheless sneered that the British resembled "monkies" in having "the same ungenteel custom of smelling [their] food before partaking of it."[78]

As the rebellion began, the metaphors of touch changed. The British had believed that Indians clung to them for reassurance and security.[79] Now hand was raised against hand, evoking the betrayal felt by the British and the violence that they faced and with which they responded.[80] "The great mutiny octopus now gradually enfolded cantonment after cantonment," wrote Robert Young, "and city after city, in the deadly embrace of its huge tentacles, till most of the N. W. Provinces and some parts of Bengal and the Punjab were in its grasp, and it seemed, for a time, that the greater part of India would follow suit."[81] India had become a dangerous animal that threatened to suffocate the civilized presence in its midst.

Battle was hard on the skin and the body overall. Soldiers on the march or in the field were even more exposed than usual to the harsh Indian summer. The intense heat was unrelieved by the high winds, "which set in about 10 o'clock daily and last until sunset," and "are all but intolerable, charged as they are with dust of a revolting nature, which fills every pore and fires the blood,—which seems to penetrate the internal mechanism of the body, as it does in reality force its way into the works of a watch."[82] British soldiers were overdressed for the terrible heat they encountered. In July 1858 twenty-two of them died from sunstroke, and the 1st Dragoon Guards rode at Lucknow in brass helmets that burned their necks and scalps; the soldiers "claimed that they could toast bread inside them."[83] To the list of outrages committed against British women and children in Cawnpore was added the heat they suffered when confined to tents or the small house in which they were imprisoned.[84] There were the additional bodily discomforts of riding or walking long distances in the hope of escaping capture, of cramped hiding places provided by sympathetic villagers, of skin that prickled uncomfortably after days without a bath or a change of clothes, and of the need to sleep on the ground.[85]

Worse were violations or penetrations of the skin: bullets fired into vital organs, wounds opened and left to bleed or suppurate, shot and shrapnel blasted into bodies. Survivors complained about insult done to the body. "Our blood is roused," cried an officer. "We have seen friends, relations, mothers, wives, children, brutally murdered, and their bodies mutilated frightfully."[86] The Joint Magistrate of Banda mistakenly rode into the village after it had been taken by the rebels. He was killed and, according to a colleague, the local nawab "allowed [his corpse] to remain stripped and exposed all the day before his gateway, and at night it was dragged away by the sweepers and thrown to the dogs." The next day, several Britons, including two women, were dragged out of a house in which they were hiding and killed. "Their bodies were stripped, thrown into a field, and left a prey to the vultures and jackals."[87] In June, six British officers were killed by a mob. The dead were "mercilessly hacked to pieces," then "stripped, there [*sic*] effects carried off—and there poor remains left to become the prey of jackalls, vultures, and other 'noisome' scavenger beasts abounding in the country."[88] From Calcutta, a correspondent reported on the "upcountry horrors" of the rebellion: "Mothers pelted with bits of their murdered infants, young English ladies led perfectly naked through the Bazaars under a scorching sun, children, their toes and fingers lopped off, and the wounded limbs exposed to a slow fire, infants wrenched from their mothers' breasts, seized by the legs and torn asunder, boys and girls compelled to eat morsels cut from the bodies of their parents, slaughtered before their eyes. Horrors yet more awful and revolting our countrymen and women have undergone, but decency demands that over these we draw a veil."[89] Here the outrages were visual, gustatory ("compelled to eat morsels"), and most of all haptic, featuring bodies violated, dismembered, and mutilated.

The British also accused the sepoys of raping European women. Rumors of rape were of course highly inflammatory, and the allegations were taken seriously by the Governor General, Viscount Canning, who in late 1857 ordered an investigation. A number of officials wrote with their impressions to William Muir, head of intelligence for the North-West Provinces. None found credible evidence of rape having occurred. The explanation, in several cases, was that the sepoys' blood lust had led them straight to murder, without stopping to contemplate the "humiliation" that rape would have inflicted on their oppressors. Other correspondents, however, argued that Hindus and Muslims, for different reasons, preferred to avoid contact with white women altogether. One thought that "the colour of European females is repugnant to the oriental taste." C. B. Thornhill claimed that "Hindoos, except of the lowest grade, would have become outcastes had they perpetrated this offence," and that Muslims, while perhaps not opposed to rape, would have found its public practice, at least, "repugnant to the feelings and habits of the country." In the end, the rebels had come to kill Britons, atrociously. Rape would have seemed a distraction.[90]

The rebellion ended as it began, district by district, town by town. The British meted out a version of justice to perpetrators and suspects according to the anger and contempt they felt for their enemies, and on the principle that the haptic traumas they had suffered ought to be returned to Indians in kind but a hundred fold. Flogging was one form of punishment used by the British, meant to inflict terrible pain and lifelong evidence of criminality borne on the flesh. "Camp followers" of the rebels were flogged, given a rupee each, and sent home.[91]

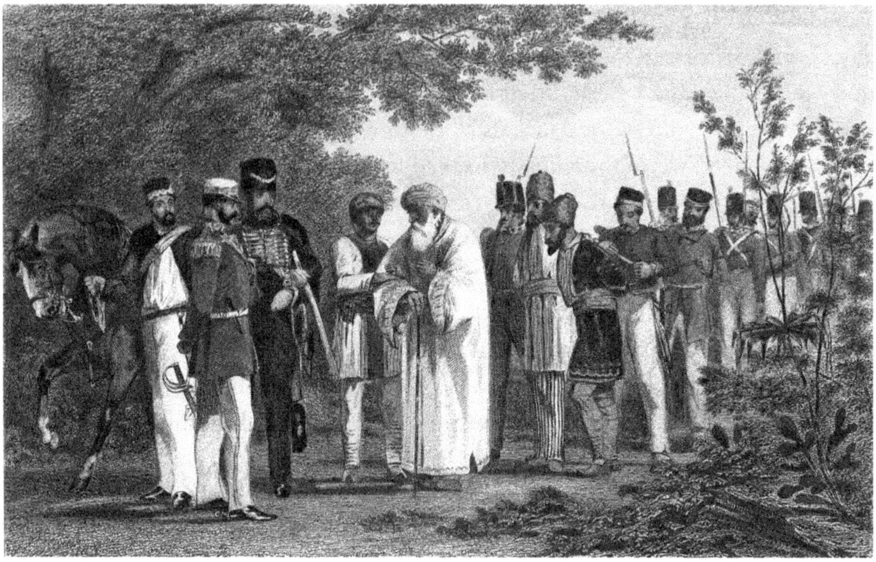

Figure 2.2 King Bahadur Shah, the last Mughal emperor, was taken captive following the taking of Delhi in early September, 1857. The King was exiled to Burma and died five years later. His three sons, also captured, were shot. Courtesy of the Anne S. K. Brown Military Collection, John Hay Library, Brown University.

John Nicholson, who led the storming of Delhi, suggested that the city's surviving resisters be impaled, burned, or flayed alive; the former governor-general, Lord Ellenborough, proposed castrating every remaining male there and renaming the city "Eunuchabad."[92] The Nawab of Farrukhabad was tied to a cot, covered in pig's fat, flogged, then hanged.[93] Scores of rebels were "blown from guns," a practice the British adopted from the Mughals (the Muslims who ruled India for over four hundred years prior to the Raj), in which the prisoner was tied to the mouth of a cannon and the gun was fired. A group of "mutineers," having fled Lahore, was captured and brought back to the city, where they were court-martialed and blown from guns while the brigade looked on.[94] On the afternoon of April 12, 1858, Chardin Johnson "went to see a Sepoy of the 12th Native Infantry who had mutineered [*sic*] and shot his havildar [sergeant] . . . blown away from a gun. It is the best and speediest way of taking life I have seen—this man was in little pieces all over the place in less than an eyewink."[95] Thus did the utter disintegration of the body, by the most powerful and hideous form of touch, pronounce the end of the Great Rebellion.

Taste was the final sense challenged by the rising. It was of course the fear of bodily pollution through the ingestion of cow or pig fat that sparked the rebellion. Metaphors of fealty and betrayal had to do with consumption. A common expression in India had it that "natives" were loyal because they had "eaten the

Company's salt." Those in rebellion were called *nimak-haráms*—"traitors to their salt," while some of the British hoped, early in the rising, that if they showed restraint their sepoys "would gladly lay down their arms and eat the Company's salt again if permitted to do so."[96]

Soldiers and civilians suffered from the gustatory privations of war. Having participated in the sieges of Delhi and Cawnpore, Chardin Johnson hoped that the provisioning of the army would improve. Instead, food continued to be hard to secure, and what was available was well below standard. "The men have had nothing but rum and biscuits for 2 days and grumble at so much hard work on empty stomachs and no wonder, but it cannot be helped," he wrote from the bank of the Ganges in late November. Three weeks later, he visited a nearby rifle brigade. He found them "exceedingly miserable. The officers have no mess or stores of any kind. . . . All they have to live upon is their rations of beef and mutton and that of indifferent quality."[97] Often liquor, relatively easy to obtain, became a substitute for food or water, which many Britons regarded as tainted.[98] Captives were deprived too. At Cawnpore, Amy Haines wrote that her younger brothers and sisters "were dying from hunger and would have eaten the most loathsome thing. . . . Our stress for water can be imagined when on one occasion we were obliged to drink it, mixed with human blood which had fallen into our vessel from the wounds of an Ayah who was close by it when the bursting of a shell carried away both her legs."[99] "Food, which in happier times would have been turned from with disgust, was seized with avidity and devoured with relish," wrote two historians of the rebellion. "To the flesh-pots of the besieged no carrion was unwelcome. A stray dog was turned into soup. An old horse, fit only for the knackers, was converted into a savory meal."[100] As the rebellion collapsed, the British retaliated for such episodes by withholding food from Indians or causing them to "lose caste" by force-feeding them forbidden meats, humiliating men whom they planned to kill anyway—often with a thrust of sword or bayonet to the abdomen, known as a "Cawnpore dinner."[101]

As the Great Rebellion ended and the British set to the task of consolidating formal rule over India, the United States was on the verge of violent sectional conflict. Its aftermath would require resetting national priorities, which came to include large-scale growth in manufacturing and agriculture, growing concentration of capital, greater interest in trade, and a more assertive posture toward the world. Americans sought inroads in Europe, Latin America, and East Asia. By 1890, the United States was building a new navy to help protect trade routes to the Pacific. It had secured island bases in Hawaii and Samoa and purchased Alaska from Russia. There was serious talk in Washington about an isthmian canal through Central America. Its leaders eyed the empires of Britain, France, Germany, and Japan with apprehension and envy.

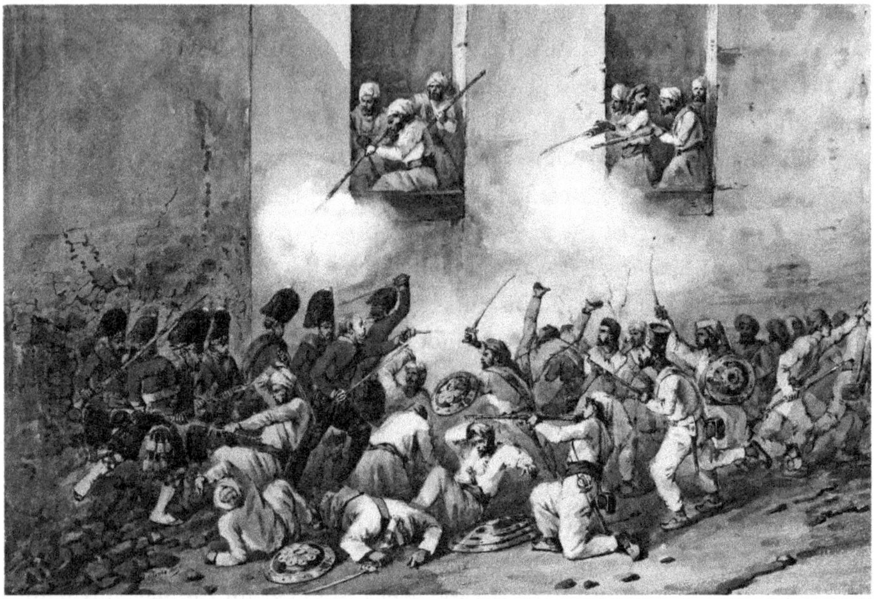

Figure 2.3 The siege of Lucknow. It required a protracted siege by the British to rescue comrades confined to Lucknow's Residency. This drawing shows the storming of the walled garden of Secundra Bagh in late November 1857. As they attacked the British soldiers shouted, "Remember Cawnpore!" Courtesy of the Anne S. K. Brown Military Collection, John Hay Library, Brown University.

When Cubans rebelled against their Spanish rulers in 1895, most Americans sympathized with the Cubans. Spanish repression of the rebellion, brutal enough in fact but much exaggerated by American newspapers, increased public anger toward Spain and raised pressure on the government to act. President William McKinley hoped to avoid American involvement in the conflict and urged Spain to come to terms with the rebels. There was some movement in this direction in late 1897. But a combination of Spanish indiscretion, the destruction of the US battleship *Maine* in Havana harbor in February 1898, allegedly by a Spanish mine, and the ongoing uncertainty of business conditions in the hemisphere further inflamed public opinion, and the reluctant president sought and got a Congressional declaration of war with Spain on April 21. US troops hurriedly trained then headed south to help the Cubans achieve their independence—though on North American terms.

Cuba was not the only Spanish colony of interest to the United States. The navy had previously surveyed the harbor at Manila, the Philippines, for strategic and economic reasons. Intrigued by potential ties to the China market and concerned about the assertiveness of Britain, Germany, and Japan in the Pacific, the Americans could hardly overlook the archipelago's location. On

February 25, 1898, Theodore Roosevelt, the assistant secretary of the navy, ordered Commodore George Dewey, whose squadron was based in Hong Kong, to prepare to strike the Spaniards in the Philippines should war come. Three days after the declaration of war, Dewey was told politely by the British governor of Hong Kong that as a belligerent in a war in which Britain was neutral, he must depart. Dewey asked Washington where he should go. "Proceed at once to the Philippines," the Navy Department (with McKinley's consent) replied. "Commence operations against the Spanish squadron. You must capture or destroy. Use utmost endeavors."[102]

Dewey fulfilled his duty. On May 1, his nine ships dispatched the Spanish fleet with startling efficiency, sinking three Spanish ships and scuttling six others. Spain suffered 161 dead and 371 casualties overall; nine American sailors were wounded. But matters in the Philippines were far from resolved. Dewey did not have the men to occupy Manila, far less the country in its entirety, and at that point it was not clear what McKinley wanted to do with the islands. Spanish soldiers remained in their positions in Manila. Although it was little remarked upon by the Americans, a Filipino independence movement had taken root in the country. While its leaders, primarily Emilio Aguinaldo, celebrated Dewey's victory over Spain, they were not interested in replacing Spanish rule with American.

At first, they did not imagine having to do so. Inspired by José Rizal, the nationalist Andrés Bonifacio had founded, in 1892, the Katipunan, dedicated to the ritual purification of Filipinos and the ousting of the Spaniards from the islands. The Spaniards learned of the presence of the Katipunan in 1896 and suppressed it by arresting and executing hundreds of its members or suspected members. In response Bonifacio declared war, but he was no soldier and led his men disastrously. Rizal rejected the course of the Katipunan; he was nevertheless hanged by the Spaniards later that year. But the movement was embraced by Aguinaldo, who quickly proved its most capable officer. Inflicting several defeats on Spanish troops in his native province of Cavite, Aguinaldo rose in esteem among Filipinos, infuriating Bonifacio and leading to a falling out between the men. In May 1897, after Bonifacio had conspired against him, Aguinaldo captured his rival and ordered his death. He then offered to negotiate with the Spaniards and even accept their rule, as long as the hated Spanish friars left the Philippines and the islands gained representation in Madrid. Unable to finish him, Spain chose talks. The two sides reached an agreement in late 1897, by which Spain paid an indemnity to Aguinaldo and agreed to make reforms. Aguinaldo disavowed the rebellion and left the country for Hong Kong. There he would meet George Dewey.

Despite the deal, Spain had no intention of lessening its control of the Philippines, and Aguinaldo continued to see a future for himself as a fighter for independence. The arrival of the Americans complicated the plans of both sides. Having gone to war to free Cuba from Spain, the Americans, whatever their ultimate intentions in the Philippines, did not count among their options leaving Spain in charge. Neither did they consider allowing Filipinos to govern themselves. At minimum, they envisioned garrisoning Manila, supplanting Spanish troops and thereby disrupting any Filipino plans to assume power. Aguinaldo, who had been encouraged by the American consul in Hong Kong and had been summoned by Dewey to join the expedition to Manila, hoped that the Americans would install him in a position of authority and soon leave the islands to him. Once in the Philippines, however, Aguinaldo declared the islands' independence. Dewey was invited to the ceremony but said he was too busy to attend. As units of the US army began arriving in Manila in late June, Aguinaldo remained publicly optimistic about the prospect of independence. To his group of advisers he added more moderate *ilustrados*. He introduced a new flag, of red, white, and blue, hoping to please the Americans, and he stopped calling himself "dictator" and used instead the title "president." Key members of his coalition urged him to permit US sovereignty over the islands for the time being, for they feared the mob even more than the presence of the imperialists. Aguinaldo counseled patience—"never forget," he told his officers, "the Americans are our friends"—but he watched apprehensively as well over ten thousand US troops arrived in the Philippines by the end of the summer. As the Americans replaced the Spaniards in Manila, the Filipinos withdrew to positions just beyond the American lines, still hoping for discussions leading, eventually, to their autonomy. Then, late that year, McKinley announced that the United States, under the guise of "benevolent assimilation," would annex the entire archipelago.[103]

Incidents of taunting, name-calling, shoving, and beating followed, nearly all initiated by the Americans. Senses on both sides were taxed. Americans and Filipinos saw each other every day, an affront to vision. The streets of Manila were noisy, hot, crowded, and stank of garbage and excrement—"a more filthy place I never saw," wrote a soldier. "The stench is something awful"—and made worse by the sudden influx of Americans. The Americans called Filipinos "gugus" and "niggers." US soldiers, mostly white and often from rural areas, casually used violence against their perceived inferiors, and hundreds of Filipinos, including women and children, were roughed up in the street, struck with rifle butts or shot. As the new year dawned, shooting on both sides occurred with greater frequency. General Elwell Otis insisted on extending American lines into areas claimed by Aguinaldo. On the night of February 4, Private William Grayson of the 1st Nebraska encountered four Filipinos, just to his front, likely drunk and possibly armed. "Halt!" shouted Grayson. The Filipinos laughed and shouted back. Grayson fired twice, his friend Orville Miller fired once, then both men ran

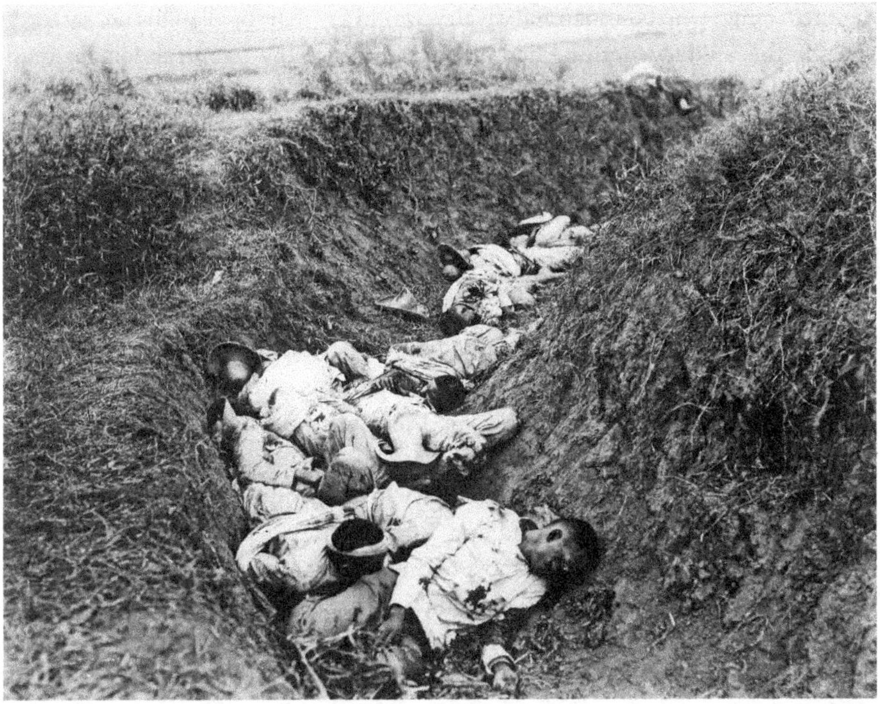

Figure 2.4 Filipino soldiers died in their trenches outside Manila at the onset of fighting the Americans, February 4–5, 1899. National Archives and Record Administration ARC Identifier 524389.

back toward American lines, as Grayson yelled, "Line up, fellows, the niggers are in here all through these lines!" With that, war began.[104]

The Americans at first seemed shocked at the determination of Aguinaldo's forces to resist them. The battle for position around Manila spread to the countryside, then beyond Luzon south to other islands. US naval units shelled villages near the shoreline and transited rivers in search of an elusive enemy, while infantry and cavalry slogged inland, occupying villages and trying to capture the fighters, their arms and supplies, and above all their leaders, without whom, the Americans believed, the "insurrection" (as they called it to avoid the international and legal complications involved in fighting a "war") would soon collapse. Aguinaldo recognized that he lacked enough troops to resist the expanding American force and in November 1899 called for a guerrilla war. From the mountains and jungles his soldiers employed hit and run tactics against Americans trained to fight pitched battles. General Thomas Anderson, who came to Manila in April 1898, recalled that "I had never heard of Aguinaldo at that time, and all I knew of the Philippines was that they were famous for hemp, earthquakes, tropical diseases and rebellion."[105] US Brigadier General

Samuel Young, who commanded cavalry, would say that for all of his nearly forty years in the military, nothing had prepared him for the "tropical deluges mud and water, the swimming, bridging and rafting of innumerable streams, most of which were not on the map."[106] In June 1900, William Howard Taft arrived in Manila to take charge as civilian governor. General Arthur MacArthur, who was military governor, dismissed the possibility that civilians could control the situation in the Philippines and resented Taft's insistence that the military stick to fighting and leave the civics to him. Something of a turning point in the conflict was achieved when Aguinaldo was captured in March 1901, though in fact by that time the Americans had gained the upper hand throughout the archipelago. Aguinaldo surrendered graciously, urging his compatriots to give up the fight and cooperate with the Americans. The fighting nevertheless continued for well over a year. Theodore Roosevelt declared the insurrection at an end on July 4, 1902. The president praised the military for its "courage and fortitude." The United States suffered 4,234 dead and 2,818 wounded. Filipino casualties ran into the hundreds of thousands, most of them civilians.[107]

Both sides committed atrocities. Aguinaldo insisted that prisoners be treated well, and on the whole they seem to have been, though as his position grew more desperate it became harder to ensure the welfare of anyone in camp, including that of captives. American soldiers nevertheless reported bitterly that

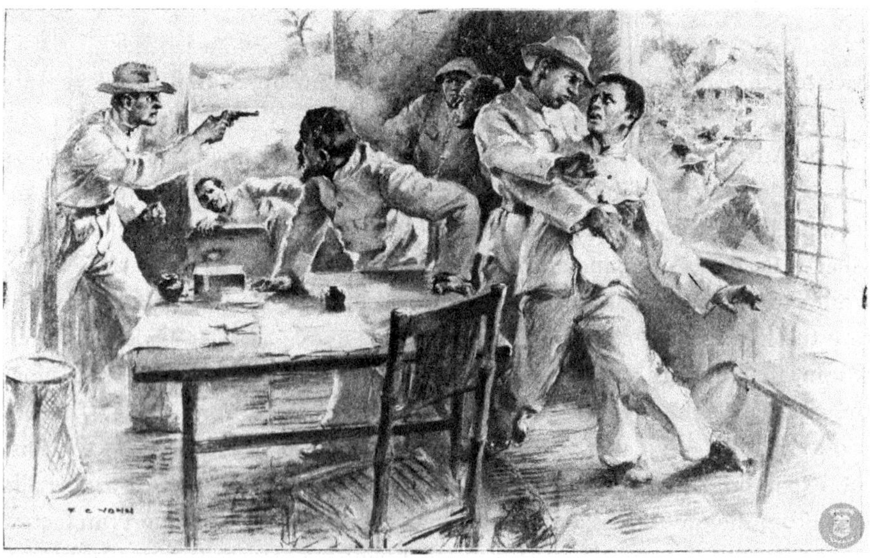

Figure 2.5 Led by Filipino Macabebe scouts and with help from a ruse, Brigadier General Frederick Funston captured Emilio Aguinaldo at his headquarters at Palanan, March 23, 1901. Aguinaldo accepted his capture gracefully, and it was a turning point in the war. From Aguinaldo Presidential Museum and Library, Manila.

their comrades had been tortured and mutilated. American cruelties were more systematic. "Any army that is required while waging war to observe the gentle rules of ping-pong will become a laughing stock at home and abroad," General Young told an audience in late 1902. "We were engaged in war against a cruel and vindictive lot of savages, who were in no way related to us," which made harsh measures seem only logical.[108] Matthew Batson, who trained and led Macabebe Scouts against the insurgents, wrote his wife that "at present we are destroying in this district everything before [us]."[109] Colonel Benjamin Cheatham suggested that his men "burn pretty freely and kill every man who runs"; William Brown spent an August 1900 evening with General Frederick Funston "discussing affairs . . . and his plans for exterminating the Goo Goos."[110] The Americans notoriously practiced the "water cure," which involved prying open the jaws of the victim and pouring quantities of water down his throat, to simulate drowning.[111] Reports of burning, drunkenness, and looting by Americans came frequently to Taft, who seemed genuinely uncomfortable with them and who reported them to influential friends in Washington as a way to gain leverage against MacArthur.[112] Even Taft thought it necessary to edit comments by Major Cornelius Gardener, the Governor of Tayabas Province in Luzon. US troops, Gardener complained, had been burning whole villages "in trying the lay waste to the country so that the insurgents can not occupy it," and "torturing . . . natives by socalled water cure and other methods. . . . Almost without exception, soldiers and also many officers, refer to the natives in their presence as 'niggers' and natives are beginning to understand what the word 'nigger' means."[113]

Atrocities are violations of bodies and abuses of the senses. They may be triggered by perceived acute threats to the senses, in which case the individual is overwhelmed and may react by lashing out in violence. Henry C. Rowland was acting assistant surgeon in the Army when he arrived in the Philippines in 1898. In a *McClure's* article published in 1902, he tried to explain why some soldiers had committed atrocities, or "the psychic reversion to atavism by which, in a few weeks' time, a civilized individual can hark back to a primitive state of savagery." He described a column on patrol through the jungle: "Heat! Heat! Heat! Hot noises, hot smells, dry hot baking vegetation that rustles crisply against their thighs. In the impalpable powder beneath their feet creep creatures stifling to see; lizards breathing dust, insects whose lurid glow is like an ember. Hot smells of dust and scorched weeds burn their throats and nostrils. Over their head comes the droning hum of insects that sound like an overdose of quinine, and might be. From a dead tree a bell-bug strikes his clear, ringing note." Two men stray, and are murdered and mutilated. When the company captures Filipino "bolomen," they execute them without hesitation. "Each man thinks of the headless corpses on the mountain side. . . . They have seen savage sights; they have eaten the food of savages; they have thought savage thoughts; the cries of savages

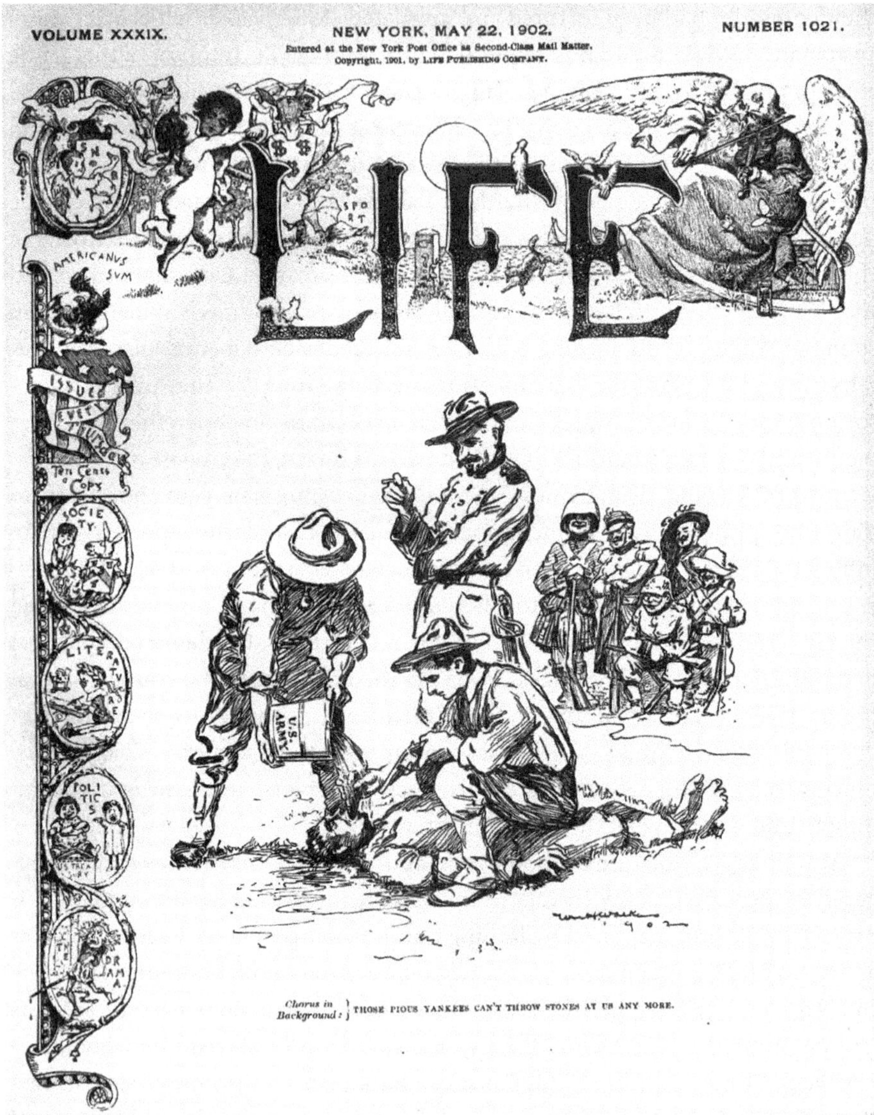

Figure 2.6 This *Life* magazine cover from May 22, 1902, drawn by William Watkins, depicts the American "water cure" against a suspected insurgent. Representatives of other empires look on, grinning with satisfaction: "Those pious Yankees can't throw stones at us any more."

are ringing in their brains. In all their surroundings there is not one single object to remind them that they belong to an era of civilization."[114] Torture is different, but equally derives from the senses. The torturer aims to inspire fear with visual threats (look: this is what will happen to you if you do not cooperate), aural threats (hear the screams of those being tortured), and may involve smell, for instance, the odors of sweat or of shit released out of fear. The water "cure" was an instance of forced ingestion, overwhelming in volume. Mostly, atrocities were haptic violations, involving pain inflicted on the skin, penetration, or dismemberment. Unlike the British, the Americans did not blow men from guns. Like the British, they flogged their enemies, dozens of them in the town of Laoag, Ilocos Norte, in May 1900; the local judge wrote Taft "that the place where these castigations occurred reminded one of a slaughter house in a country town, and all from human blood."[115] They shot, knifed, burned, and hanged Filipinos. They confined them behind untouchable barbed wire.

Atrocities represented the most extreme practices of war. Even in their absence, the Philippine-American War, like the Great Rebellion in India, was a war of the senses. Confusions of vision set in for American soldiers even before they arrived in the Philippines. Soldiers were brought to San Francisco's Camp Merritt, where they were thrust together with unfamiliar comrades and could hardly see through the fog. Then they boarded ships for weeks at sea. Many had never traveled by water, and the vast emptiness of the ocean awed and troubled them. They looked slovenly, as they admitted, clad in "an assortment of blue wool, brown canvas, and white linen" that passed as uniforms.[116] Visual confoundings only got worse as they began fighting. "The friends at home would hardly be able to recognize their soldier boy in his field clothes, unshaved and often unwashed," wrote one man. "The uniform consists of a variegated assortment of shirts and greasy pair of 'cast-iron' pants deeply dyed in the rich mud of the Philippines. All are bronzed, the hair uncut, the beard untrimmed; fine, healthy, robust men, in their wild appearance not unlike the portraitures of Robinson Crusoe."[117] They found Manila hideous, "the dirtiest, most tumble down place I ever saw. It is nasty," concluded Ernest Tilton.[118] There were better sorts of Filipinos, men and women who, the Americans admitted, bathed frequently and wore clean clothes, though the men spoiled the effect by wearing their shirt tails outside their pants, and otherwise respectable women wore rice powder "so thickly on the arms and faces" that "they looked as though they had been dipped in the family flour barrel."[119] On the whole, Americans found Filipinos unattractive, even repulsive. They were "the dirtiest, ugliest, and poorest people on earth," according to the infantryman Charles Fischback.[120] "I hate the sight of the niggers and, although they are always bathing and are cleanly as a people as far as washing goes, in other ways they are filthy. I avoid them like the plague," Robert Carter wrote his father.[121] Whites regarded dark skin as dirty and ugly in and of itself.[122]

Like the British in 1857, Americans in the Philippines in 1899 had trouble telling friend from enemy. Filipinos, said the Americans, had a talent for appearing innocent even while they plotted violence. "Experience taught," wrote Emily Conger, who accompanied her soldier son to the islands, "that the most guileless in looks were the worst desperadoes of all."[123] The racist term "gook" (or "goo-goo" or "gugu") likely comes from the expression "goo-goo eyes," which meant feigned innocence concealing murderous intent.[124] "It is going to be very difficult to start a government for these people," wrote Ernest Tilton. "They are utterly incomprehensible to me. They are a cross between a child and an animal of some sort. It seems a pity to kill them but they are treacherous."[125] He summed it up: "I won't trust them as far as I can see them."[126]

Vision in battle was occluded, distorted, and fraught. The country was poorly mapped.[127] Sudden downpours of rain and enveloping dark made it impossible to see even at close quarters, which led nervous and trigger-happy men to fire promiscuously at the enemy, civilians, comrades, even animals.[128] Clenard McLaughlin described a doctor standing up recklessly to fire at Filipino lines. "I said to him later on, 'what were you standing up for?' 'Well,' he said, 'I couldn't see anything to shoot at and I was looking.' And I said, 'Did you hear anything?' 'Oh,' he said, 'I heard something go whish.' So lots of the times you didn't see what you were shooting at, but you knew they were in there because they were firing."[129] The visual treachery Americans ascribed to Filipinos generally could be fatal when practiced in battle, and the problem, the Americans complained, became acute once the insurgency degenerated into a guerrilla war. The *insurrectos* hid out in "mountain fastnesses" and "bamboo thickets," from which they darted out suddenly to ambush small groups of American soldiers.[130] "We scout, scout, and the enemy is harder to find than the proverbial fleas," wrote Lt. Lee McCoy, and an exasperated soldier complained that "the Filipino soldier is not very large but what he lacks in size is made up in agility; now you see him and then he is gone."[131] One officer referred to the US army as "a blind giant."[132] When a group of *insurrectos* encountered an American force, charged Henry Hoyt, they would "vanish in the jungle and 'presto change'" into white coats and pants, and thus "emerge innocent amigos clad in white."[133] The Americans were not delicate in their attempts to expose the enemy. They searched Filipino women for knives, making a habit of checking for weapons hung from the waist, between the legs.[134] When the fighting started, Americans found, to their chagrin, that the Spanish Mauser rifles the Filipinos used were smokeless when fired, while their own Springfields betrayed their owners with a billowing puff every time they were discharged.[135]

The casualties of war were dismaying to see, even when they were Filipino. *Harper's* reporter John F. Bass recorded a scene "which burned into my memory, and which I cannot forget if I would. A middle-aged grizzly-headed native sat bolt-upright. A bullet or a piece of shell had passed through his neck, and completely shattered his jaw. He was perfectly conscious, but he showed no evidence of suffering. He did not even moan but sat upright, and looked at us with expressionless face and ghastly, staring eyes."[136] Bass later witnessed a slaughter of insurgents who wore charms called *anting-anting*, which were said to make their bearers invulnerable. They launched a suicide charge; many of the dead were boys.[137] For the Americans, seeing their own dead was worse. General Funston witnessed the death of Private Charles Pratt, who had been shot through the brain, and "for some time his body lay there, a grewsome [*sic*] spectacle for those who had occasion to pass near the company and were not yet used to such sights."[138]

The Philippines sounded different from the United States. Few Americans spoke Spanish, as educated Filipinos did, and almost none spoke Tagalog or any other Filipino language. Tricks of the eye were augmented, in American ears, by deceptions of the tongue, just as the British had claimed in India decades earlier. Filipinos never spoke the truth; it had "little value in their eyes," according to Dana Merrill, while Guy Henry concluded that Filipinos "are the most deceteful and bigest liers [*sic*] on the face of the earth and that is saying a good deal."[139] "How strange our advent and actions must seem to them," Samuel Young wrote in his diary. "They are certainly a race of most cheerful liars."[140] There were times of quiet, near silence, and these moments, soothing to civilians, were agony for soldiers uncertain of enemy positions. While the Americans, loaded down with weapons, ammunition, and equipment, clanked through the countryside "rattling and tinkling," "the barefooted enemy, knowing every by-path, can slip through the jungle as soundlessly and rapidly as wild animals."[141] Mostly, though, the Americans found the islands cacophonous. They brought noise with them, as Manila's bars throbbed with the sound of drunken idle soldiers, bands playing, and men celebrating, whoring, and brawling.[142] When they sought silence, they were betrayed by their environment. Troops attempting to leave the town of Siniloan under cover of darkness set the dogs barking, and monkeys shrilled warnings of men approaching through the jungle.[143] The quinine soldiers took to prevent or combat ubiquitous malaria made their ears ring.[144]

Mostly, after February 1899, the Philippines sounded like war. Men cried out, in jubilation, fury, and pain. The Americans were urged by their commanders to yell as they attacked.[145] On the night the war began John Bass could see little, but his ears were attuned to the sounds of battle. "The rattle of musketry broke the stillness of the night," he wrote. He made his way through the streets of Manila, "where only the tramp, tramp, tramp of companies going to the front, and sharp challenge of sentries at every corner, broke the silence." Two miles from camp the insurgents' bullets "began to hiss and rattle on the tin roofs along the road." The Americans frantically deepened their trenches and dug new ones: "Pound, pound, pound went the picks into the dry, hard, earth." At midnight, "bang! ping! the ball opened again for half an hour. The Mauser rifles of the insurgents made hardly any flame in the night, and their presence was known only by the sharp cracks and whistling of bullets overhead." The Americans' Springfields "made a deep round sound." After a time, "a great shouting came across the

San Juan River from the Filipinos, and one distinctly heard: 'Viva la Republica Filipina! Americanos mucho malo!" The sides exchanged artillery fire; "a roar from the right of San Juan Hill" indicated the position of a Filipino gun, and when the Americans fired a shell back, "one could hear it panting all the way. A sharp crack . . . told of its arrival."[146] Bass later witnessed a battle from the gunboat *Laguna de Bay*. "The guns boomed, the shells hissed. Then we remembered the doctor's directions to put cotton in our ears, keep our mouths open, and stand on our toes. The din was awful, shaking the iron plates all around the deck like a gigantic storm behind the scenes of a Bowery melodrama. Below, it was a regular pandemonium, like being shut up in a barrel with a bunch of exploding giant firecrackers."[147] "We used shell and shrapnel and the noise of the bursting shells was worse than any Nutley thunderstorm you ever heard," Ernest Tilton told his wife.[148] Fire, caused by shelling or deliberate burning, had its own sound, and when it burned bamboo it "pops off like a Mauser," one of "dozens of camp sounds [that] keep one on the qui vive all the time."[149] Colonel Fred Funston fought at Caloocan, twelve miles from Manila, on February 10, 1899. The Filipinos had evidently pulled back, but "there was some delay in finding a trumpeter to blow 'Cease firing,' and in the meantime one of our men was hit, and gave a shriek that was heard almost the length of the regiment. In an instant the men were beyond control." They fired at will, making a "deafening" sound through the smoke and gloom, until at last every trumpeter blew the cease fire and officers resorted to "blows and kicks . . . to bring the men to their senses."[150] Men on both sides were meant to respond to bugle calls, but these were difficult to hear, and Walter Cutter claimed that insurgent buglers, scattered widely among the enemy's troops, tried to deceive the Americans into thinking "that they faced us in large numbers."[151]

Every Philippine town had church bells, and these figured heavily as war engulfed the countryside. Some Americans found the sound of the bells uplifting, a reminder of home. Others thought them a nuisance. Bell ringing signified more than piety or an effort to annoy the interlopers. Those sympathetic to the insurgency rang bells as the vanguard of an American patrol reached the town church, then ceased once the column had passed: "The number of men could be judged by the time it took them to pass."[152] The Americans made other kinds of bells work for them, fastening small ones to fences that enclosed prisoners or civilians who had been "relocated" to camps, thus ensuring that a tinkling sound would alert them to any escape attempt.[153] Like US army units, every Philippine village also had a band, a legacy of Spain, which was largely brass, but might also include guitars, violins, and instruments made of bamboo. They greeted the Americans as they arrived to "liberate" towns, and some soldiers admitted that they enjoyed the bands' renditions of American songs, nearly always including "Hot Time in the Old Town Tonight."[154]

The Americans tried to control the soundscape of war, and in part they succeeded. The guns fell silent, concrete stilled the squeaking iron wheels of the Philippine cart, or *carromata,* and the brass bands were disciplined by American officials. Yet there was a curious harbinger of hybridity to come in the postwar soundscape. Americans in the Philippines increasingly picked up phrases of Tagalog, or a pidgin version of it. Thus, observed George Brandle, wherever US troops were stationed and in contact with local people a linguistic "mixture" emerged, "a cross between all." So " 'die-die' means dead; a 'boom boom' anything from a pistol to a cannon; 'chow-chow' or 'son-son' anything to eat."[155] Brandle seemed surprised or amused that such mixing had been adopted. The lesson may be rather that sound is less susceptible to dominion, and in fact more catching, than many would imagine.

The American soldier's sense of smell was challenged from the time of his training stateside. His food smelled bad, and men lived at close quarters in camp and aboard ship, making it hard to keep clean and thus intensifying the odors of bodies. In the Philippines the smell of the street and the native was, said the Americans, often repellent, while the smell of battle was sharp and distinctive, even to veterans of other conflicts. Manila stank of waste, sweat, urine, and spilled liquor. "Filthy odors arose from the beach, which is the dumping ground for the refuse matter of the surrounding district," wrote one correspondent. "When the tide is out the black mud is tinged green with a disgusting slime, and the stench is horrible. No one but an Oriental or a very Orientalized European could abide in such a locality."[156] Among the Filipino dead and dying at an American *reconcentrado* camp in Samar, an officer complained that "the corpse-carcass stench wafts in and combined with some lovely municipal odors besides makes it slightly unpleasant here."[157] Americans objected especially to the Filipinos' use, or overuse, of coconut oil on their skin and hair, which they found "rancid" and "repulsive."[158] The military humor magazine *Jolo Howler* included a poem called "The Belle of Jolo," which contained the following verse: "Her long, dark, floating tresses / Are sweet (?) with oil of cocoa / I know full well, its fragrant smell / Will surely drive me loco."[159]

In a series of letters to his wife, Lottie, George Telfer described conditions for the soldiers and the odors they produced and encountered. He complained that the men could not bathe for lack of water and proper tubs. (They were told not to bathe in the sea because of the presence of "poisonous fish.") Dried sweat clung to them for days. Their leather pouches turned redolent with mold, and their clothes "sour[ed] as soon as [they were] worn." The omnipresence of excrement particularly disgusted him. "Calls of nature are attended to wherever . . . it is the most convenient—indoors or out of doors," he wrote. "It is worse among the rich than among the poor for the former confine the deposit to their houses—while the latter go out into the street. Capt. Prescott has been on smelling detail among the monasteries near us. He is a very robust man, but he has to excuse himself from the balance of the party now and then—to vomit." He asked her to imagine Manila, where people shared their homes with horses and emptied chamber pots from second floor windows into the street below. "Think of all the bad smells you ever ran against—combine them (in your mind) and you may have some idea of a Spanish city," Telfer wrote. They were trying, he said, to clean things up: "We have a large street cleaning department and every foot of street is swept daily. Twice a day carts gather garbage from dwellings. This with disinfectants is lessening the smells a little." To these smells was added on the battlefield the odor of death. "It is great fun for the men to go on 'nigger hunts,'" Telfer wrote. "The air would be delightful were it not for the odor from dead niggers which have been left unburied."[160]

As in the Great Rebellion, the Philippine War was particularly hard on the skin, and it thus made Americans acutely sensitive to feel and touch. Aboard ship, crossing the Pacific then waiting to disembark, soldiers' mattresses became soaked with sweat and had to be destroyed. Lice drove them mad with scratching.[161] The tropical air was hot and moist and alive with insects, slowing movement and irritating flesh. James M. Smith claimed that "it is so hot in this country that a man has to keep his mouth shut to prevent the sun's rays from warping his teeth."[162] Despite the heat, men were advised to wear woolen undershirts and "stomache bands," cinched tight around the waist and reputed to prevent cholera or "the mulligrubs"—"a griping of the intestines" leading to "a despondent, sullen, or ill-tempered mood."[163] The various insects that crawled or flew were at best a nuisance. "I am on guard," George Telfer wrote from Manila. "It is night, very warm and I am trying *not* to notice mosquitos, prickly heat, red ants, little rivulets of perspiration running down my back, fidgets in my feet, and dozen or more other small things which make life in the tropics interesting."[164] Albert Sonnichsen spent his 21st birthday as a prisoner of the Filipinos. Held in a hut thatched with nipa leaves, he was miserable as rain trickled on his chest all night, and "insects . . . sought shelter about my person, and seemed to be fighting among themselves for the best places."[165] "Insects are thick," Robert Carter told his father. "One becomes extremely nervous when they first live here—sweat, sweat, sweat, bugs, bugs, buggier."[166] The land itself defied movement with haptic resistance; "it was as if nature had taken sides with the insurgents." Men ascribed their rampant dysentery to their moist bodies and despaired as rain turned to mud the roads and paths along which they tried to march.[167] The soldiers fought in swamps and jungles, impeded by thorns and vines and thick stands of bamboo that also concealed their enemies. Samuel Young recalled that nothing in his long military experiences "had prepared him for the 'tropical deluges mud and water, the swimming, bridging and rafting of innumerable streams, most of which were not on the map.'"[168]

The friction of the environment against Americans' skin was uncomfortable and could be dangerous. They experimented with clothing that would soothe rather than rub. Soldiers argued the merits of cotton khaki versus wool undergarments, though in truth both fabrics were coarse and irritating. The army tried putting men in underwear dyed reddish orange, thinking that it might cool the body, but a scientific study debunked this theory and in any case the men resisted wearing such lurid colors.[169] Many Americans, among them Governor Taft, imported softer cotton underwear. Even that did not always help: Taft developed a rectal fistula—aggravated, if not caused, by friction against his skin—that would require three surgeries.[170] Nearly all suffered from sores, ulcers, severe rashes, blisters, boils, and scabs that would not dry out. Many of these the men blamed on "*dhobi* itch," an affliction also claimed by the British in India, where those who washed clothes were called *dhobis*. Its exact cause was then unknown, though westerners believed variously that it was caused by the polluted water in which the *dhobis* washed clothes, insufficient rinsing that left soap in the creases of the garments, a small worm or parasite that infiltrated the clothes during drying in the open air, the ink in tags used by *dhobis* to identify the owner of the clothes, or a disease imparted by the *dhobis* themselves.[171] Walter Cutter wrote that "many of the men had dhobie itch so badly that their feet resembled chunks of putrid meat. They could not wear their shoes, and went around barefooted or in loose canvas shoes."[172] Robert Carter was hospitalized with sores on his feet, then experienced swelling in his ankles and his groin that "had to be reduced by poultices and hot water"; he was, during his stay, "cleaned out of a bucket of hard puss [*sic*] through boils and running sores everywhere." The treatment failed to solve the problem. He wrote his father: "After my work is done, I drop on a cot and endure agony from my feet and veins of my ankles which I have again. . . . The feet feel to the touch like stoves and are green, purplish red and pain and throb like I imagine gout does." He got *dhobi* itch too, which made riding agony and refused to respond to any sort of treatment, including a daily bath with carbolic soap. "It is on the legs," he wrote, "and will drive a sane man to drink."[173]

Physical contact between American soldiers and Filipinos was at all times fraught. There were moments when Americans relied on "natives" to carry them bodily across streams or through the surf to shore, and the Americans admired the strength and stamina of the men dwarfed by them but at least as strong.[174] George Telfer noticed the physical affection shown by Filipino men for their women and children, and observed that older children were not shy about touching Americans, which he found both charming and threatening.[175] Journalist John Bass claimed that people living in a village near Manila approached him and other Americans seeking cures by touch. "An old man with stomach trouble put his hands on my ribs, and an old woman with a swollen nose wished to touch our noses. The lame, the blind, and, worst of all, lepers pushed their way towards us."

Bass and the others fled.[176] The Filipino habit of kissing the hand of a benefactor, or a social superior, discomfited Samuel Young.[177] Filipinos and Americans came to grips during battle, with "hand-to-hand work in indescribable confusion, the opposing elements commingled" in the fight for Manila—the only time, recalled Frederick Funston, that he saw bayonets used.[178]

The Americans who fought would say that Filipinos had tough, coarse skin, a sure sign of a low level of civilization. Many believed that dark skins were thicker than light ones, which meant that Filipinos and other people of color were less sensitive to heat and other haptic stimuli than were Caucasians. Dark skins seemed impervious to harsh, prickly clothing, including that made of maguey, bamboo, and the starchy piña lace favored by many Filipinas.[179] Yet Robert Carter insisted that "the niggers are always scratching. They perpetually itch."[180] The "natives" were "nearly all suffering from leprosy or some skin disease or worse."[181] "Keep this to yourself," Ernest Tilton advised his wife, but "as we found the Krag bullet does not stop them we have had to come down to dumdums"—bullets, developed in India, that expanded on impact—"and the result was terrible. No wounded lived to tell the tale, they were blown all to pieces"; here was the only possible way to stop men with thick skins, and therefore justified.[182] As the conflict ended, American officials hoped to persuade local people to work with them on building governments and making public improvements. Efforts were stymied by officers such as Capt. John Ketcham, who refused to shake hands with town of Hilongas dignitaries: "I did not want any *d—d nigger* to put his hands on me, so I drew my revolver and called the detachment which had stacked arms outside."[183]

Yet Americans did touch Filipinos, visiting prostitutes almost as soon as they arrived in the islands and, according to testimony from soldiers, committing rape. Dreadful as this was for Filipinos, the act of intercourse, whether paid for or demanded by force alone, troubled American officials only insofar as it invited illness in their men. Many American soldiers came to the Philippines having already contracted venereal disease, but their officers chose to ignore that and exclusively blamed prostitutes. The military sent prostitutes to hospitals for examination, for which they were charged up to a dollar, and isolation if they were found to be carrying disease. Commanders decided against physical examination of the soldiers because it would involve intrusive touching that was unworthy of white gentlemen.[184]

Americans had different standards regarding the tactile needs of their Filipino enemies and subjects. US officers provided no beds for Filipino prisoners, whom they regarded as having renounced all human rights.[185] Villagers were packed into *reconcentrado* camps, their bodies pressed against each other. The Americans abused Filipino bodies with beatings and torture. They discovered Filipino haptic practices that puzzled or annoyed them, including a prohibition against touching the body of someone who had been killed in battle.[186] At least once, this sort of ignorance had fatal consequences for the Americans. In late September 1901, the Americans occupied the town of Balangiga, at the south end of the island of Samar. Capt. Thomas Connell ordered between eighty and a hundred Filipinos into two tents meant to hold sixteen each. Some of those confined were *insurrectos*, and their plight made it easy for them to recruit and organize a counterstroke. On the morning of September 27, the Filipinos surprised the Americans in their quarters, killing fifty-nine and wounding twenty-three men.[187]

American soldiers in the Philippines were supplied with rations by the military, and as long as supplies could reach them they were assured of some nourishment. The quality and appeal of the food were different matters. The standard ration included hardtack, coffee, bacon, flour or corn meal, and canned tomatoes. There were beans in abundance; experts worried that soldiers ate the beans without cooking them and reported the battlefield aphorism, "beans killed more men than bullets."[188] Butter and condensed milk came in cans. Dry foods, including oatmeal and macaroni, were susceptible to infestation by "weevil."[189] If the soldiers were lucky, they got potatoes and onions, and if very lucky, a bit of beef.[190] Men were encouraged to find fresh food in the countryside, which they were supposed to buy but often stole. Occasionally, they feasted. The journalists John Bass and John McCutcheon stumbled into camp one evening to find a pair of officers presiding over a "bewildering sight . . . : roast chicken, and plenty of it, bread, butter, jam, tomatoes, cheese, potatoes."[191] When soldiers settled into garrison, they grew, or appropriated, fresh vegetables, among them corn, radishes, and tomatoes.[192] Often there were chickens and eggs, and Ernest Tilton ate so much chicken that he threatened to divorce his wife if she served him the dish once he got home.[193] Men ate well on holidays. On New Year's Day 1900, Walter Cutter had "roast duck, mashed potatoes, layer cake, cranberry sauce, peaches and cream, peas, [and] cocoa," though the peas were canned and the cream evaporated. Thanksgiving featured two kinds of potatoes, young onions, and pumpkin pie, while Christmas brought three good meals, including steak, doughnuts, oyster stew, chocolate, and apricot pie.[194]

These were exceptional times. Americans were for the most part wary of eating Filipino food, or eating like Filipinos, as they feared doing if they remained too long in the country. "If we eat like natives," warned an American officer, "we will become as stupid, frail, and worthless as they are."[195] Samuel Young worried that his men would be undernourished by the food they could find and cook while on the march, and, more pointedly, that it was not just nutritionally but racially inadequate: "A diet of half-cooked rice, with an occasional piece of carabao is not proper food for white men under any circumstances, but is especially bad for American soldiers marching and fighting on foot, in mud and water and rain, day after day."[196] Everything George Brandle ate and drank tasted like garlic; bacon turned soggy in the moist climate, rice was dirty and undercooked, and meat and fish were impossible to keep fresh.[197] Men lamented what seemed to them a loss of civility around meals, understandable in wartime but nevertheless unsettling, and made worse by life in the tropics. "We are becoming perfect barbarians," George Telfer told his wife. "One would think we were all from the frontier; refined conversation and table manners—gentlemanly acts of all kinds are forgotten. It is curse, swear, drink, and gamble from morning until night. And at table—it turns my stomach to see men eat. We have reached the hardened stage which follows bad treatment, neglect, and disappointed hopes."[198] "You ought to see us at meal time," John Doyle wrote to his hometown newspaper. "We are issued our rations raw, and each one cooks his own meal. Have been living on chickens and pigs most of the time, but the supply is about exhausted, and we have to fall back to bacon and hard tack now."[199] They drank too much "bino" or "tuba," the local liquors.[200]

They must not eat like the "natives"—yet of course, they did. Americans disparaged Filipino tastes, even while recognizing that in some measure they came to share them, and, perhaps guiltily, to enjoy them. They grew to love mangoes and pineapples, which they were unlikely to find at home. Even as they scorned some Filipino foods—the "little rice cakes, thin, hard, and indigestible as bits of slate," or the dogs and insects consumed by people upcountry—they acknowledged that many Filipinos avoided these things too.[201] Insofar as they may have wondered why many Filipinos mistrusted them, they might have examined their own reputation for gustatory practices. Far more often than Filipinos, the Americans put prisoners on lean rations, such as rice and salt for weeks at a time.[202] Puzzled as to why so many of the inhabitants of Catbalogan had fled with the arrival of American troops in early 1900, Ernest Tilton discovered that the villagers had been told that the Americans killed and ate Filipino children. "Think of that," Tilton wrote. For whatever reason, the rumor seemed credible to local people.[203]

Filipino senses were differently engaged during the "insurrection." They were fighting and living in their own environment and were well adapted to the sights, sounds, smells, haptic stimuli, and tastes of home. They were not in their own eyes duplicitous, as the Americans saw them, but interested in surviving, and thus intent on hiding if threatened and willing to say what they thought the armed strangers wished to hear. Their inability to speak English was hardly an act of defiance. That they smelled of coconut oil was a sign of cleanliness; the unbathed American soldiers were revolting. Filipinos knew how to live with the heat and the rain, and the lightness of their clothing made their skins a good deal more comfortable than those of the white men. Rice and fish struck them as far more wholesome food than the canned corned beef and condensed milk the Americans ate.

Yet there were ways in which Filipinos and Americans shared sensory challenges, for both, after all, were at war. This is made evident in the journal of Simeon Villa, a medical doctor and colonel who served with Aguinaldo. The darkness in which the Filipinos traveled and fought was as profound for them as it was for the Americans. Men in the column were frequently forced to hold hands, relying on touch to avoid becoming separated. Like the Americans, Filipino fighters contended with sickness, especially malaria, borne by mosquitoes that pestered them constantly. There was quinine for the Americans, but Aguinaldo, on the run almost from the start of war, had none, and his men suffered terribly. A third of them had malaria, Villa estimated, and they could only "rely upon the protection of a Divine Providence" in the hope of surviving. Pursued by the invader, and exposed at all times to betrayal by frightened villagers, Aguinaldo's men made silence a priority—though when they felt safe and needed to let off steam, they held exuberant *bailes* (dances), featuring bands that played on instruments fashioned from bamboo, and speeches by Aguinaldo designed to raise the morale of his followers. Facing great scarcity, they were obsessed with food. A handful of rice and a few *camotes*, similar to sweet potatoes, were often all they got, though when they happened upon cattle they slaughtered the animals instantly, and cooked and ate them "without either salt or rice, as we, being desperately hungry, stood upon no ceremony and ate as long as we were able, until our bellies were filled. This heavy feed of meat after our long fast gave the majority of us an intestinal inflammation." The hazards to the senses encountered by the Filipinos soldiers would not have been unfamiliar to the Americans in the same circumstance—and here, perhaps, was basis for a glimmer of understanding between the sides.[204] When Aguinaldo was captured in March 1901, he was taken aboard an American ship bound for Manila. Assigned to mess with American officers, the Filipino general surprised his captors with his civility. Following his second meal (which he ate with knife and fork), Aguinaldo "made a neat address, expressing his appreciation of the courteous treatment, which he had been accorded by his captors. His quiet, dignified and courteous demeanor kept him on good terms with all of us."[205]

In the aftermath of the Great Rebellion, the British sent many more troops to India and recruited Indian soldiers carefully among the "martial races" who had largely remained loyal, especially the Sikhs. They paid special attention to the sites of rebellion. In Cawnpore, the British created a memorial to the slain European women and children. It was guarded day and night by a British sentry, and no Indian was permitted to approach.[206] In Lucknow, the capital of Oudh where the mutiny had begun, the local ruler Maun Singh in early 1859 put on a festive entertainment and dinner, meant to affirm the restoration of British control of the area. The event stimulated all the senses. Triumphal arches, covered with silver leaf and lights, rose over the entrance to the city, and a golden shield proclaimed "Victoria, Queen of India." There were rockets and fireworks, which frightened the elephants assembled for the occasion. Inside the great hall there was a *nautch*, a dance by two young women supported by an orchestra, and an English reporter present remarked on "their songs, those strange, not unmusical cadences. . . . The noise of fiddles and drums from these various parties [of musicians] is overwhelming. . . . As to the general effect, the mass of fizzing, crackling, sparkling lights set in a framework of black faces and white turbans was picturesque, and ever varying, full of wonderful shade and life." Then came dinner, with an array of foods including meats—both ham and beef—apparently chosen to satisfy the British while offending all Muslims and Hindus present. Maun Singh had not quite got his etiquette right. The table settings were mismatched; "officers drank champagne out of soup plates." Nor had the British got their etiquette right. Late in the proceedings, an uninvited British captain asked Maun Singh to "take his cap off his head, and . . . clapped it on his own. Now, to uncover the head of an Asiatic is a great insult"—and touching a royal article of clothing was a blatant breach of manners. Such were the sensory tensions that were to be projected much larger than before, as the British prepared to administer India and discipline its people.[207]

As E. M. Collingham has argued, 1857–1858 brought a change in British bodily practices in India. Before the rebellion, officials of the East India Company had permitted themselves partly to adopt Indian customs and habits. They wore Indian clothes, ate Indian foods, smoked the hookah, and bathed far more often than they would have done at home. Their households included servants and possibly an Indian mistress, thus making fluid the boundaries between European and Asian identities and flouting proscriptions against "race-mixing" that their compatriots took on faith. They were Anglo-Indians, *nabobs*. After 1858, persuaded that such hybridizing practices had weakened them and left them vulnerable to attack, the British hardened the boundaries between themselves and their subjects, creating an " 'affective wall' which distanced the British body from India." There would be no more Indian dress or food; of these commodities the British would supply their own. In this way, Collingham writes, "the British grounded their authority in the bodily difference between ruler and ruled, thereby ensuring that the body became the central site where racial difference was understood and reaffirmed in British India." Displays of sight and sound—the great *durbars*, or assemblies of the late nineteenth century—would represent British authority. The British would attempt to isolate themselves against the foul odors of India or would attempt to eliminate them. They would try, with limited success, not to touch Indians or allow Indians to touch them. Their efforts to avoid the allegedly debilitating effects of Indian curries would prove almost comic and finally futile. In short, they would withdraw, as best they could, from India's sensorium.[208]

Unlike the British in 1858, the Americans had no prior experience living among the people they would attempt to manage after 1898. They came to the Philippines with bodies already tightly closed against what they believed was the malignant influence of a tropical environment and the mysterious, dangerous people it sustained. They wanted no part of living like Filipinos. To look, sound, smell, feel, or eat like them seemed a ludicrous proposition. They might exploit them sexually, but they told themselves that such contact would not lower their level of civilization, for surely it was the prostitute, the Filipina, who bore responsibility for luring them to bed and for infecting them with venereal disease. Filipinos made "goo goo eyes" to deceive them and concealed themselves in the jungle. They were loud, their voices and instruments discordant. They smelled foul, had a harsh climate and coarse, dark skin, and ate strange foods rudely. Americans were, or did, none of these things, and would never descend to the level of their uncivilized subjects. Or so they told themselves.

A writer for a lively English-language newspaper in Manila saw things differently, as early as May 1899. The city of San Fernando, just north of Manila, teemed with American soldiers. These men, the reporter observed, were living "very much as the natives did." They spent days resting in the shade, smoking and "washing their much worn and only suit of clothes. At meal times they dip into the erstwhile family pots and squat about the late Filipino tables, to take their chow. . . . After dark, the rude native lamp shines from every bamboo hut, and American soldiers write letters home on insurrecto paper, with insurrecto pen and ink, upon insurrecto tables—the tables which have turned. You may walk down the narrow streets and hear, to the twang of insurrecto mandolins and guitars, the most unforgettable of American songs."[209] If the Americans were to control the Philippines, body and soul and all five senses, they would have to do so on terms that were not exclusively their own.

3

Governing

Subjects and States Envisioned

> Call it gut instinct. Call it a sense. Call it experience. Call it what you will, but acknowledge that it is there—we judge others when we look at them.
>
> —Sharrona Pearl, *About Faces* (2010)

> No history of imperialism is complete without heeding the constitutive capacity of visuality, and correspondingly, no history of modern visuality can ignore the constitutive fact of empire.
>
> —Sumathi Ramaswamy, *Empires of Vision* (2014)

Smoke clears in the aftermath of war. But the end of fighting invariably does less than victors hope to reveal the landscape and the minds and bodies of the defeated. New subjects—in this case Indians in 1858 and Filipinos in 1902—do not willingly show themselves to their conquerors. Once the land has been pacified, the guilty have been punished, the dead buried, the wounded forgotten, and the damages of battle addressed, ruling must begin, and it must start with making legible empire's subjects. It is therefore fitting to begin this account of empires with the sense of sight. Who were the people of India and the Philippines? How many were there, where did they live, what did they look like? How were Britons and Americans to organize them into a visible, thus governable, community? However sudden its genesis, empire was—or would become—a *vision* of imperial dreamers, in this way consistent with their growing reliance on the sense of sight to locate, represent, classify, and judge others. Agents of empire would generate thousands of documents about their subjects, and administrators formed their impressions of how it was all working by reading these documents, even in offices far from where they could hear, smell, feel, or taste India or the Philippines. With paint, ink, and film they attempted to represent their subjects in images. Disconcertingly, subjects gazed back at imperial officials, sometimes admiringly, perhaps mockingly, and often with the critical eye of the distressed or aggrieved or angry. Together, rulers and subjects shaped what historians have called a "scopic regime," constructed of unevenly mutual perceptions and misperceptions.[1] The eye revealed everything—except when it did not.

The administrators of empire were alive to signs that the men and women they had determined to rule were capable of being civilized and ultimately self-governing. Vision became a way in which one vital sense could help determine whether people were well behaved, clean, and neatly dressed, with pleasant, open expressions and without deformity or other visual flaws that prevented them from transcending their alleged racial incapacities—in short, whether they, or rather some of them, could be made respectable to the imperial eye. The British had long experience of looking at Indians, but the Great Rebellion forced them to reconsider their gaze. Men whose appearance they had trusted had betrayed them. The obligations of formal governance demanded more careful scrutiny of their subjects, and the new administrators who arrived in India for the first time after 1857 were there to impose order and discipline. The British acknowledged that many Indians were enlightened, educated, and sophisticated; these were the *bhadralok*, the natural political and cultural leaders of society. Yet most of them were Bengali men, whom the British no longer trusted: they were, said the British, wily, devious, and unmanly. Given the weaknesses of their presumed leaders, it would be some time before Indians could rule themselves, if the day would arrive at all. The Americans read Filipinos somewhat differently. There were, they said, deceivers among them, and the depravity of those who lived in the forests and mountains and villages of the hinterlands could not be doubted by anyone who saw them, with their skimpy clothing and the repulsiveness no amount of clothing could conceal. But there were also the bright young men of Manila and other towns, the *ilustrados* trained in manners by the Spaniards, men capable of visual grace, intelligent conversation, and cultural aptitude generally. They were not civilized yet, but they were relatively closer to managing their affairs than the British believed the *bhadralok* were. These remained empires bent on civilizing their subjects, though they were anxious about whether or how they would be able do so. They knew in any case that they must first make their subjects visible, then render them visually respectable.

In the nineteenth-century West great importance was placed on seeing others and measuring them by what was seen. A growing reliance on sight did not necessarily mean the eclipse of the other four senses, in the metropoles of empire or especially in its subject nations. The four other senses retained their influence: when sight was blocked or unreliable, when agents of empire sought to quiet people, suppress their odors, cure or control their bodies by touch, or consume their food and drink. Civilized men and women were meant to respect all the senses.[2] Nonetheless, the advent and wide distribution of typed text was one sign of sight's increased importance.[3] While the growth of urbanization and industry in Europe and the United States clouded vision with air pollution, the era also witnessed the eye sharpened by improvements in the telescope and microscope, the gaze made panoramic with the advent of photography and landscape painting, the gaze made to wander, with the *flâneur*, along bustling city streets and through shopping arcades, his way illuminated by gaslight or electricity, the gaze made clinical by the advent of the x-ray at century's end.[4] The eye had gained agency, subtlety, and the ability to appraise others at a distance. It required no noise, ugly sniffing, inappropriate touching of others, or tasting what was handled by others to do its work.[5]

Vision became an increasingly important indicator of individual and group character in both Britain and the United States. The eye could teach its owner about class and status, especially in cities, where the bustle of crowds in the street made swift assessment vital to safety and self-definition; the undifferentiated masses who walked the urban pavements were difficult to register and sort out. Britons and Americans read the same popular etiquette manuals, often written in Britain then reprinted in the United States, and learned from them the importance of making a respectable public appearance—neither slovenly nor showy, quietly self-contained, open in expression yet without excessive eye contact—in short, properly middle-class.[6] The eye imposed its own discipline. "Indulge in no facial contortions, as they rapidly become habits difficult to break and usually leave their traces on the face in lines impossible to efface," advised Maude Cook in *Social Etiquette* (1896). "Lifting the eyebrows, rolling the eyes, opening them very widely, twisting the mouth and opening it so as to show the tongue in talking, are all disagreeable habits, that, once acquired, can only be broken by ceaseless vigilance."[7] In London and New York the science of physiognomy, connecting facial traits to character, emerged as a principal means of classification and distinction, a way of identifying the Self in a bewildering world of Others. The size and position of facial features, the slope of the jaw, pitch of the nose and ears, were read as signs of character. Eventually so were voluntary forms of self-presentation, including dress, hair style, and make up. At first meant to classify individuals, physiognomy became "a way to talk about groups . . . and to paint communities with broad strokes rather than in specific detail," according to historian Sharrona Pearl. These characterizations were generally derogatory. In the United States, immigrants and people of color were subjected to searching physiognomic examination predicated on contempt; in Britain, such classifications were imposed with particular force on the Irish and Jews.[8]

What began in the metropolitan centers of London and New York continued on the streets of cities and towns in India and the Philippines. The science of physiognomy was readily deployed by the agents of empire, anxious in their positions, eager to know their subjects by their appearance and intent on affirming their visual superiority over them. Anne Wilson, the author of a manual read widely by British women on their way to India, thought it best "to have pleasant things to look at . . . instead of ugly ones," as attractiveness had "a greater influence on one's spirits than is perhaps consciously recognized," and advised that when hiring servants, "you must finally trust to your own knowledge of physiognomy, that unwritten language which is writ so plain, and judge by it if the man is capable, well set up, and on the whole trustworthy."[9] The journalists who published, in 1858, a historical atlas of India sought to debunk the theory that Hindus were, like Britons, Caucasians. This was, they wrote, "a fantastical notion, for which there is hardly even so much as the shadow of a foundation. The only three points in which any analogy has been discovered between the Hindoo and the European are the oval form of the face, the shape of the head, and traces of a certain community of language. In every other respect the points of contrast are incomparably more decisive than those of resemblance. The European is white, the Hindoo black. . . . The European is taller than the Hindoo, more robust, and more persevering. Even in the rudest stages of civilization, the European has exhibited a firmness, perseverance and enterprise, which strikingly contrast with the Hindoo."[10] So did Americans in the Philippines contrast themselves physiognomically to their subjects. In September 1899, a reporter for the *New York World* described the physical features of Admiral George Dewey, hero of Manila Bay. The paper provided detailed sketches of Dewey's eyes, nose, an ear, chin, mustache, and hands, which revealed "the Admiral's high-strung spirited nature best of all." Dewey's face, the article continued, "might be called classical. It is just a trifle too heavy, perhaps, for an Apollo Belvidere, but it would be a mighty good face to trust."[11] Eighteen months later, following the capture of Emilio Aguinaldo by (among others) Frederick Funston, the *New York Evening Journal* assessed the facial features, all of them pictured, of captor and captive. Funston's eyes were "deep set, and [their] softness changes to sternness when he has a difficult job on hand. He is a man absolutely without fear." Aguinaldo's eyes were "most remarkable"—"almost of hypnotic power and at times savage. They are coal black and piercing. He has the power to control men with them." Evidence of the temperament of the two men emerged also from the shape of their mouths and chins. Funston's mouth indicated "determination. It is strong in every particular. His jaws come together like a bulldog's. A man who knows him well, describing his chin, said—'God almighty knew what he was about when he put that chin on Funston.'" In contrast, "Aguinaldo's mouth denotes the savage. His lips are red and thick. The lower lip hangs down heavily. The upper lip turns up coarsely. His brutality is plainly shown."[12]

Keeping up appearances, looking after one's own physiognomy, in the empire required effort—and money. Subalterns, servants, and ordinary Indians and Filipinos were, the Anglo-Americans assumed, scrutinizing them carefully, expecting officials to look respectable and authoritative. One trope of Raj literature and memoir was the conceit that staining the skin dark and having a knack for the local language could fool Indians into thinking that a Briton was one of them.[13] In fact, Britons were embarrassed when their appearance was suddenly or accidentally altered. When Hilda Bourne removed her blouse to have a bath, she recalled, "I found to my horror that I was bright scarlet all over my neck, arms, and shoulders, except where my stiff collar and tie had been, and there I was pure white."[14] Whatever antipathy or contempt for Indians the private British self harbored, he must never show it.[15] Military men had a full complement of well fashioned suits and uniforms. "The first task of the new ADC [*aide de camp*] was to fit himself out for all the different occasions which would arise," explained Frank Pearson. "A three piece lounge suit—£10 and I needed four; grey morning suit—£13, and a black one—£11; dinner jacket suit and evening tails, together with shirts, etc. Uniform was much more expensive but these I got second hand. Heavy box cloth scarlet coat with gold facings, dark blue frock coat, evening tail coat with light blue silk facings—these were the main items with caps and helmets to match. The white dress helmet topped with a plume of scarlet feathers. Very impressive outfits as befitted the impressive ceremonial of which one was a small part."[16] For civilians, and especially women, British catalogs offered a variety of products—furniture, linens, fancy hats, and infant bibs that said "My Pet" or "Baby" on their front—to help maintain a respectable-looking household.[17]

In the Philippines, the Americans tried, as the British did in India, to extend the lessons of middle-class civility they had been expected to master at home. They were to appear coolly in control, which meant visibly clean and well groomed and with a friendly, pleasant mien. Officials should look their subordinates and subjects in the eye, yet they must also avoid any hint of condescension. As in the United States, their appearance and their gaze at others must not convey rudeness, what historian John Kasson has described as "a kind of social obscenity, a violation of the codes of civility in such a way as to make public that which should remain private, to single out for special attention that which should remain inconspicuous, or else to cast public actions, conduct, and individual actors in an unworthy or degrading light.... Indeed, rudeness threatened not simply in words but in the slightest expression—a gaze held too long, an insolent gesture, an overly familiar smile, an unwelcome touch."[18] Americans had to dress appropriately. This directive presented particular challenges in a tropical climate. When he first arrived as Governor in 1900, William Howard Taft was determined to maintain the dignity of his office by dressing formally, as he would when he undertook official business at home. Accordingly, in July, Taft and the other American Commissioners put on frock coats and silk top hats and ventured out to make calls on several important Filipinos. They returned to their offices "heated throughout and dripping with perspiration," and at Taft's insistence, they decided immediately that formal attire would never again be required

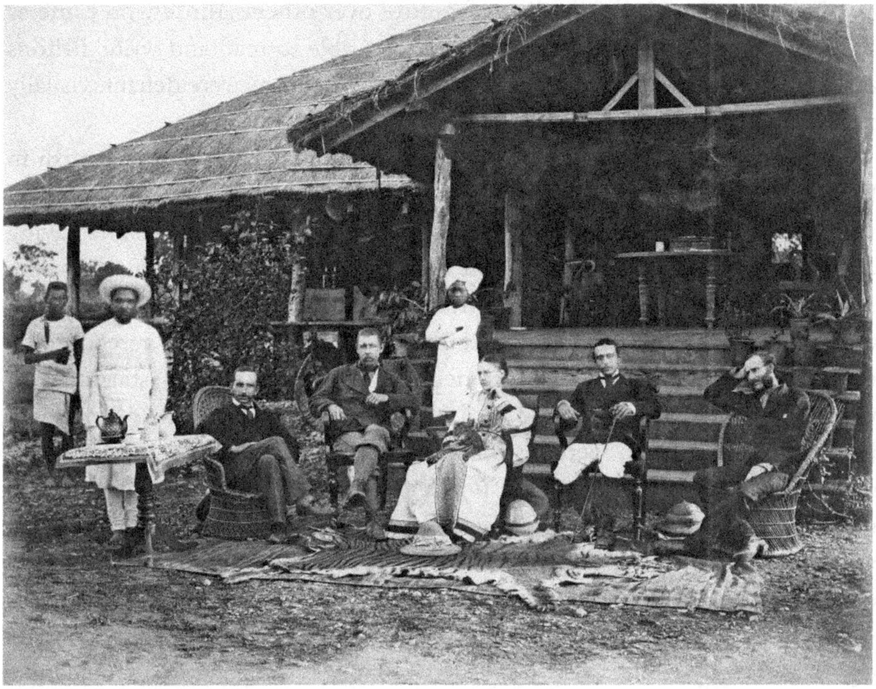

Figure 3.1 Four British men and a *memsahib,* with servants, in northwest India, 1876. They mean to show how one conducts oneself in front of the camera: at leisure, taking tea, but firmly in charge. The woman holds a baby tiger on her lap, perhaps the offspring of the adult whose skin lies at their feet. Mansell/The LIFE Picture Collection/Getty Images.

of them.[19] Taft and most of his colleagues and successors settled instead on wearing white cotton or linen clothes, along with white hats, shoes, and socks.[20] Three years later one of the Commissioners, Benjamin Ide Wheeler, chose to ignore these instructions and insisted that he and incoming Governor Luke Wright dress formally for Wright's inauguration in Manila. "They paid dearly for their fancy," wrote T. H. Pardo de Tavera to Taft, "because the Philippine climate punished their caprice making them perspire under their coats as if they had been in a Turkish bath."[21]

Britons and Americans had in common their etiquette manuals, and they tried for the most part to obey their rules of seeing and being seen. Imperial officials came broadly from the same classes: once soldiers had largely given way to civilians, they were at the top ranks aristocratic political appointees with independent sources of wealth, and below that level professional civil servants, missionaries, teachers, and sanitation engineers. While they did not all come from or work in crowded cities where their gaze had to be trained and tested, all were members of ocularcentric societies that valued sight as the maker of first impressions and the first line of control over others. Those who came as administrators to the outposts of empire were able to read and write. Britons and Americans agreed, finally, that their imperial subjects were defiant, visually and in other ways.

Differences concerned the political mission undertaken by the British in India and the Americans in the Philippines, and more significantly the type of social system they encountered in the countries they occupied. Despite having considerable doubts about the fitness of Filipinos to rule themselves, the Americans more quickly than the British began building political institutions to be shared with their subjects, and ultimately, the Americans agreed, to be ceded to them. They created government from the grassroots up, starting with villages, moving to regions, and, in 1907, supervising elections to a national legislature. The British were less eager to admit by 1900 that the time had come to construct a homegrown political system in India, though they did institute modest self-rule for Indians in big cities. This difference of approach existed in good part because the Americans found in place a number of highly educated Filipinos who had learned about European ways from the Spaniards, were Catholic, spoke Spanish, and were determined to assert their political rights, as they had done in the last years of Madrid's rule. There were of course thousands of well-educated Indians by 1900, but they were not yet sure of their political direction, were split along religious lines, and were divided especially by caste. While Filipinos had their own ways of seeing and being seen, a combination of often disconcerting directness and a tradition of performing spectacle, these were not unfamiliar to Americans nor altogether condemned by them. The British, by contrast, struggled to understand the significance of the Hindu practice of *darshan*, Sanskrit for "seeing." While technically reserved for the gods, *darshan* spilled frequently into the realm of the secular, and it was meant to be reciprocal: one saw and was seen. It enabled authority but required mutual respect.

The Deceitful Subject

Imperial subjects in several ways confounded the occupier's eye. Some of these confoundings were probably unintended. Others indicated a desire by subjects not to be seen and thus known by their would-be masters; these were calculated. During their military conflicts, the Anglo-Americans insisted that their subjects were deliberately tricky or deceitful. It was understandable, if maddening, that combatants would try to fool each other, and if the British and Americans hardly forgave those who had hidden from them or masqueraded as innocent during war, they were not inclined to think such behavior was extraordinary or to take it personally. Once war ended, though, such deceptions must end. That they evidently did not was a source of abiding frustration. In India, the British concluded that deceit was a cultural or even a genetic feature of the people, or some group of them. There were liars in the marketplace, where Hindu merchants were notorious among the British for using false weights to measure grain, or of holding their scales in ways that overestimated weight so cleverly that it was "not detectable even by the sharp-eyed customer."[22] Beggars were "snake-eyed Asiatics" who had, thought Joseph Salter, mastered the arts of "artifice and deception."[23] A British assistant collector at Nasik had trouble visually differentiating and identifying Indians who came to his office to receive their pensions, until he devised a document listing the facial characteristics of each man. One pensioner had "eyes like a cat's and a deceitful expression," as he came each month to receive his cash payment.[24] Rendering justice in an Indian court, where the judges were British, was made nearly impossible by the alleged Indian facility for lying, even while appearing sincere. "The offender never fails to look so placidly innocent," wrote Marianne Postans, "that the inexperienced judge is often disposed to question the truth of evidence."[25] Dangerously concealed inside Indian bodies were deadly diseases to which the unsuspecting British were vulnerable.[26] The counting and classifying of Indians that started with the East India Company became far more extensive under the Crown, but it proved frustrating for the bureaucrats who undertook it. Under the surface, the "placid, timid, forbearing exterior of the Indian," forensic pathologist Norman Chevers discovered a "strange combination of sensuality, jealousy, wild and ineradicable superstition, absolute untruthfulness, and ruthless disregard of the value of human life." "The old racial stereotype of the docile Indian gave way to a new one of a creature whose mildness was a façade behind which lay a morally flawed character," writes historian Lawrence James. "He was, in short, a natural deceiver."[27]

The British were intrigued and appalled by *zenana*, the practice of secluding Indian women in areas of the home off limits to men who were not family members. British men regarded the removal of women from their gaze as part insult, part challenge; they eroticized the *zenana*, and their fantasies about what went on behind closed doors ran unchecked. The unseen Indian seemed to them both an attempt to deceive and a provocation. Male British doctors were rarely permitted into women's quarters, and they and other men complained that their lack of access prevented Britons from knowing all their subjects, and thus from taking care of them.[28] British women were from time to time allowed into *zenana*. Some imagined their admission as an invitation into India's domestic soul, and looked forward to it. Others found experiencing a glimpse of the forbidden disappointing, as did a Mrs. Weitbrecht, who described *zenana* as a "collection of dirty courtyards, dark corners, break-neck staircases, [and] filthy outhouses."[29] Either way, the concealment of women was one more trick, another effort to deceive the European eye and thus prevent the civilizing work of empire from going forward.

Then there were the tricks played by the magicians and performers who meant to delight audiences with the seemingly impossible, but who frequently struck the British as intending only to fool and torment them. The practice of magic depends for its success on the trust and good humor of those watching it. If the audience is not altogether voluntary, and by its own definition meant to be part of an apparatus of social control, it is unlikely to find pleasure in being fooled. If, moreover, British viewers regarded the Indian trickster as a synecdoche for Indian society as a whole—if they believed, in other words, that all Indians are tricksters and thus in on the joke that they themselves don't get—they will suspect that they are being played for fools, or, even worse, being set up for a shock as unexpected as the Great Rebellion.

Magic seemed to be everywhere in India. The British called its practitioners "jugglers" and remarked on it constantly. Snake charmers appeared in public gathering places and at tourist sites, able to tame dangerous cobras with beguiling music or the movements of their bodies. Mango trees burst out of nowhere, decapitated boys were suddenly made whole again, *faqirs* lay placidly on beds of nails.[30] In May 1879, Mrs. Robert Moss King and other women put on a carnival for children and invited "some first-rate jugglers. They performed the famous mango trick . . . with spectators in front and on all sides of the jugglers then they put one of their people into a trance, and during the trance put a skewer through her tongue, and finally with great deliberation cut a piece off and handed it round for us to see. It certainly was flesh, and had we not known that we were there for the sole object of being imposed upon, we should have sworn it was a piece of her tongue, and that we had seen it cut off, and could still see her tongue hanging out and with the end gone. How very little we can trust the evidence of our own senses!" These, she went on, "had been cheated in the outrageous way we know they may be cheated." It could not have happened. Yet "the evidence of our eyes" told them that it had.[31]

The Indian rope trick mystified and vexed Britons more than any other act of magic. Testimony as to its authenticity circulated in Britain starting in the late nineteenth century. Some of it was quite precise; this came from a woman who claimed to have witnessed it:

> One of [the magicians] threw a rope into the air which hitched itself up to apparently nothing in the sky above; one could see the

> rope going straight up as far as one could see anything . . . A small boy then swarmed up this rope, becoming smaller and smaller, till he likewise vanished from sight, and a few minutes later bits of his (apparently mangled) remains fell from the sky, first an arm, then a leg, and so on till all his component parts had descended; these the juggler covered with a cloth, mumbled something or other, made a pass or two, and behold! There was the boy smiling and whole before us.

The trick was variously attributed to mass hypnosis, the use of drugs by or on the audience, the jugglers' discovery of laws of nature as yet unrevealed in the West, or the credulity of a few people who simply did not know a hoax when they saw it. All these interpretations led to the same conclusion: Indians delighted in deceiving people. They were naturally tricky.[32]

Americans did not find accomplished jugglers in the Philippines; when Ruth Hunt saw a "native . . . sleight of hand performance" she found it poor, though she noted that the Filipino audience loved it.[33] Yet the Americans in general were as certain as their British counterparts in India that their subjects were intent on deceiving them, making their vision unreliable and thus thwarting their attempts to take control of the people and land of the archipelago. They found Filipinos endlessly performative, even flamboyant, masking their honesty by excessive display. Filipino showiness was one thing. Their insistence (said the Americans) on lying outright was another.[34]

They were not magicians, but Filipinos, said the Americans, were performers and purveyors of spectacle. Many commented on the facility with which Filipinos musicians picked up tunes and rated them highly as instrumentalists and singers; Filipinos played with a "rhythmic buoyancy" and their children were "by nature endowed and by environment encouraged to respond to music and to participate in it."[35] George Telfer wrote from Manila in late 1898 that he had gone to a Filipino circus. There were "good" gymnasts, then a "pantomime," and since the "people are natural born actors as well as musicians," it came off well. "They also have a high sense of humor," Telfer concluded. "So their pantomimes are worth seeing."[36] American officials who traveled across the islands to organize local governments were treated to elaborate welcoming ceremonies, featuring newly built arches decorated with flowers, banquets lavishly laid on, and always a dance, or *baile,* to which the local people came in their finery and danced with their visitors. "It was a procession, a meeting, a *banquete* and a *baile* every day for nearly seven weeks," recalled Taft's wife, Helen, of one of their extended sojourns through the archipelago. At the end of their journey, she reported, the party was exhausted, yet gratified.[37]

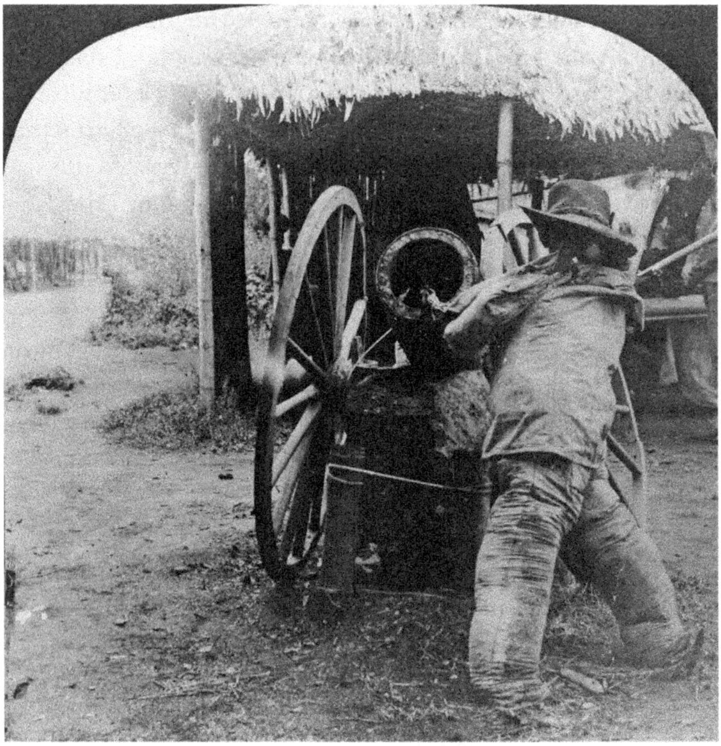

Figure 3.2 Outmanned and outgunned, Filipino insurgents resorted to deception to slow the Americans down. This photograph depicts a "dummy cannon with scarecrow gunner," erected by Filipino troops. It was the sort of deception to which Americans hoped to put an end. Courtesy of the American Historical Collection, Rizal Library, Ateneo de Manila University.

For the most part, American complaints about the deceitfulness and perfidy of Filipinos echoed British sentiments about Indians. Governor Taft thought that the Filipino "was disposed to conceal his real feelings," especially "when in opposition to the person whom he is addressing," and while Taft urged forbearance, other Americans, who identified the same trait, were less inclined to be forgiving.[38] Nicholas Roosevelt concluded that Filipinos simply did not "value integrity as we do," displaying instead a "cheerful indifference to the correlation between statement and fact."[39] Like Indian bodies, those of Filipinos concealed dangerous organisms that they refused to treat, probably because they could not see them, and the "peasants" who were sick "remained invisible" to health care providers until their situations had turned grave.[40] Men and women looked handsome—until they opened their mouths to reveal teeth reddened by chewing betel or blackened from decay.[41] They buried their dead in secrecy, under cover of night, hoping to hide the harsh truth that a contagious disease had claimed a loved one.[42]

The Hideous Subject

What Asian subjects revealed the British and Americans often regarded as unkempt, filthy, ugly, or deformed. Dark skin was, according to westerners, coarse, impenetrable, and dirty—signs of the mark of Ham. Deformities prevalent in Asia included cleft lip, kyphosis (hunchback), elephantiasis, the amputations of leprosy, or self-inflicted distortions such as those undertaken by Indian *faqirs* or *sadhus* (holy men). These marked bodies as pathetic and worthy of sympathy, but witnesses still recoiled in revulsion at the sight of them. It went beyond that. Slovenliness, the failure to keep up appearances, was rude, a sign of poor breeding, bad habits, or disrespect, especially when evinced by servants or subordinates. It was not innate but a choice made by those who knew better, because they had been taught how to behave but refused to do so. Sloppiness and ugliness were not just offensive but subversive of the visually civilized order of things.

The British knew Indians with light skins who dressed well and kept themselves clean. But these, they said, were relatively few, and they were not immune from committing visual offense. Chewing betel nut seemed nearly universal, staining and distorting the teeth of those who practiced it, and covering the pavement with what looked to many like blood.[43] Servants showed contempt for their employers by appearing coatless, or by wearing their shirts untucked or the ends of their turbans dangling recklessly behind them.[44] Hindu *faqirs* appeared everywhere, and their image—emaciated, sparsely clad in rags, and with filthy, matted hair and fingernails untrimmed and never cleaned—was popularized in India and Britain on postcards and through "magic lantern" slide shows.[45] The streets of cities teemed with poor people afflicted with diseases and deformities sadly common among the very poor. Safe within the "cocoon" of his first class railway carriage, a British captain reflected on life on the Bombay pavements: "I might still shudder at the sight of the poor, skinny spindle-shanked, emaciated, filthy diseased," and on a trip to get his laundry he saw an "old grey man, half-naked, emaciated asleep on the ground, and the small baby on a box, its thighs quite shrunken to a chicken's wing, flies crawling over its penis; outside Lloyd's Bank, a woman advanced in pregnancy lying prone on the pavement, her swollen belly exposed, her naked breast clutched by a baby sprawling naked beside her."[46] To leave the city was no escape from the monstrous assault on the eye. "Indians all look the same class once outside the big towns like Bombay, Calcutta or Delhi, mostly rather ugly and very dark-skinned," Carol Hyde wrote her parents in England. Their eyes were "rather blood-shot," and nearly all wore "dirty white sort of garments—a cross between trousers and a skirt—with a messy looking shirt with the tails invariably worn outside." Women distorted their features with "rings or clips in their ears or noses and stained red or yellow marks between their eyebrows."[47] Saddest and most repulsive of all were the bodies of polio victims, usually beggars, "with the[ir] withered twisted limbs knotted under them," and the lepers, armless and legless or with "their hands and feet nearly all disappeared."[48]

Americans in the Philippines put a great deal of effort into classifying their newly acquired subjects by race, and that meant by skin color. This was part of the process of sorting people out in preparation for governing them. In 1903 Daniel Folkmar, who would later become governor of Bontoc Province, used inmates in Manila's Bilibid Prison to create a racial taxonomy for the country as a whole. Each "provincial type," he decided, had "differentiating characteristics" based chiefly on pigment. Cagayans were "reddish-brown," Pangasians "yellowish," Tagalos "yellowish-brown," Igorots "vermillion," and the Manobo "burnt umber, approaching burnt sienna."[49] Tagalos, who were the majority of Manilans, Catholics, and had dealt most closely with the Spaniards, often appeared respectably dressed and turned out, sometimes in "western" clothes, and even the "lower classes" were for the most part clean and garbed in cotton shirts and trousers, though, like their Indian counterparts, they did not wear proper shoes and could not seem to keep their shirts tucked in—this last was regarded as a serious transgression in both countries.[50] Others, clumped variously together as "Malays," "Chinamen," "Negritos," and "the wild tribes," were far less mannerly and physically attractive. The first Philippines Commission, which studied the "race" issue carefully, posited a three-tiered system of classification. At the top of hierarchy were "Indonesians," whom the Americans judged "physically superior" to their compatriots. "They are tall and well developed, with high foreheads, aquiline noses, wavy hair, and often with abundant beards. The color of their skins is quite light. Many of them are very clever and intelligent." More numerous were the "Malayans." They were of "medium size," had browner skin than the Indonesians, and noses that were "short and frequently considerably flattened." The men had "straggling" beards that appeared "late in life." At the bottom of the scale were "Negritos," "weaklings of low stature, with black skin, closely-curling hair, flat noses, thick lips, and large, clumsy feet. In the matter of intelligence they stand at or near the bottom of the human series, and they are believed to be incapable of any considerable degree of civilization or advancement."[51] Edith Moses claimed that "many of the Negritos live in trees, and look almost like animals."[52] The first group was educable and to some extent already literate; from its ranks political leaders could be drawn. Caution was needed, because nearly all Filipinos shared some undesirable traits. The men were lazy, showy, emotional, and lovers of vice.[53] W. B. Wilcox thought that the process of civilizing the Filipinos would be slow. "The native will remain with a Malaya tinge for generations," he wrote, "and I quite believe it will be as difficult to change the Tagalo as a Hindoo."[54] "One of the most difficult, one of the most necessary, points in thinking of the Filipino is to remember quite clearly and all the time that, whatever his individual training and gifts, he is not a dark-skinned white man but a Malay," claimed the writer Katherine Mayo.[55] Appearances, including a "Malaya tinge" or "dark skin," would remain a marker of difference and a predictor of incompetence.

So would habits, practices, and conditions that revolted the Americans as surely as they did the British in India. Like Indians, Filipinos of all classes chewed and spat betel.[56] Even Filipino elites could get their clothing wrong, as Edith Moses discovered when "a number of ladies" tried to "transition from the charming mestiza costume to the European dress. It is ugly," she declared, "a tucked waist of silk, with lace and ribbons, and over this a neckerchief, while flowers and bows decorate the shoulders."[57] The alleged ugliness of dark skin was made worse by other distortions of physiognomy and attire. Albert Sonnichsen, held captive for ten months during the insurrection, described one captor who had "a complexion . . . but a shade lighter than ebony," with teeth that "protruded between thick and prominent lips, and so conspicuous was the upward slant of his eyes that in his anger he bore a strong resemblance to a Chinese Joss." He wore "a pair of soiled white trousers and an unwashed shirt the tail of which fluttered in the fresh breeze that came in through the open doors and windows." A second guard had an "appearance [that] was far from prepossessing. Being unusually black, he was [also] short of stature, thick-lipped, and pock-marked, a typical full-blooded Filipino."[58] The further Americans ranged upcountry, the greater the insult to their eyes. Among the Ifugaos in 1910, Governor-General William Cameron Forbes witnessed the slaughter of a carabao. The water buffalo "was hacked to pieces by a hundred men who fought for the pieces and came out a mass of gore, bearing their prizes, a very hideous spectacle so degrading that I shall see if I can't have stop put to it."[59] Alice Kelly, a school teacher of Igorots in Baguio, found her students "filthy . . . clad only in a 'gee string,' and that usually a piece of pliable bark wound round their bodies."[60]

Sonnichsen's "pock-marked" Filipino was most likely a survivor of smallpox. Disease took many lives or left living victims with its mark. After visiting the smallpox ward of San Lazaro hospital, John Bancroft Devins promised that "the reader shall not have even a word picture of that face, which frequently comes before the writer when thousands of miles separate him from the hospital."[61] William Freer went to a leper hospital, where he found the patients "pitiable": "their faces were swollen and blotched, the bridge of the nose was usually sunken and sometimes lacking, arms and legs were withered and deformed and all had raw sores. Many had lost fingers and toes, the scars having healed over; some had their feet tied up in bandages, evidently to prevent further loss."[62] Emily Conger recorded that one day, the wife of her Filipino cook turned up unannounced. Conger found her hideous, with "one eye crossed, a harelip . . . mouth and lips stained blood red with betel juice," and "screamed at her to run away." "The diseased, the deformed, the blind, the one-toed, the twelve-toed, and monstrous parts and organs are the rule rather than the exception," she concluded. "These things are true of nine-tenths of the people."[63] That was doubtless exaggerated, but it suggests the extent to which Americans found reason to distance themselves from men and women they found visually loathsome.

Such reactions were immediate and visceral, meant to categorize Others as fundamentally different from Selves. To appear hideous was rude, and it could be prevented—there was no need to dress badly or chew betel—or it threatened the civilized body with an optical violation or contagion. Still, the ugly could be made less loathsome, taught better habits, cured, isolated if a cure proved impossible, or even got used to, as in the case of the wife of Emily Conger's cook, who despite her appearance soon became a household fixture.[64] The Americans also meant to correct the Filipino sense of sight. In 1911, at the behest of the recently established Bureau of Education, Alice Fuller published in Manila an etiquette manual titled *Housekeeping and Household Arts*. In it, and among other things, she urged teachers to "take the[ir] class sometimes to the market and the native shops and call their attention to any unsanitary conditions which may exist, as well as other common sights which appeal to the observing person as contrary to the laws of life." She had in mind "food, exposed to dust and flies; people handling the food and spitting about the market place; half-starved dogs poking their noses into food receptacles; youngsters going about in the cool season with one little garment, a cough, and a troublesome nose; thin peevish babies chewing on impossible things." She also advised readers to treat others with visual sensitivity. It was vital to show "good manners." "It is most unkind," she wrote, "to stare at or comment upon the infirmity of any one, or call another's attention to it. People who are lame, ugly, cross-eyed, fat, or peculiar in any way, are sure to be over-sensitive; and they do not like to have their peculiarities noticed. Many who are afflicted with birthmarks of some sort are so sensitive that they do not care to go among people; and left by themselves, they live lonely, unhappy lives. We can make such people much happier by helping them to forget that they are not just like the rest of us."[65]

The Overexposed Subject

The annoyance and fear of the Anglo-Americans that their subjects tried to frustrate western vision by refusing to reveal themselves—the deceptive Other—had a flip side: too often Indians and Filipinos offended their rulers by revealing too much, allowing the overexposure of their bodies. "The naked body, the absence of clothing, were profoundly powerful symbols of difference understood physically as well as culturally, intellectually as well as economically: material proof of the need for a firm colonial hand," as historian Philippa Levine has written about British India. Nakedness meant indifference to decorum, an absence of shame, brazen sexuality, defiance of the civilized eye; it was "principally a symbol of savagery."[66] Victorians were appalled at its ubiquity, especially among the lower classes. Bare breasts were titillating but "indecent," a word that observers used frequently to describe their reaction to nudity.[67] The proximity of naked Indian bodies to their own alarmed Britons no end. In the 1880s authorities in Calcutta banned Indians from the Eden Park bandstand because of British complaints about the Bengalis' "transparent clothes" offending the women who walked there during the evening. Mary Carpenter was struck especially by the flimsiness of male clothing. "They seemed to consider that a black skin supersedes the necessity of raiment, and in this respect the lower orders appear perfectly devoid of any sense of decency," she wrote. "I never became reconciled to this, and believe now, as I did then, that living thus in a sort of savage state in the midst of a civilised people increases that want of proper self-respect."[68] The British regarded servants as the worst offenders. "There is something in the idea of gentlemen who never wear any clothes picking the fruit you eat which is not at all appetizing," argued Florence Marryat.[69] The *malis* (gardeners) hired by Ethel St. Clair Grimwood tended the grounds in the nude. She gave them bathing trunks hoping to "inculcate decency," but soon found them wearing the trunks on their heads against the sun.[70] Servants, including men, were expected to tend to their masters and mistresses in the intimate settings of bath and bedroom, and the skimpy clothing worn by the servants at best took getting used to.[71] The British admitted less often to the erotic charge they felt in the presence of naked or nearly naked servants, but an occasional confession of excitement slipped out, as it did in a letter Carol Hyde wrote to her parents in early 1933. The Hydes were traveling, sleeping each night in a tent. One night a snake got in. The servants rushed in to find it, "with lamps and torches to help them in their search, gleaming on their brown bodies and in their rolling excited eyes. I was thrilled with the scene—and nervous too, those snakes are deadly poisonous—but couldn't help appreciating the scene inside the tent with the wind howling and the rain pouring down, the men all looked so dark and wild, their black curly hair all tumbled with the wind, their naked bodies glistening with the rain, and their bits of loin cloth all bedraggled."[72]

"It gives one just arriving from America a bit of a shock, as he drives about the streets of Manila, to see children running around clad principally in their brown birthday suits," wrote John Bancroft Devins. Working men, he added, often wore little more than a loincloth, though women in the city were more modestly dressed.[73] Americans in the Philippines were perhaps less shocked than the British in India about their naked subjects, and if this was so it is likely because fewer Americans had servants, and the officials who did have them were mainly in Manila and insisted that they work fully clothed. Outside the city there was more nudity, especially among children and those who lived in the remote places of the archipelago. "There is little fear of exposing the naked body," observed Frank Laubach.[74] Americans noticed that many of the people upcountry bore large, vivid tattoos on their bodies—distractions from nudity though hardly substitutes for clothing.[75] The American episcopal bishop in the Philippines, Charles Henry Brent, had a prurient curiosity about whether Igorot women covered their breasts when he was present.[76] Because they were not mannerly or civilized, claimed Americans, Filipinos showed an ignorance of social codes concerning bodily exposure. Americans generally found this amusing; they expected little else. Ralph Buckland stared at women weavers who kept hiking up their skirts, "exposing their brown nether limbs." "They were not overstepping any rules," he admitted, for "they would have not have known modesty had they come face to face with her beneath a glaring noonday sun."[77] In 1908 Dr. Victor Heiser, director of health in the Philippines, accompanied his Filipino colleague Dr. Felipe Calderón to the United States to discuss public health issues in the islands. Heiser kept close watch on Calderón, who seemed not to understand that he could not undress in public and should not wear pajamas to a train's dining car.[78] Laubach was writing a letter home from Davao one day in 1915 when "a fine muscular specimen of manhood passed the house, wearing nothing but a cloth about his loins, and a very large paper hat on his head."[79]

The Blind (or Blinding) Subject

The supposed lack of civilization among Indians and Filipinos was itself a form of blindness, according to their conquerors. These were, after all, subjects who relied too little on seeing things clearly, too much on their "lower senses" to apprehend their environments and decide how to act on them.[80] Blindness was not solely a metaphorical problem. In India, smallpox epidemics often left survivors sightless—authorities attributed seventy-five percent of blindness in India to smallpox.[81] Working at close quarters in factories or plantations, Indians contracted contagious diseases with terrible regularity. Some, including conjunctivitis, were treatable, but many victims had no access to medical care, mistrusted British doctors, or preferred their own remedies. Along with other eye diseases, cataracts were "common" in India, recalled Sir Ernest Bradfield, who, as Surgeon General of Bombay, removed "thousands" of them.[82] Margery

Hall was told by her Indian doctor that his son had had an eye plucked out by a crow. Such occurrences, he reported sadly, were common.[83]

The British suffered much less from blindness in India, but they too struggled to see through obstructions or overcome shocks to their vision. They were stunned by the powerful tropical sun. "When you walk out . . . into the sun of India it hits you like a blow," recalled a British officer. "Every time you walk out of doors during the middle of the day you feel as if you've been hit by something."[84] The effect was exaggerated by the darkness of British interiors, where men and women strained to read by dim kerosene lamps.[85] When the monsoon came the water sluiced down in torrents; "it's like living under a waterfall," said Rosamund Lawrence.[86] The vivid colors of the landscape frequently overwhelmed them. Once in a while, a Briton, usually a woman, acknowledged that blindness in India could be self-inflicted. One day, Iris Macfarlane, who lived on a tea plantation in Assam, had a revelation while writing. "I couldn't believe I had been so blind. Once a week I had driven to the club through villages I had never entered, past people whose language I couldn't speak, living lives I knew nothing of, dancing and singing to unknown tunes. I had not, honestly, thought of them as people; they were a brownish blur, like the greenish blurs of the rice and bluish ones of the mountains." She resolved thereafter to learn Assamese and to look at her surroundings more carefully.[87]

As in India, disease literally blinded Filipinos, with smallpox and leprosy taking a considerable toll. Governor Forbes's personal assistant shuddered to tell of "the horror that stayed with him from seeing a lepress whose eyes had rotted away."[88] A "psychopathic ward" was established on the island of Corregidor for American soldiers blinded by the intense summer sun and maddened by their sightlessness.[89] Blindness was metaphorical, too, which had graver implications for the colony's future. The people needed the Americans to guide them on the path to freedom and self-government. Lacking such help, the people would, according to the Commissioner Dean Worcester, "be left to stagger along alone, blind in their own conceit under the keen and watchful eye of another powerful nation, hungrily awaiting their first misstep."[90] Worcester felt sure of his capacity to lead; other Americans, finding their own vision blurred in the islands, were less certain. The colors and features of the land dulled Americans' vision with their monotony, causing the gaze to grow weary and falter.[91] Filipino politicians with whom the Americans had chosen to work tried always to "pull the wool over our eyes."[92] More vexing to the Americans was Filipino showiness, called in Tagalog *palabas*. Usually regarded as harmless, sometimes charming, it could also serve to distract Americans, and Filipinos themselves, from the seriousness of the archipelago's problems. According to Katherine Mayo, the Filipino "loves dress and luxuries . . . . the dearest and the showiest always," which left him wanting life's necessities and perpetually disappointed when he fell short of his own material desires.[93] Ruth Hunt went to the market in Manila to get material for a dressing gown for her husband. The silk sellers showed her "lurid and ghastly materials," and when she insisted on something more subdued "they at once lost interest." "These people," she concluded, "like more glaring and atrocious color schemes in their clothing than the American Negroes."[94] The lavish melodramas performed for official audiences in Filipino villages, and the garish décor splashed throughout banquet halls in towns too poor to afford indoor toilets, seemed to them the result of this peculiar national trait.[95] It was all flash and spectacle, and it left them as if blinded by its brightness.

The Asian Picturesque

The British and Americans insisted that deceptions, occlusions, the ugliness of Indians and Filipinos, and their startling self-exposures distorted and impeded their imperial vision and thus inhibited the clarity needed for enlightened rule. Yet the agents of empire had another impression of their possessions overall: whatever the aesthetic or moral challenges to their vision, they often described the land and people of India and the Philippines as "picturesque." Contemporaries seem to have defined the term shallowly, "suggesting something that was pretty rather than profound, appealing to the eye rather than troubling to the soul, worthy of being made into a picture but otherwise of little arresting importance," as historian David Arnold has written.[96] It was landscape, both natural and of the built environment, that diarists, artists, and photographers most often took as their subject—the nineteenth-century British photographer Samuel Bourne listed as "features of the picturesque . . . lakes, rivers, streams, 'rustic bridges,' 'ivy-clad ruins, trees, and mountains' "—but the concept could also include people, especially those who confirmed Anglo-American stereotypes of Asians as quaint, authentic, or primitive.[97] Those who described the Asian picturesque saw Asia as sensual, erotic, emotional, heathen, an uncivilized place of schoolbook fantasy. What made the colonies picturesque to western observers was exotic, raw, and yet stubbornly tethered to familiar aesthetic categories in a way that made them seem manageable and reasonably safe.

It was the form of India's landscape that first caught the eye of Fanny Parks. "This river is very picturesque," she wrote, with "high cliffs, well covered with wood, rising abruptly from the water: here and there a Hindu temple, with a great peepul-tree spreading its fine green branches around it: a ruined native fort: clusters of native huts: beautiful stone ghats jutting into the river." She admired people (and their handiwork) and animals as they moved though nature: "the native women, in their picturesque drapery, carrying their vessels for water up and down the cliffs, poised on their heads. Fishermen are seen with the large nets; and droves of goats and small cows, buffaloes, and peacocks come to the river-side to feed. But the most picturesque of all are the different sorts of native vessels; I am quite charmed with the boats."[98] "The common sights along an Indian road, too, are always picturesque," wrote Mrs. Robert Moss King in 1878. "The wide plains, with great herds of smoke-coloured, delicate-limbed cattle being driven slowly home for the night, accompanied by troops of ungainly, fierce-looking buffaloes, and flocks of goats and black long-tailed sheep. Then gangs of wayfarers clad in every colour and degree of costume, from the simple suit of ashes of the Fakír to the gorgeous combination of white and coloured raiment of some rich man who has just dismounted hurriedly from his carriage, drawn by a pair of white humped oxen, to salaam to Robert," and the indigo workers, their loincloths and skins dyed blue from their work.[99] "The bazar [*sic*] is a feast of colour," recalled Kate Platt. "The booth-like open shops filled with many-hued wares, gay silks and cottons, and piles of luscious fruits, with the brilliantly coloured garments of the passers-by and of the loungers (for in the East there is no hurry), make the native city a joy to the lover of colour. The effect would be garish, but with the background of closely set fantastic buildings, the sunny lights and deep velvety shadows, the picture gives joy and satisfaction to the onlooker."[100] Erica Farquharson was taken to the bazaar as a girl. "How I loved it," she remembered; "so full of colour and movement and laughter and all so kind and friendly to the 'missee-sahib.' The little shops were brightly lit by flaring lights. We went at night. There were bright cloths, rolls and rolls and lengths handing in the open front. There were craftsmen fashioning brass and silver goods, delicate silver filigree ornaments for hair, or bracelets, or the heavily worked bowls and dishes . . . . The bazaar was a magic cave, glistening and sparkling."[101] A "feast of colour," a "magic cave"—here was the stuff of fantasy and desire. But as Platt went on to remind readers, the bazaar did not bear "close inspection," for the "state of sanitation is such that diseases when introduced spread with incredible rapidity. It is not without reason that the European residential quarter is built at a considerable distance from the fascinating but dangerous native city."[102] In the presence of the picturesque, the British eye could be beguiled.

The Americans encountered similar sights in the Philippines. After the shock of arrival in Manila wore off, the capital seemed to lose some of its exoticism, so nearly all of the Americans' experience of the picturesque came in the provinces: "The wild tribes and the Moros are certainly more picturesque than the Europeanized . . . natives of Manila," declared Edith Moses.[103] The land was harsh but often beautiful. Americans remarked on the majesty of the

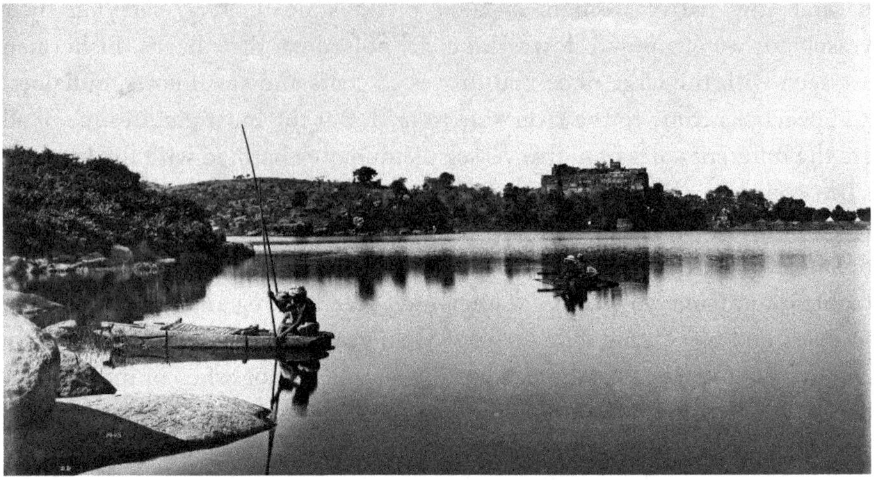

Figure 3.3 An example of picturesque India, the natural and tranquil beauty of Barwa Sagor (generally Sagar, or Lake), near the city of Jhansi. All is calm as two Indians row across. Courtesy of British Library, Asian and African Studies.

sea, the green mountains of the cordillera, and the jungle. "A beautiful tropical country," wrote Moses. "The groves of mangoes, cocoanuts, and other trees, with a thick undergrowth of brilliant flowers and bushes, make the jungle of our imagination."[104] Mostly, as in India, it was the attire of the people that stimulated the western eye. Even in Manila, Helen Taft was charmed by the reds, yellows, and the "calicoes of extravagant hues and patterns" worn by the locals.[105] The surprise and delight were greater upcountry. In Jolo, "the bright colors of the turbans and trousers, with that of the women's sarongs, produced a gay effect against the green trees and a brilliant white wall as a background"; among the Moros at the Dansalan market Frank Laubach saw a "medley of brightly colored clothes," "a sea of red fezzes, hats of purple, pink and green," blankets "patterned with red, magenta, green, yellow, purple, blue and black—a dizzy riot of gaiety"—not to mention the women who "dye their teeth in order to make them a brilliant black, and color their lips red."[106] "The little Igorrote was an odd and picturesque sight," observed William Freer, either because he wore a "red calico blouse and yellow calico knee-trousers" or nothing at all, while the "costumes" of the Bogobos of Davao were made of "bright colored cloth covered with fine bead work." Freer, who was traveling with Governor Taft and the members of the Philippine Commission, noted that Taft asked members of the party not to buy clothes off the bodies of the Bogobos until Dean Worcester had had a chance to photograph their owners.[107]

Seeing and Organizing Subjects and States

Given all these tricks of the eye, the deception, blindness, and splash of the picturesque, how could westerners "see" imperial subjects and make them legible by state apparatus, with the purpose of controlling their bodies and remaking their institutions? The state must know who and where its people are, and it must record their presence to make them visible. It is one thing if the center's rule can be shallow or haphazard, reliant solely on local authorities to govern in the absence of its interest in mobilizing resources or asserting control. But if the state seeks effective intervention, if its "objective requires changing the daily habits (hygiene or health practices) or work performance (quality labor or machine maintenance) of its citizens, such ignorance can well be disabling." The task of the (imperial) state is to fashion what anthropologist James Scott calls an "administrative grid of its observations," and then to bring into conformity the "social reality beneath it." "Legibility is a condition of manipulation," Scott concludes. "Any substantial state intervention in society—to vaccinate a population, produce goods, mobilize labor, tax people and their property, conduct literacy campaigns, conscript soldiers, enforce sanitation standards, catch criminals, start universal schooling—requires the invention of units that are visible."[108] A shallow, sightless state is an invitation to chaos, such as the British recognized from 1857 and the Americans after 1899.

Anglo-American ambition began with control, but it did not end there: India and the Philippines were targets for the forces of civilization, and therefore energetic state involvement, in the absence of which there could be no genuine progress. Left unobserved, Indians and Filipinos would persist in the indolence and mischief of centuries. How to make colonial societies legible? "Interlinked with one another . . . the census, the map and the museum illuminate the late colonial state's style of thinking about its domain," explains Benedict Anderson. The colonizing power sought to create a flexible "classificatory grid" to impose control over people and their efforts at meaning-making. Its effect was "always to be able to say of anything that it was this, not that; it belonged here, not there." It made societies "countable."[109]

The British and Americans were not, of course, writing on blank slates. India and the Philippines were vast land masses that contained diverse multitudes. Part of India had been to an extent controlled by the British East India Company, and the Philippines had been a possession of Spain since the sixteenth century. But many of the people in the two countries were indifferent to European control and existed outside of it, governed by local princes or *dattos* who demanded loyalty, taxes, and occasional conscripts and otherwise left them alone. Wary of attempting to control large, unfamiliar populations, the British and Americans pursued at first a cautious approach to governing. In India, the British extended their authority over those areas that the company had ruled, but had no plan for full state governance.[110] In the immediate aftermath of the Great Rebellion, for example, Governor Canning confiscated the lands of Oudh, then returned to their former leaders control of nearly all of the villages in the state. Canning's hope was to make the local aristocrats agents of the empire, despite their recent disloyalty, and on the whole the plan succeeded.[111] The British faced a demographic reality: though they had flooded India with troops during the rebellion, they would never have enough soldiers or civil servants to rule by force or fiat. The census of 1891 showed a European population in India of 166,000. Of these, 85,000 were British members of the military, including families. There were 287,000,000 Indians. There were almost 700 native states, containing 63,000,000 people and covering an area of 700,000 square miles across the country.[112] The British remit did not run smoothly there; they needed collaborators. In big cities, the British permitted local corporations to make vital decisions, and by the 1870s Indians controlled those bodies in Bombay and Calcutta. To increase "political and popular education," in 1882 Viceroy Lord Ripon expanded municipal boards and extended them to larger districts. These legislatures were empowered to raise taxes, run schools, and oversee dispensaries.[113] Native states were tied to the government by a variety of arrangements. Some dealt directly with the Foreign Office. Others were loosely overseen by an agent of government or the Political Department of the Bombay Presidency.[114] In Punjabi villages, the British mandated registration of land, in the process lowering over them "a grid of official categories" concerning many aspects of social organization and allowing the British to establish in the countryside the "basis for a new rule of law" and enabling them to better visualize their subjects.[115]

The Americans, who inherited a rebellious elite but no deeply embedded princes, moved more quickly than the British in India to plant the seeds of self-government in most Philippine localities. This did not mean that Governor Taft believed the Filipinos were ready to rule themselves. They were, he wrote Senator John Spooner in September 1900, "as unfitted for self government as it is possible to imagine. The mass of the people are ignorant and superstitious, and they are controlled by a small number of Tagalog politicians, crafty, deceitful, ambitious, and insanely jealous of each other, who would lead their people into anarchy and chaos were they given a free hand."[116] Yet the process of conferring some measure of responsibility on the Filipinos had already moved forward. In 1899, the First Philippine Commission, led by Jacob Gould Schurman, had heard extensive testimony concerning the racial character, and thus, they felt, the suitability for self-government, of Filipinos. Witnesses agreed that while the "wild tribes," who still practiced head hunting and other acts of savagery, were not close to being able to manage their affairs, the "educated Filipinos,"

Tagalos and mestizos, might soon be of help, perhaps to "be intrusted [*sic*] with a larger and more independent share of government—self-government, as the American ideal, being constantly kept in view as the goal."[117] Before Taft and his Commission arrived in Manila in June 1900, the US military had accepted a plan drafted by the *ilustrados* Felipe Calderón and Cayetano Arellano that called for the creation of municipal councils with latitude for legislating on local issues, subject to oversight by the ranking American military officer in the area. Taft's Commission strengthened the councils, adding to their powers municipal tax collection and budgeting.[118] This authority was elaborated in February 1901 when the Commission approved the Provincial Government Code, which extended political power outward from municipalities to provinces, establishing the position of governor, who was first to be appointed by the Commission, then elected the following year by Filipinos on the basis of limited suffrage, and a provincial board consisting of the governor, an appointed treasurer, and a supervisor of public works. Days later, members of the Commission, along with cooperative Filipino politicians, began traveling through the archipelago, carrying the new code from town to town, explaining its provisions, and making appointments to office as needed. The provinces held elections in February 1902. Nearly two-thirds of the Commission's gubernatorial appointees won office. Later that year Congress approved the taking of a census in the islands—a necessary step toward finding and counting eligible voters and preparing for land surveys and tax assessments—two years after which a national legislature was to be formed.

In the meantime, Taft settled the tangled issue of what to do with lands held by the Spanish friars. Just before Christmas 1903, and by agreement with the Vatican, the Americans paid the church $7.2 million for all but 10,000 acres of the friars' lands, to be transferred to the Philippine Government.[119] The census was published in 1905. Accordingly, elections were held in 1907 for the new Philippine Assembly. To the Americans' dismay, the Nacionalista Party, which advocated immediate independence, won a solid majority, but the Commission became the upper house of the legislature and the American governor-general retained his position. And none of the political reforms applied to the "non-Christian tribes" upcountry, who remained subject only to the governor.[120]

The Philippine census, essential to making society legible, preceded the devolution of some political power and the assembling of the collaborative imperial state. This was true as well in India. Surveys of Indian cities were carried out in the early nineteenth century. The first national census was scheduled for 1861, but it was postponed because of the "dislocations" of the rebellion, and so it happened only a decade later, and thereafter every ten years. The censuses, along with official gazetteers, annual reports of various agencies, architectural surveys of Indian monuments, and various illustrated volumes, were intended to count heads, but also to classify them. The British were hoping to figure out what made an Indian an Indian, and their answer, increasingly, was appearance. Yet not all of them looked alike. Differences in physiognomy indicated to the British ethnographic differences and therefore caste differences too, and both categories were ways of organizing people subject to Britain's control. [121] Caste, observes anthropologist Bernard Cohn, was "a 'thing,' an entity, which was concrete and measurable; above all it had definable characteristics—endogamy, commensality rules, fixed occupation, common ritual practices . . . . This way of thinking about a particular caste was useful to the administrator, because it have the illusion of knowing the people . . . . India was a sum of its parts and the parts were castes."[122] In the late nineteenth century, the science of anthropometry—the comparative measurement and evaluation of human bodies—became, along with the study of physiognomy, more and more racialized. British anthropologist H. H. Risley was the leading advocate for "reading" people this way. His observations convinced him that the racial divide between Aryans, Caucasians who had moved into India from the north and thus resembled Europeans, and the "native" Dravidians of the south and "Mongoloids" in the east, persisted, and could be seen in the physical characteristics of the various peoples. These included "stature and proportions of the head, features, and limbs," and the "nasal index" of those pictured. Into the early twentieth century, Risley's anthropometry proved influential in the work of colonial authorities, for whom it offered "a convenient guide to India's complex social order." [123] Only if the authorities knew the location, appearance, caste, and number of Indians could they plan to govern and civilize them, to provide them with sanitation and health care and schooling.

The US census of the Philippines, undertaken in 1903, had similar purposes. Like its Indian counterparts, it followed previous efforts to catalog newly subject people, including the report of the first Philippine Commission, which classified its subjects by means of a racialized physiognomy and anthropometry.[124] Its completion would provide the basis for creating the next iteration of the colonial government by including in its legislature a Filipino Assembly. The Philippine census was modeled on the recent Cuban and Puerto Rican censuses, but it was more complicated given the size and diversity of the archipelago. Because of these difficulties, the director of the census, retired Major General J. P. Sanger, brought the Filipinos administering the survey to Manila in January 1903 to receive instruction on how to approach their work. They and their "enumerators" were to be the eyes of the central government, recording on forms they were given the "name, age, sex, race, or tribe, whether native or foreign born, literacy in Spanish, native dialect or language, or in English, school attendance, ownership of homes, industrial and social statistics," and any other information of interest that was particular to the place being surveyed.[125] Sanger assumed that gathering material from the Christian tribes would not be hard, but collecting it from the "non-Christian tribes" would be far more difficult, owing to these populations' "savagery," shyness, remoteness, illiteracy, and resistance to answering questions put to them, even by "tribal" colleagues, in the name of the government.[126] In the end, Sanger was pleasantly surprised at the high rate of response from the population overall. As the Americans had hoped, the census yielded conclusions vital to governing the islands and the people. It found, for example, that the "proportion of defectives"—"the insane, blind, deaf, and deaf and dumb"—was much higher than that in the United States. An impediment to progress was "the superstitions which seem to permeate the entire race," though Sanger was optimistic that these would vanish as "the people become more intelligent and rational" by exposure to American institutions. Education and greater contact with each other would result in the desirable homogenization of Filipinos over time. And despite frequent "epidemics of cholera, bubonic plague, and smallpox, the prevalence of tuberculosis, malarial fever, dysentery, beri-beri, and leprosy," the Philippines, Sanger averred, "are not unhealthful."[127] The text, tables, graphs, and maps that constituted the census put the islands on paper, in black and white, in numbers and in English, and made it possible to move ahead with the colonial administration of the islands.

Equally vital as a way of visualizing colonial subjects was mapping their land. The British had been drawing maps of India for years before they carried out their first full census. Fine-grained accuracy was not always possible; as Lord Salisbury observed, "We have been engaged in drawing lines on maps where no white man's foot ever trod; we have been giving away mountains and lakes and rivers to each other, only hindered by the small impediment that we never knew exactly where the rivers, mountains, and lakes were."[128] Yet accuracy was not the only task of the cartographer. By mapping the land, the British were asserting their legitimacy as its rulers, turning land into territory and establishing their claim to it and their control of access.[129] If mapping turned land into territory, surveying territory made it property and established ownership. Modern survey techniques replaced Indian systems of marking boundaries with stones.[130] Land that had looked "naked" to British travelers because it lacked enclosure appeared properly "dressed" once it was bounded.[131] This kind of work came together on plantations overseen by J. L. H. Williams in the Western Ghats bordering Madras and Travancore states in South India. Williams was putting in tea, cinchona, and coffee, claiming his plots from old growth forest. Lacking theodolites for surveying, he used compass and chain to demarcate the land, then felled trees and burned the undergrowth to open areas to planting. "As soon as the ground was cool enough—usually about a week later—work started on lining for pits for the tea plants and roading and putting in miles of inspection footpaths," he recalled. "I opened a 320 acre clearing in this way." He "had to cut off the whole of the top of a hill to build a factory" for processing products—"a very full but a very satisfying job."[132]

The Americans found few detailed maps when they arrived in the Philippines, and their census-takers ran into immediate difficulty when they tried to define "enumeration districts" for making their surveys.[133] The military had relied on a combination of Spanish maps, more careful "reconnaissance maps" drawn by its engineers when they could get them, and more often rough sketches made by officers or soldiers.[134] These would not do for officials looking to read the fine print of Philippine society. In April 1903, Taft received two boxes of maps from the Bureau of Insular Affairs.[135] Thereafter, Americans, like the British in India, conducted surveys for roads and railroads, assessed the friars' lands for purchase then division, and provided town maps in an effort to establish ownership for purposes of taxation (cadastral maps).[136] It took the Philippine Assembly until 1912 to pass a Cadastral Survey Law, much to the impatience of American authorities; the sticking point was Filipino insistence that some number of the surveyors involved be Filipinos, "known to be utterly incompetent," fumed Dean Worcester.[137] An American missionary named Peter Lerrigo bought land near Capiz for a mission house and school in 1906. "Having fenced the land, our next task was to make it accessible to ourselves by running through it a series of roads," he wrote. "This was done for us by an American contractor who possessed some strong Australian horses. What a wonderful difference it made when the brush was cut down and the roads put through. It began to assume the aspect of civilization and cultivation."[138]

The American hill station at Baguio, championed by governors from Taft onward but the project especially of William Cameron Forbes, was designed to provide its well-connected residents with vistas commanding mountain landscapes and the Igorot population. As conceived by its architect, Daniel Burnham, Baguio's government buildings and official residences were to be placed on the highest ground, where they would "dominate everything in sight," allowing clear sightlines along the town's streets and ensuring the ready visibility of American power. A subsequent project to divide residential Baguio into individually held parcels of property displaced Igorot cattle grazing. Property owners who built in these new neighborhoods were far easier to count and otherwise manage than itinerant farmers who had roamed more freely through the district.[139]

Figures and maps aside, there was no substitute for laying eyes on the people and the land, and British and American officials spent a good deal of their time traveling to all points of the empire to examine conditions for themselves. In India following the Great Rebellion, the British considered it especially important for officers to surveil with care the Indian soldiers they recruited and trained. Agents embedded with the princes, for "vigilance was vital," writes Lawrence James, "even though it was physically impossible to keep a close eye on the inner workings of every state." Reckless or indolent behavior observed by British residents was cause for deposing a prince.[140] Authorities sponsored archeological tours of Indian monuments, such as those undertaken by Alexander Cunningham from 1861–1865.[141] In 1902, the Viceroy, Lord Curzon, visited the Nilgiri Hills in India's south. The governor of Madras arranged for twenty Toda women and men, representatives of the local "tribe," to attend Curzon at his tent while he had "a little refreshment" so "you will be able to look at them."[142] British magistrates or collectors, members of the Indian Civil Service, traveled constantly throughout their often far-flung districts. They oversaw tax collection, the administration of justice, and personal disputes among local people, who regarded them with deference real or imagined. Sitting in front of a tent or under a shade tree, magistrates received their subjects and meted out judgment, usually with a good deal of improvisation. They were the eyes of the empire and the objects of observation by those who came before them.[143]

So did American officials travel throughout the Philippines, observing in person their experiments in pacification, government, and education. They inspected everything, from Filipino architecture (in the hinterlands indicative of "savagery") to incarcerated lepers in Vigan ("not sanitary," wrote Victor Heiser).[144] Taft established the practice of touring, and each of his successors followed his example. The people were "anxious to catch a glimpse of" the Commission, thought Daniel Williams, who accompanied the Taft group in 1901. They were impressed by the sheer "size and avoirdupois of the Commissioners," who averaged two hundred and twenty-seven pounds.[145] Taft remarked repeatedly on the warmth of the reception the commissioners received, where the "houses of the humblest people were decorated in our honor," and they were heralded by flower-covered arches and welcomed with speeches, banquets and balls.[146] Following another journey in 1902–1903, Taft thanked one of his hosts, the *presidente* of Lilio: "We shall never forget the fine band so gracefully clad, the splendid pagodas and uniformed carriers, the magnificent Eiffel tower, the bright eyes of the ladies, the bounteous banquet and the pleasures of the ball which we had in your hospitable mansion."[147] William Cameron Forbes visited throughout the archipelago as acting governor general in the summer of 1909. "I've accomplished a lot on this trip," he recorded in his journal in July. "I know conditions and people better . . . . I believe in government after seeing—and seeing with my own eyes."[148] More than a decade later Manuel Roxas, speaker of the assembly and no friend of the American occupation, nevertheless admitted that Governor-General Leonard Wood's energy in inspecting conditions "all over the Islands have produced remarkable results in the improvement of the government service. The people and the officials feel that he knows what they are doing and that he has a personal interest in it."[149] It was important for both peoples to see and be seen.

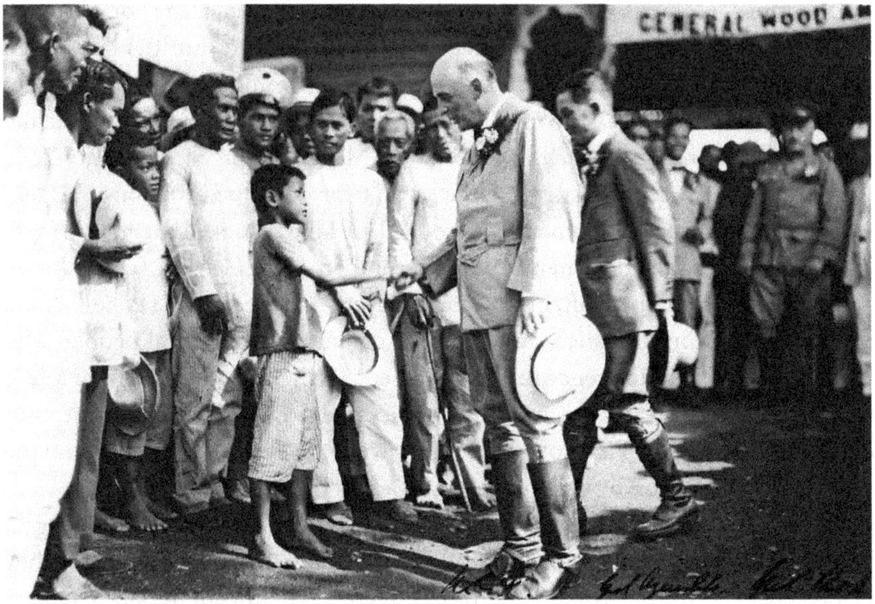

Figure 3.4 Believing that it was important to see and be seen, American officials traveled throughout the archipelago to present themselves to their subjects. In this photograph, taken ca. 1910, Governor W. C. Forbes tours with Emilio Aguinaldo, the former leader of the Filipino insurgents, in order to demonstrate American forgiveness and the attractiveness of cooperation. General Leonard Wood is in the background, right. Courtesy of the American Historical Collection, Rizal Library, Ateneo de Manila University.

But these strategies could not fix vision in time and place. Once out of sight, colonial subjects might resume behavior inimical to their control by the government. Censuses and maps might do figuratively, but seeing by means of them meant reducing others to print on the page, and did not permit extended visual examination of individual faces or amount to embodied knowledge. To do these things would require making images of subjects and their environments, perhaps by drawing or painting but preferably by taking photographs.[150] The British and Americans embraced photography as a way to record the landscape as territory, and to capture on film their "native" charges as a means of studying them for purposes of classification and control. The landscapes they intended to depict were at once wild and exotic yet capable of being tamed. Those whom they captured on film were individuals in a limited sense only, for individual subjects were, inevitably, collected and seen by photographers and viewers of photographs as members of a group, a racial or ethnic type. John William Kaye, who was Secretary in the Political and Secret Department of the East India Company until 1874, wrote that "to represent India by mere word-painting is an almost impossible task.... Only a vague, unsatisfactory idea of the objects, represented by the printed page, is left on the reader's mind ... It is only by the great exponents, form and colour, appealing to the fleshly eye, that truthful impressions can be derived of a country, which differs so essentially from all that is made known to us by the teachings of European experience."[151] His words described equally well American thinking about the Philippines.

Daguerreotype photography, begun in France in1839, moved quickly to India and the Philippines. By 1854, the East India Company was directing that photographs should replace drawings or paintings of the cave temples in western India; a Spanish government agent named Sinibaldo de Mas opened a portrait studio in Manila in 1841.[152] Photography expanded quickly in both places. Its alleged accuracy meant it could be used for record-keeping and surveillance. In India, provincial governments were instructed to gather photographs of their "races and classes" to be placed on exhibition in Calcutta. Authorities in Lucknow proposed in 1862 that prostitutes carry photo identification stating whether or not their bearers had venereal disease.[153] Working in Kashmir and the Himalayas during the 1860s, Samuel Bourne shot landscapes that were, in his own terms, "picturesque," balancing the play of light and shadow on stone and minimizing the presence of "unsightly objects" or "industry" in the foreground of his compositions.[154] By "unsightly objects" he meant "people." Bourne was contemptuous of the porters who hauled his heavy equipment up mountainsides and quickly grew frustrated with subjects who refused "to stand or sit in an easy, natural attitude. Their idea of giving life to a picture was to stand bolt upright, with their arms down as stiff as pokers, their chin turned up as if they were standing to have their throats cut."[155] Bourne also photographed Barrackpore, where the Great Rebellion had begun, and commemorating the sacrifice of Britons during the uprising became a practice of other artists as well. Hugh Fisher was sent to photograph India in 1907 for a lecture series to be given by Halford Mackinder, of Oxford University. Fisher took pictures of the pockmarked Baily Gate in Lucknow and the Memorial Well at Cawnpore, which Mackinder used as magic lantern slides for lectures he gave across Britain.[156] And, beginning in the late nineteenth century, picture postcards were printed of Indian subjects, of monuments or the lower castes at work, to underscore the civilizing effort to be undertaken.[157]

Above all, photography would become in India a tool of caste and racial classification.[158] The best example of this work was the eight-volume *The People of India,* a collection of photographs edited by John William Kaye and John Forbes Watson and published between 1868 and 1875. The project had modest origins: the Governor-General Lord Canning and his wife Lady Canning wanted a souvenir of India "which might recall to their memories the peculiarities of Indian life." Ultimately, sensing the magnitude of the project, Canning referred it to the government's home secretary for completion. The enterprise employed dozens of photographers, amateur and professional, with James Waterhouse among the most prominent. He had complaints from the start. He worked in a tent, and by the time his often tardy subjects arrived to be photographed it was often too hot for his equipment to function. The Raja of Ratlam could not hold still "for the duration of the exposure"; some subjects were shy; Waterhouse got sick; and the Mahrattas he photographed were "impertinent . . . always on the look-out for an opportunity of saying or doing something unpleasant to an European's feelings, and never thinking of offering any assistance whatever." The editors admitted that the photos had not been collected systematically, and that the volumes were thus produced "without any definite plan." Yet certain tendencies were clear. Some subjects were featured for their loyalty to the British cause during the rebellion. Others appeared for their peculiarities, or their seeming hostility, among them Shair Ali Syud, a Muslim who exhibited "the obstinacy, sensuality, ignorance, and bigotry of his class. It is hardly possible, perhaps, to conceive features so essentially repulsive."[159] The physiognomy of a Pachada man, according to the text, revealed his proclivity for "rapine, murder and robbery on a large scale. . . . His countenance is extremely forbidding, and is perhaps an index to the lawless and unreclaimed nature of his tribe. . . . These and people like them, are bad elements in the general population of the North-West provinces, and need constant watching."[160] Yet the impression left by *The People of India* was of individuals as representative of the frequently problematic whole, with its goal to shape and reinforce categories of Indian people.[161]

In the American Philippines, photography both fixed the image of Filipinos and marked them as racially distinct from each other and inferior to their occupiers. The Kodak camera appeared in 1888, and with its relative portability and ease of loading film, it quickly found widespread use in the Philippines.[162] Soldiers with cameras took pictures of their exploits in war. Albert Sonnichsen noted that the men had a penchant for photographing dead insurgents, and for captioning their pictures with triumphant sentiments: "Can the d—-d Regiment boys shoot? You bet they can. Count the dead niggers."[163] American soldiers sought to have their pictures taken before leaving the islands, and regarded shots of Filipinas as bonuses. A newspaper advertisement for a Manila photography studio in 1908 imagined an exchange: "'Hello Billy! Where are you going?' 'Well, Jack, I am in a hurry. Before we leave I want to have my photo taken at the PERTIERRA STUDIO, STERNBERG BROS.—105 ESCOLTA STREET, same entrance as the Hotel de France. They make, indeed the best and cheapest photos in Manila, and will give me, free, a nice photo of a Filipino woman as a souvenir of the Philippine Islands.'"[164] Gilbert Grosvenor, the editor of the fledgling *National Geographic*, received from Taft photographs taken by census enumerators and published 138 of them in the April 1905 issue, which proved extremely popular.[165] In the name of science, officials took photos that were by any definition prurient. Victor Heiser photographed naked people reading the Montgomery Ward catalog, and later built a museum in Manila that included an abundance of photographs.[166] "The wild people were photographed at regular intervals," he wrote, "showing the stage of civilization to which they had arrived year by year."[167]

Views differed as to whether Filipinos liked being photographed or not. G. D. Rice claimed they did. "The natives have a great love for photographs," Rice wrote, "and they will pay high prices for two or three inferior pictures of themselves in best attire. They also crave for views of their homes, and will squander considerable money in this line."[168] William Freer, however, found the Moros at least resistant to having Americans point cameras at them. Freer hid behind a tree near a Moro market and quietly shot a roll of film "unknown to the passers-by."[169] In 1914, the Philippine Legislature passed a law directing "that anyone who 'exploit[ed] or exhibit[ed] tribal people' would be fined five thousand dollars or be imprisoned for not more than five years."[170] This was followed by a proposal by the Filipino Director of Posts to prohibit from the mails all "photographs, engravings, lithographs, books or any kind of printed material depicting any inhabitant of the Philippine Islands belonging to the so-called non-Christian tribes." The director contended that such materials damaged prospects for Philippine independence when they appeared in American newspapers or libraries. Governor-General Leonard Wood rejected the proposal, arguing that it would deny the "non-Christian tribes" the ability to send photos of themselves to friends or families and prevent the mailing of "any scientific or ethnological work concerning them." Wood thought the proposal "intolerant." It would, in addition, suppress vital information about the Filipino people, such that "not only reveals the fact that the Filipinos are not one people but that many of them are primitive and addicted to strange customs and costumes."[171]

Here again, and as with the British in India, was the heart of the matter: photographs made manifest the differences among Filipinos and the unsuitability of many of them for self-governance. The first compendium of photos, *Our Islands and Their People as Seen with Camera and Pencil* (1899), contained images of Cuba, Puerto Rico, Hawaii, and the Philippines. Captions beneath photos of Filipinos dismissed any possibility of early independence for the islands. The description of a "group of the better class of Filipino women" notes that two of those pictured are "Mestizos," who have "a more agreeable cast of countenance . . . inherited from their Spanish father." As for the others, "the Malay predominates," showing "plainly in the rather unpleasant scowl of their faces." "It is rare to see a pleasant face among these people," read a caption under a photograph of people at a Manila restaurant. "As a race, they are vindictive and treacherous—just the kind of people that all good Americans desire to keep away from." A group of schoolchildren, many with an "African cast of countenance," were "hardly up to the mark" as American citizens. When "bright-faced American boys" entered the scene, they were "out of place in such company."[172] The collections of photographs of Filipinos for "ethnographic" purposes portrayed them as hopelessly divided, dark-skinned men and women without clothes, pierced, tattooed, or otherwise appearing a stunted version of humanity. Such depictions undercut those who imagined them ready for independence and justified the continuation of American control. Photographs of Filipino census takers and *presidentes* might stand in contrast to those of "tribals," with the former shown in front of buildings and with "the symbols of 'civilization' conspicuously displayed (the hats, the canes, the pocket watch chains, the bow ties)," the latter in the bush, staring uncomprehendingly at the photographer.[173] The Americans believed in the faithfulness of photographs to depict subjects without distortion or bias; the camera did not lie. Anthropologist Daniel Folkmar photographed prisoners at Manila's Bilibid Prison in preparation for the 1904 Louisiana Purchase Exposition in St. Louis. The prison, Folkmar wrote, provided "an unexcelled collection of the leading [*sic*] peoples from Northern Luzon to Mindanao." Propagandizing for the retention of the Philippines from 1913 to 1915, Dean Worcester showed American audiences lurid photos of non-Christians, insisting that they remained savages and therefore incapable of governing themselves and subject to abuse by their Christian compatriots, and proposed to make a series of films that might be useful for the same purpose.[174]

Subjects and Nations Displayed

The actual work of governing subjects required their cooperation. It also demanded greater resolution on the part of British and American audiences at home to accept the responsibilities conferred on them by their empires. They must see Others displayed as in need of guidance, discipline, and correction, in ways both benign and coercive. They must believe their eyes that their intervention in far-away places was the right thing, their duty to those who might otherwise succumb to the aggression of outsiders or to their own ignorance. Immediately following the Great Rebellion and the defeat of the insurgency in the Philippines, Britain and the United States embarked on parallel efforts to display their power to their subjects and to display their subjects, in all their merits and (mainly) foibles, to Britons and Americans who would by their agreement sustain their new empires. Both did this by appropriating ceremonial forms they found in place on arrival. Both assumed their subjects' affection and aptitude for spectacle. The British more thoroughly made Indian ceremonial display their own, while the Americans created their biggest performance not in the Philippines but in the American heartland, nevertheless making sure that Filipinos were a vital part of the proceedings.

Both Britain and the United States had previous experience with grand exhibitions at home. They mounted fairs meant to display their prosperity and power to their empires and would-be rivals. London's Hyde Park hosted the Great Exhibition of 1851 at the Crystal Palace, which featured innovations in industry, technology, and science, and a popular India exhibition containing the Koh-i-Noor diamond, the largest in the world. Chicago was the site of the World's Columbian Exposition in 1893. There Henry Adams found himself awed by the Great Dynamo that powered the fair, and visitors heard Swami Vivekananda discuss Hinduism at the World's Parliament of Religion. Empire more fully demanded its due thereafter, as the British and Americans established formal control of India and the Philippines. The impresario Imrie Kiralfy staged the Empire of India Exhibition in London in 1895 and 1896. It featured a stage show purporting to present a millennium of India's history, including Gilbert and Sullivan-inspired faqirs: "Cursing, crying, flesh chastising, / See us Fakirs, martyrising." Outside the theater Kiralfy built an Indian street scene, including mosques, a curry restaurant, artists at work on handicrafts, and of course jugglers and snake charmers. An estimated twelve million people visited the exhibition.[175]

The most important displays came in India, where after 1858 the British revived the durbar, a coming together of British authorities and local Indian rulers. The Mughals had long maintained the practice of using such ceremonial meetings to emphasize their authority and demand obedience from local leaders. In 1858 the British discarded the old political order, putting on trial and then exiling Bahadur Shah II, the last Mughal, and proclaiming Queen Victoria's sovereignty over the country. Now-Viceroy Lord Canning toured the north, to be received by Indian princes and others who had stood by Britain during the rebellion. To them, he offered "honors and rewards," conferring on his favorites titles such as Raja and Nawab, special clothes and emblems, land grants, and pensions. The Duke of Edinburgh came to India in 1869; the Prince of Wales toured for six months in 1875–1876. Indians were meant to see these men, in all their royal splendor, as representatives of British authority. Large imperial durbars were held in Delhi in 1877 (formally, an "assemblage"), 1903, and 1911. They aimed at what *The Scotsman* called "the susceptibility of the Eastern mind to spectacular glitter and scenic display," for "Orientals" were, like children, "dazzled by the mock splendours of panto."[176] Even the aristocracy, claimed Viceroy Lord Lytton in 1876, was "easily affected by sentiment and susceptible to the influence of symbols to which facts inadequately correspond." The events were elaborately choreographed. "A code of conduct was established for princes and chiefs for their attendance at the durbar," Bernard Cohn writes. "The clothes they wore, the weapons they could carry, the number of retainers and soldiers that could accompany them to the Viceroy's camp, where they were met by British officials, the number of gun salutes fired in their honour, the time of the entry into the durbar hall or tent, whether the Viceroy would rise and come forward to greet them, where on the viceregal rug they would be saluted by the Viceroy, where they would be seated, how much nazar [gold coins] they could give, whether they would be entitled to a visit from the Viceroy, were all markers of rank and could be changed by the Viceroy to raise or lower their rank." All of this was meant to make the British "insiders" by establishing the writ of their monarch throughout the part of India they ruled, and even to the princely states beyond.[177]

At the 1877 assemblage, the Viceroy's tent was surrounded by servants bearing mare and yak tail whisks, markers of authority, and a mix of British and Indian soldiers. Gas lamps illuminated the camp. Lord and Lady Lytton arrived at the Delhi train station, greeted throngs of well wishers, then departed for the durbar in a silver howdah mounted on what was said to be the largest elephant in India. A British civil servant designed coats of arms for the princes, including his ideas of their genesis, the gods they worshipped, their histories, and "topographic features of their territories." Lord Lytton noted that the Indian soldiers who lined the processional presented "a most striking and peculiar appearance . . . a vivid and varied display of strange arms, strange uniforms, and strange figures." Sir Dinkar Rao, prime minister of Sindhia, was impressed: "If any man would understand why it is that the English are, and must necessarily remain the master of India he need only go up to Flagstaff Tower [the highest point overlooking the camps] and look down upon this marvelous camp. Let him notice the method, the order, the cleanliness, the discipline, the perfection of the whole organization and he will recognize at once the epitome of every title to command and govern which one race can possess over others."[178] The 1903 durbar, held to honor the succession of King Edward VII and Queen Alexandra as Emperor and Empress of India, was Curzon's glory, featuring a vast tent city with exhibitions, ceremonies, and grand balls. The 1911 event aimed in various ways to puncture the growing Indian nationalist movement by justifying the empire "to Indians, the British, colonial populations and even peoples elsewhere."[179]

Neither Americans nor Filipinos had a tradition quite like durbar, but display and exhibition were nevertheless part of their practices. Filipinos greeted American officials in their towns with elaborate presentations of gifts, formal speeches, profusions of flowers and offerings of food and drink, and elegant *bailes* at which they appeared grandly dressed and danced the *rigodon* with American partners. Manilans celebrated *carnival* in February each year. The Americans were uncomfortable with some of the events associated with *carnival*, which struck them as hedonistic, erotic, and expensive. In late 1921, Governor General Wood summoned the director of *carnival* to his office "and had a short talk with him concerning the coming Carnival; [I] told him that while we wanted it to be lively and interesting, we did not want any immoral displays, pictures or other things which tend to break down the decency and morality of the people."[180] Such performances confirmed to Americans what they referred to as the Filipino love of spectacle. In their view, a little of it went a long way.

The most prominent example of American efforts to display Filipinos for the broadest possible audience was the Louisiana Purchase Exposition in St. Louis in 1904. The fair was a showcase for ethnography, and none seemed to its organizers more timely or fascinating than that of the newly pacified archipelago. W. J. McGee, head of the exposition's Department of Anthropology, believed that exhibiting Filipinos who fell all along the evolutionary spectrum would prove educational and lucrative. "It is a matter of common observation," he wrote, "that the white man can *do* more and better than the yellow, the yellow man more and better than the red or black."[181] Where on the color spectrum to place the varied peoples of the Philippines was unclear; to exhibit them alongside each other would offer observers a chance to decide for themselves. Working with the ethnologist Albert Jenks, who had done research among the Igorots for several years, McGee assembled a forty-seven acre Philippine Reservation, consisting of as many as 1,200 Filipinos "living" in villages built along Lake Arrowhead. Fairgoers entered the exhibition by crossing the Bridge of Spain into a simulated Manila, a reminder of the islands' recent and civilizationally liminal past as a Spanish possession. Close by was the Visayan village, inhabited by Christian and Hispanicized people. Beyond the center were the villages of the non-Christian "tribes"—the exotic, racially indeterminate yet surely uncivilized Igorots, Moros, Bagobos, and Negritos. Behind them lay encampments of Philippine Scouts and members of the Constabulary, who had collaborated with the Americans at home and were now entrusted to patrol the reservation and even to appear throughout the grounds of the exposition; the well-regarded Constabulary band opened the fair each day. The spatial configuration of the reservation was meant to indicate the relative possibilities of civilizing the various groups.

The Philippine Reservation quickly became the fair's leading attraction. Intending to showcase the progress made by Visayans and Scouts under American rule, the exhibition instead inspired voyeurism at the villages of the non-Christian Igorots and Negritos.[182] Controversy arrived almost instantly over the scarcity of clothing worn by some of these peoples. Worried that bare chests, loincloths, and G-strings would confirm the impression that all Filipinos were savages and therefore unready for any form of self-government, Taft, reflecting President Roosevelt's position, urged fair organizers to require men to wear "trunks" and women "shirts or chemises of some sort." Anthropologists involved with the display refused, arguing that "to put pants on [the Igorots and Negritos] would change a very interesting ethnological exhibit which shocks no one into a suggestive side-show." With admissions to the reservation soaring, the administration backed down.[183] Largely confined to their exhibition villages, the non-Christians remained an ethnological sideshow, perceived as the essence of the Philippines and its most authentic embodiment. Negritos, the "blackest" of the people on display, were "primate-like," a "distinctive race" who were the "lowest grade of human creatures" under American jurisdiction. The Igorots danced and sang, to the evident delight of the crowds. The Bontoc Igorots ceremonially killed and ate dogs, which scandalized observers even as they flocked to witness it. Moros from Samal dove for coins visitors threw into the lake.[184] Such spectacle far outstripped interest in the Visayans and other "civilized" groups, much to their irritation. When the Scouts ventured out into the fairgrounds, as they were invited to do by St. Louis schoolteachers, they were first taunted as "niggers," then assaulted by packs of Marines who objected to their presence in the company of white women. The specter of racial mixing at the fair was too much for the St. Louis *Post-Dispatch,* whose editors feared that when the Scouts departed the United States, they might leave behind them white "American brides . . . , as American soldiers returning from the Philippines" had done with women there.[185]

As with durbars in India, the messages conveyed in St. Louis were meant to go both ways. Racism was made manifest to the Scouts who wandered beyond the fences of their village. Also present at the fair were *pensionados*—young men and women who had been sent to the United States at Taft's behest starting the previous year. They were students, speakers of English and well versed in American customs, and they served as guides to the Philippines Reservation. Other fairgoers were uncertain what to make of them, these dark people "clad in neat, fashionable clothing." The *pensionados* themselves voiced dismay at the way they were regarded. "How ignorant people are here," one complained, and another expressed disgust that a woman had "asked me if I liked wearing clothes."[186] Little is known about how the "villagers" felt about the gaze directed at them day after day that summer and fall. Some appeared to welcome attention, and resented other Filipinos who in their view "hogged the limelight." Moros were either shy or actively hostile to having their picture taken.[187] When the Exposition ended, most Filipinos returned home, some of them bearing American-style clothing and crafts. Items the Filipinos had produced at the fair were sold off or given to the Museum of Natural History in New York. A few Igorots were hired by carnival impresarios to appear on state fair midways and in vaudeville shows.[188]

Subject Gazes: Indians

In certain ways, Indians adopted, or adapted to, British visual practices. Eighteenth- and nineteenth-century British patrons commissioned miniature paintings from Indian artists who had long experience with the medium. These "Company School" paintings, done in watercolor rather than the gouache the artists had previously preferred, blended Indian craft with a British aesthetic. Photography came to India with British practitioners and was soon taken up by local photographers. A society of Bengal Photographers was started in 1862. Members produced popular *cartes-de-visite,* a requirement for the best sorts of Indians and Britons, which placed their subjects in photography studio settings widely used in Europe.[189]

In other ways, Indian optical practices departed from those of the British. Britons in India felt this acutely. They believed Indian vision to be unreliable, at best untrained; they reported that Indians tended to look at pictures upside down.[190] The British also found the Indian gaze intrusive and disturbing. Everywhere, they said, Indians watched them intently. When Anna Leonowens attended a dinner party in the early 1880s, she noticed the servants who were not waiting on table at the edges of the room, standing "with arms folded across their breasts under the shadows of doors and pillars . . . so still and motionless . . . that they might almost, save for the glitter in their eyes, have passed for bronze statues. . . . With those dark, restless eyes watching every turn, motion, and expression of our faces," Leonowens felt uneasy and "anxious to escape. If I laughed or talked or moved, those dark eyes seemed to observe me, even when they were seemingly fixed on vacancy." She longed for the meal to end.[191] Mrs. King was stared at by women in her train carriage in Punjab with the "curiosity with which we might watch a family of gorillas," and in the bazaar in Srinagar by "young street-Arabs."[192] Britons resented attempts by Indian women especially to avoid their eyes, as in *zenana,* and observed with amusement the discomfort shown by Indians confronted with British bodily exposure. Indians seemed offended at the sights of Englishwomen playing tennis in shorts, men and women in bathing suits, and clothes that revealed a woman's shoulders and arms, including dresses with narrow shoulder straps.[193]

A late sixteenth-century account by Tahir Muhammed includes his observations of the "Franks" in India: "They wear very fine clothes but they are often very slovenly and pimply. They don't like to use water. They bathe very rarely. Amongst them, washing after relieving oneself is considered improper."[194] Offended as Britons often were about the visible habits of Indians, complaints concerning unkempt and unwashed Europeans were common among Indians, who placed enormous significance in their visual perceptions of others, and in their own apprehension of others' visual habits. More than one Briton recalled being told by an Indian servant that he or she looked at people improperly, or that there was something wrong with their eyes. Hilda Bourne once reached out to cuddle "a darling little dark baby," only to be stopped by her nurse: "No, no, they think Missus bring evil eye."[195] Irene Bose found that Indians made "a fine distinction between the persons who meet them upon their own level and those who 'look at us,'" presumably with disapproval or condescension.[196] A group of Brahmins from Jodhpur petitioned the Viceroy to remove from office the civil servant Sir Leonard Reynolds, because he had, they said, "pig like eyes set in an arrogant face."[197] Much different was the encounter between Sir Pratap Singh of Jodhpur, a leading Rajput and well known in England, and Queen Victoria, on the occasion of the Queen's golden jubilee in 1887. As Singh recorded it, Victoria summoned him, "and in obedience I presented myself. Reaching near her, I made my salute, Indian fashion, placing my sword on the ground: then, coming closer, I kissed her gracious hand, extended in English style; and immediately I raised it to my eyes. All English officers present were astonished at the eccentricity of this salutation: and after the reception was over they asked me about it. I explained that, according to Indian ideas, it was thought ill to salute one's master bearing arms. So I laid down my sword. Further, after kissing Her Majesty's hand, I raised it to my eyes, because there is nothing dearer to a man than his eyes. This explanation seemed to satisfy everyone."[198]

Vital to Hindu—and, some would argue, Indian Muslim and even secular Indian practice—was the concept of *darshan*. The word means "seeing" in Sanskrit, and it pertains in the first instance to viewing a representation of a god. Hindus will travel a great distance to gaze upon a divine person or godhead, the *lingam* of Shiva or the image of Brahma, a custom that is central to their worship. The witness is said to "take *darshan*," while the deity reciprocates by "giving *darshan*," or presenting "himself to be seen" by onlookers. The mutuality of this act of seeing is of vital importance to those engaged in it.[199] Outside of devout Hindus, the practice is reflected in perceptions of persons or images who are divine only in the loosest sense. So, for instance, did Indians regard people of great power or importance with both reverence and expectation: they would gaze at such people, and in return they hoped their gaze would be met by a look of understanding and compassion from the object of their respect.[200] Such treatment was afforded Mahatma Gandhi long before India won its independence. M. L. Darling interviewed small farmers in Punjab in 1930 and asked about their views of Gandhi. The farmers knew who Gandhi was, but told Darling that "we have no certain knowledge of what he teaches—we have not seen him."[201] Without laying eyes on him, they were unwilling to accept his authority unreservedly.

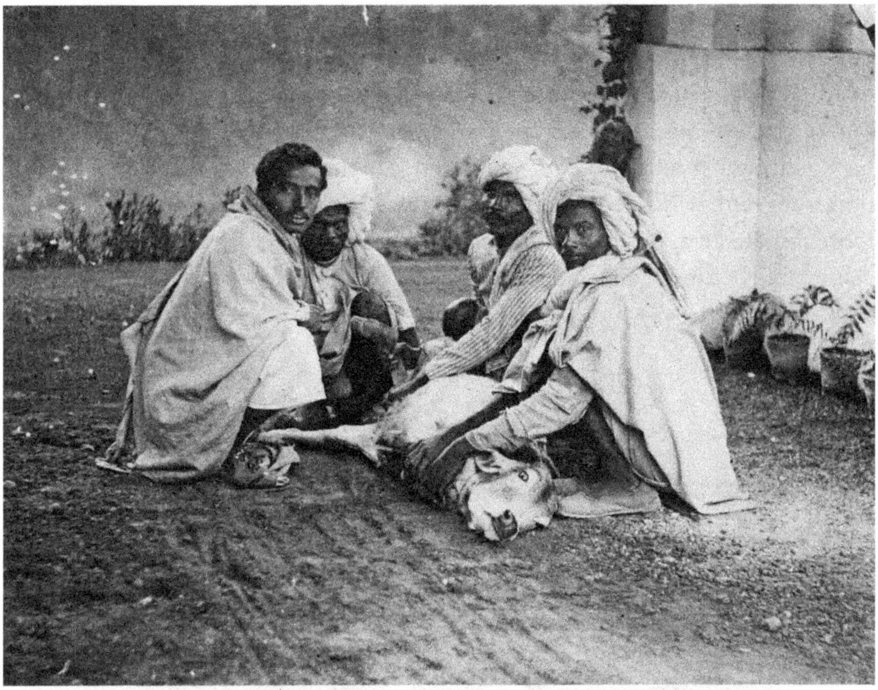

Figure 3.5 British photographers often had an eye for the exotic or appalling. Here, four Indians and their dead calf stare fixedly back, a reminder that the gaze went two ways. Courtesy of British Library, Asian and African Studies.

Subject Gazes: Filipinos

There was no *darshan* as such in the Philippines. To some extent American Protestants recognized the Catholic iconography familiar to many Filipinos, and agreed that it distinguished them more from the non-Christians of the islands than from themselves. Still, the visual practices of Filipinos outside of churches surprised the Americans and increased their suspicions concerning their charges' deceitfulness and depravity. Like the British, the Americans were discomfited when they were stared at, as was Ralph Buckland and others at the beach in Bushwang ("They seemed very much interested in our whiteness"), and Edith Moses, forced to wash her face and comb her hair in full view of a busy street in Tagbilaran, to the "intense interest" of the local people.[202] The Americans noticed that while Filipinos seemed greatly to value photographs of themselves and their finest possessions, like Indians they did always know how to look at them, frequently holding them upside down.[203] Away from Manila and the larger towns, Filipinos hid from the American gaze or appeared to dissolve in front of it. Evidently, the Moros who were shy in St. Louis behaved the same way at home. The Moro headman Ampatuan told James McColl that if the government reached too far into his country the people would "hide in the hills" and declared that he had "never seen an American who knew the 'Custombre' of the moros." If the Americans continued to demand face-to-face meetings with him he would simply refuse to come, and they could thereafter expect no cooperation from him or his people. McColl summoned a Tiruray chief from an even more remote area, but found the man too terrified to speak in front of him: "I cannot talk because I am afraid. I am afraid of the white people."[204]

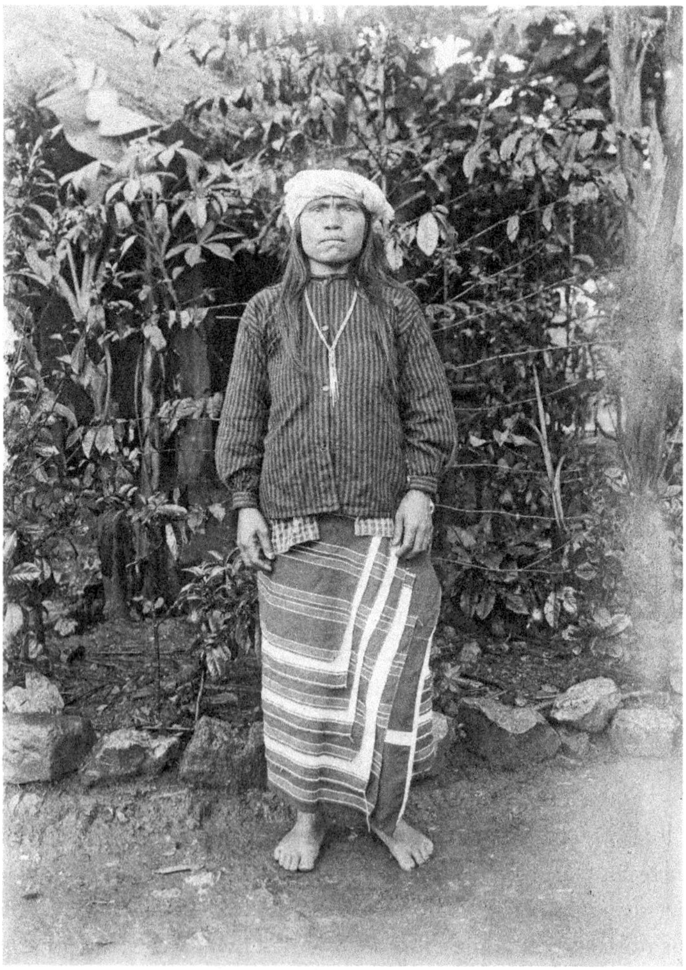

Figure 3.6 A "wealthy Igorot woman" in Benguet province, 1901. Taking and collecting photographs of Filipinos was a way for Americans to classify them. Like the Indian men in the previous photo, this woman stares back. Courtesy of the Museum of Anthropological Archaeology, University of Michigan.

Accused of performing distracting spectacle and perpetrating fibs of vision, Filipinos hurled similar charges at the Americans. In 1914, the US Congress discussed the Jones Bill, which after its passage granted greater political power to Filipinos and pledged eventual independence for the archipelago. Filipino nationalists were suspicious of the bill because it failed to set a date for independence. An American spy attending a nationalist meeting in Manila reported that speaker after speaker denounced American supporters of the bill for "deceiving" Filipinos with vague promises of full self-government.[205] Filipinos were convinced that American perfidy existed everywhere. "It seems the country has been flooded with spies of all kinds," reported the organization Pro Libertad in 1923, "with the only end of safeguarding the interests of our oppressors of their devil's soul, that colonel of bad death who in life is called Mr. [Leonard] Wood, but who perhaps very shortly will take a long voyage of impossible return." It referred to the Americans as "cuttle-fish," a reference to the squid's ability to disguise itself with ink. In the end there was little need for "vigilance," because Wood's agents were all "drunkards and degenerates who live on whiskey, cocaine and with the blackest and vilest women."[206]

Clarity of vision was vitally important to Filipinos. If there is anything comparable to *darshan* in some part of Filipino culture, it is the relationship between humans and ghosts: the former cannot see into the others' world, the latter can. Anthropologist Fenella Cannell has observed that Filipinos will apologize to a ghost, or *tawo*, if they think they have accidentally harmed one. Perpetrators of such acts explain to the *tawo* that "you can see us, but we cannot see you." Unlike the gods in India, the *tawo* has no obligation to humans, who can only plead with it to forgive them.[207] Even while US troops battled Emilio Aguinaldo in late 1899, the Philippine Commission recorded the Filipino leader's statement begging his followers "that when we observe any wrong conduct that we shall be the first to expose it, for . . . we have some companions of strange conduct, who for love of money strive to dissimulate concerning that which they have hidden or are about to hide and to divert suspicion from themselves when spoken to about it. . . . Truth will always prevail, and your neighbor has always good eyes" for seeing it. The insurrection, in short, required transparency.[208] "How can we be well governed by men who have never even seen a Filipino?" demanded a man of Albert Sonnichsen.[209] In the absence of sight there was no real knowledge; one might as well try to govern a ghost. Metaphors of sight and sightlessness came easily even to children in the Philippines. American teacher William Freer listened with gratification to a speech given in his honor by ten-year-old Lorenzo Perez. It was, the boy said, the duty of teachers to "open our eyes. Our eyes used to be shut, but now they are open, and we can see with them." Lorenzo was sure that Freer "never sleeps and never rests. Every day he travels from town to town to see all the teachers and how they teach the children."[210]

Americans were certain that Filipinos cared a great deal about appearances, the outward need for respect, or saving face. This claim offered an apparent contrast between the supposedly superficial concerns of Asians and the more profound ones of westerners, yet the *ilustrados* were angry and embarrassed when Americans represented all Filipinos as savages.[211] Theodore Friend has noted that the concept of face is expressed in all major Philippine languages, and American observers of the Philippines were convinced that face factored heavily in their relations with the people there.[212] "To the Oriental—and the Filipino is an Oriental—'face' is everything," argued William Anderson. "It is position; it is power."[213] It was especially important for Americans to perform their public functions with confidence; exhibition and spectacle were manifestations of their power. "Appearance is valued for its own sake regardless of the underlying realities, and yet 'face' is largely dependent upon strength and force," wrote Nicholas Roosevelt of Filipinos. "All the outward trappings of show are important elements in it—the position which a man occupies, his titles, his clothes, the style of his equipage, the number and strength of his followers or assistants, the splendor of his house, his wealth and his deportment."[214] When William Howard Taft arrived as governor of the Philippines in 1900, he deliberated about where he and his family should live. In the end, he chose to move into Malacañan, on the Pasig River. The imposing house was uncomfortable and needed a good deal of work, and it was infused by all the sights and smells of the river. Yet Taft felt there was no choice. The Spanish rulers had lived there, and so had American generals. "Appearances play so great a part with these people that it would certainly be unwise for the head of the Civil Government not to move into that place," Taft wrote to a friend. Whatever its discomforts, Malacañan was the house in which Filipinos expected to see him. Face required him to live there.[215]

Ralph Kent Buckland, the son of a congressman from Ohio, spent several months in the Philippines in 1904. In the end, he concluded glumly, "not one American occupying a high official position ever has the chance of seeing a Filipino town as it really is, or of seeing the native officials in their routine work, or of seeing the average native under the influence of his ordinary temperament." The official eye was inevitably fooled. Buckland's description of how this happened is worth quoting at length:

> An American official thinks of paying a visit of inspection to a Filipino town.... The Filipino's stronghold is his ability to make a good impression; so, forewarned of this visit, the town is raked from one end to the other, the tall grass in the plaza is cut, the carabaos are shooed out of sight, and the secretary, the treasurer, and the *Juez de Paz* work nights to get their books in order for a possible looking over. On the day set for the arrival, the officials of the town don their best white drill raiment

> and go forth in carriages, on horseback, or on foot . . . to meet and greet and profusely welcome the American official. Why should not the American official feel pleased and optimistic and deeply impressed? They set him down to a sumptuous banquet . . . ; they wine him, they champagne him; they toast him— . . . —then some one whose type of face leads one to conjecture that his mother may have looked twice or thrice at a Spaniard, gets up and labors through a lengthy rigamarole, not very original, not very logical, and not very elucidating, about how well fitted the Filipino people are to run their ship of state. . . . . In the evening, a gay ball is tendered the American in honor of his visit. All the *senoras* and the *senoritas* and the *senors* and the *senoritos* are out in their gala attire. A liberal application of powder, or of whitewash, has somewhat lightened the landscape; and a plentiful supply of violets or of jasmine perfumes the path of every individual, male or female, as they pass in and out through the elaborately decorated dancing *sala*. Of course, the sight is a pleasing one, and, of course, the visiting official is even more than ever won over the charms of the richly dressed women and by the brilliancy of the whole affair. He retires that night to dream rosy-hued dreams of a Philippine Paradise, where beautifully gowned women and mealy-mouthed men flit back and forth past him, begging him to decide immediately whether or not they are ready for independence. And he mutters in his sleep: "Yes, you're almost ready all right, all right. Let's waltz another round."[216]

In 1934 Vicente Rama, a member of the Philippine Assembly, wrote in the nationalist weekly *Bag-Ong* (*New*) to excoriate the new American governor, Frank Murphy. Murphy had vetoed a bill to abolish the *cédula*, a certificate of identification given to all Filipinos who had paid a required tax; the word had come to mean the tax itself. It was "a shameful and humiliating tax . . . a slavery tax, hence a cruel one, inasmuch as a man not in a position to pay it is jailed," wrote Rama. There was no such tax on Americans, Chinese, or even the "African negro" in the islands. "But Murphy is trying to have the Filipino bear the stigma of slavery, as he thinks they are not men but brutes. This is the reason why our Chief Executive laughs heartily whenever he sees a naked and filthy Filipino in the market places."[217] Here was a response to a state trying to make legible its subjects, counting then taxing them, demanding their visual respectability, then registering them permanently by issuing them documents that confirmed their subordinate status. The ocularcentric state was determined to do its job. At least one of its subjects bitterly resented it.

So was imperial vision afflicted with tension on all sides. The British and Americans tried to reveal Indians and Filipinos. Insofar as they could manage this they then worked to make their subjects, or some number of them, visually respectable—this was both a feature of and a condition for civilization and thus eventual self-government. Indians and Filipinos had their own ocular priorities, some of them intersecting with those of their masters, others at odds with them. Putting vision right was meant to be the first step in the sensory refinement of Asian subjects. If it could be achieved, with the *bhadralok* and the *ilustrados*, there would be hope that imperial pupils might learn other lessons of the body as well.

4

Educating

New Soundscapes

> By noise, I mean a broad yet imprecise category of sounds that register variously as excessive, incoherent, confused, inarticulate, or degenerate—the insistent pejorative comes with the word itself which derives from the Latin nausea, originally meaning sea-sickness. . . . Thus, to echo Mary Douglas on dirt as "matter out of place," we might call noise "sound out of place."
>
> —Peter Bailey, *Popular Culture and Performance in the Victorian City* (1998)

> Every colonized people—in other words, every people in whose soul an inferiority complex has been created by the death and burial of its local cultural originality—finds itself face to face with the language of the civilizing nation; that is, with the culture of the mother country.
>
> —Frantz Fanon, *Black Skin, White Masks* (1967)

By the turn of the twentieth century, the process of visualizing Indian and Filipino subjects was underway. Yet sight had horizons beyond which it could not go. Census figures, tax rolls, maps and photographs were all, literally, mute. To know their subjects, the agents of the imperial state also had to hear them and to understand what they were hearing. Soundscapes—the "sonic environment" that made up, writes historian Emily Thompson, "both a world and a culture constructed to make sense of that world"—were more elusive than landscapes, harder to recall or retain.[1] The eye demanded satisfaction first. But life in the late nineteenth and early twentieth centuries was also to be comprehended by the ear; hearing complemented seeing. Innovations of this period included the gramophone, microphone, telephone, and radio, the sounds of or from which were more often remarked upon than their appearances. In the United States there were campaigns against the pulling of the ears of schoolchildren, as medical practitioners cautioned against damaging the sense organ that allowed people to hear the modern soundscape.[2]

Historian Hillel Schwartz has called this era the "Age of Noise."[3] The phrase, while accurate, requires an important qualification. Noise, as historian Peter Bailey defines it, was a pejorative, constituting sounds that jarred, disrupted, or otherwise intruded on the soundscape. It meant "rudeness, wildness, primitiveness, irrationality."[4] Noise lacked pitch and meter; it was undisciplined, uncontrolled, uncivilized—"sound out of place." Sound itself was welcomed, providing as it did aural information, predicting danger, inviting delight. If the distinction between noise and sound was not always clear cut and in part a matter of taste, by 1900 middle-class Europeans and Americans had reached a broad consensus on what constituted each, and they deplored the first while valuing the second. Manners policed the line between them. Decent people, makers of sound, did not publicly shout, belch, fart, blow their noses audibly, or slurp their food.[5] Making noise was the vice of primitives or the unruly Other, including women, foreigners, the lower classes, and imagined racial inferiors. The civilized soundscape, respectable practices of listening and hearing, could not brook intrusion from noise.[6]

Sound was classical music, opera, and the marches of John Philip Sousa, so long as they were played smartly, note for note, by trained brass bands. The disharmony of "native" chanting, songs sung or instruments played out of tune, and ultimately the jazz performed mostly by African Americans, driving "the half-crazed barbarian to the vilest deeds"—these were noise.[7] So were "blaring music," the shouts of men and women crowded into the ethnic neighborhoods of cities, the braying or barking of animals, the crying of peddlers, and the honking of automobile horns.[8] Gossip, "private talk," was insidious noise, largely because it was deployed by women outside male networks of power, which it thereby threatened.[9] The soaring, crashing music in the Catholic church, no less than the exuberant call-response preaching of Southern African American Baptists, were cacophonous to Anglicans and mainstream Protestants on both sides of the Atlantic. American towns had " 'quiet' white sides and 'noisy' black sides."[10] As much as technology required greater attention to sound, in the end it helped to civilize soundscapes, replacing clamor with sound at a regular pitch, and aiding thoughtful audition. The widespread use of the stethoscope by the late nineteenth century permitted intimate listening to the body, at the same time demanding absolute quiet in the examination room.[11] And in Anglo-America, spoken English was sound; other languages were noise.[12]

The British heard noise as they expanded their empire. In Australia they put their axes to the forest in order to clear land for food cultivation. By purchasing or extinguishing land rights of indigenous Canadians and Maoris in New Zealand they removed noisy people and replaced them with what they hoped were more sonically dutiful white settlers. The Mfengu of South Africa, quiet grain producers rather than warriors like the Zulu, in 1836 swore under a tree allegiance "to God, the mission, and the British Crown," thus audibly declaring themselves British subjects, willing to do London's bidding in the conflicts that followed.[13] The 1883 eruption of Krakatoa in the Dutch East Indies was heard in Ceylon, and remarked on in the writing of Tennyson, Gerard Manly Hopkins, and John Ruskin.[14] Americans endured the cacophony of war, against Indians who inhabited the "howling wilderness" and Mexicans and between themselves, in order to secure a subdued peace, marked audibly by the transit of plows, the whirring of cotton gins, and, increasingly after 1865, the sounds of men, women, and machines at work in factories.

Yet the satisfying sounds of industry could quickly become ominous noise. In England and the United States, factories, and the cities that housed them and their workers, were by the late nineteenth century increasingly regarded as acoustic threats to the altered soundscapes long associated with civilization. The concentration of manufacturing, once considered desirable, created unsightly conurbations of buildings and people, air pollution, and noise. Cities were exciting places, but also sites of loud and unpredictable lower-class mobs, unchecked ethnic clamor, the clatter of carts and horses (later, the sounds of streetcars, automobiles, and buses, over half of which were reported as being "unfit for service" in 1907), music played loudly on street corners, the shrieks of children, the raucous laughter of young women and men, the cries of drunks.[15] Writers in London felt threatened by what the *Times* called "the noisy, dizzy, scatterbrain atmosphere" of the city; Thomas Carlyle, who introduced into English the aphorism "silence is golden," built himself a soundproof room in his Chelsea attic in the vain hope of shutting out the cacophony.[16] London streets were paved with macadam or asphalt to mute the sounds of wheels, horses' hooves, and feet, and officials directed that straw be placed outside hospitals to muffle street noise and thus speed the recovery of patients whom it made nervous.[17] Charles Dickens and other literary figures helped restrict performances by street musicians, who seemed ubiquitous. The sounds made by organ-grinders especially were likened to bad smells and said just as surely to transmit disease. More pointedly, critics pointed to the foreignness of musicians, including the Italian organ-grinders, German bandsmen, and Indian drummers. In 1864 Parliament passed a bill empowering residents to demand, even without sonic cause, that street musicians leave their neighborhoods, under threat of jail for any musician who refused to go.[18] There were thousands of automobiles and buses in London by 1910. Rubber tires meant less "clattering" than metal-wheeled carts had inflicted, but the roar of engines and constant honking of horns kept noise levels unpleasantly high.[19]

American cities were sites of noise abatement campaigns, undertaken starting in the late nineteenth century by Progressive reformers. These accompanied efforts to eliminate smoke, suppress bad smells, and reshape urban landscapes to include more open spaces.[20] Sounds of industry, once tolerated, even celebrated by the American middle class, were now heard by urban residents as dangerous to their health. Noise threatened sleep and thus efficiency and productivity.[21] "There is nothing fanciful," according the *Saturday Review of Literature*, "in the assertion that the pitch of modern life is raised by the rhythmic noise that constantly beats upon us. No one strolls in city streets. . . . Our nervous hearts react from noise to noise."[22] Some noise must have seemed relatively innocuous. A late nineteenth-century etiquette manual instructed readers: "Don't beat a tattoo with your foot in company or anywhere, to the annoyance of others. Don't drum with your fingers on chair, table, or window-pane. Don't hum a tune. The instinct for making noise is a survival of savagery."[23] Yet such habits were rude, not to be practiced in polite society, and, as in Britain, the quest to distinguish the respectable classes from the disreputable—the poor, immigrants, men and women of color—demanded enforcement of the strictest sonic boundaries. Noise was the enemy; quiet was a relief; silence was best of all. E. L. Godkin, the editor of the *Nation*, argued that "the progress of a race in civilization may be marked by a steady reduction in the volume of sound which it produces. The more culture of all kinds it acquires, the less noise it produces."[24] Various levels of government responded with alacrity to popular concerns about noise. Federal authorities forbade "the unnecessary blowing of whistles in ports and harbors" in 1907. Baltimore appointed an "Anti-Noise Policeman," who silenced streetcar bell-ringers, shouting newsboys and fishmongers, noisy schoolchildren, roosters, and cats.[25] "By 1913," writes scholar Raymond Smilor, "every city in the nation of any size or importance had anti-noise ordinances."[26]

Such were the dynamics of Anglo-American soundscapes in the late nineteenth and early twentieth centuries. They transferred readily and deliberately to sites of empire, to India and the Philippines. In both places sonic environments were more noise than sound. In their presumed resemblance to Native Americans, immigrants, ethnic and racial minorities, and the lower classes at home, Indians and Filipinos presided over undisciplined natural soundscapes abetted by their own primitive noise. Britons and Americans would try to impose their own auditory regimes on obstreperous subjects. If they could not get silence, they would at least demand quiet. They would teach their subjects not to transgress the auditory boundaries of civilization, insist that Indians and Filipinos cease shouting, clanging, clattering, farting, belching, loudly spitting and snorting, and smacking and slurping as they ate. And they would teach them to speak correct, "unaccented" English, the better to understand and thus control them. Like all imperial projects, the imposition of sonic discipline was not actually a project at all, but a series of loosely coordinated efforts undertaken by men and women made anxious by their profound sensory displacement and the ambivalence with which they ruled. As the British and Americans had watched each other's imperial progress, so they now listened carefully as their sonic regimes grew audible.

Indian Soundscapes

Britons in India did not hear throughout the country the same things or hear them in the same way. The sounds of the temperate hills and mountains and of the people who lived there were, for instance, regarded by the British more favorably than those of the plains. The birdsong was sweeter, and one could hear "the sound of the river rising as pulsating waves of air."[27] Botanist Joseph Hooker delighted to the sounds of flute-playing by the Lepcha coolies of Sikkim—"sweet and melodious," in "contrast to the hateful tom-toms of the Hindoo of the plains! Which used to drive me almost distracted on the Ganges."[28] As a girl in Lucknow, Nancy Vernede found soothing the sounds of the Indian night, the "reassuring noises of her *ayah's* soft singing and faint clash of her bangles outside the door."[29] For others night was an ominous time, when drums sounded in the distance and insects and animals, including mosquitoes, cicadas, frogs, and howling jackals, made a strange chorus; and the "Brain-fever" bird, so named by the British, had a hysterical cry.[30] The heat seemed to intensify sound. To the haptic discomforts of heat and humidity were added, remembered Emma Roberts, "a horrible discord," exacerbated by the hot weather and including "the rumbling and squeaking of a low cart, in which a child is dragged for hours up and down a neighbouring verandah, the monotonous ditty of the old bearer, of which one can distinguish nothing but *baba*, added to the incessant clamour of the *tom-tom*"—all of which made for "a concert of the most hideous description."[31]

Like Joseph Hooker and Nancy Vernede, some Britons found the sounds of India pleasing. Vernede's husband, Raymond, loved hearing the night sounds of animals, even the jackals. "Some people disliked this," he recalled. "I can't understand why. I thought it was a most enchanting sound, very comforting and familiar."[32] Anne Wilson, who had thought Indian music "repellent . . . synonymous with pandemonium," changed her mind when she heard a man playing the violin in a field outside her tent. She found his playing transformative, evocative of "the heart of the people." "For me," she wrote, "it was that evening as if the dumb had found a voice and deaf ears had gained the power of hearing."[33] On the whole, though, Britons resident in India were a good deal less smitten with what they heard. Indians made noise, not sound, and Britons regarded it as something between a nuisance and a threat. Both British and Indian observers remarked on the relative quiet of British homes in India. "It is odd," thought Erica Farquharson, "that [in] India, so essentially noisy and extrovert in its native life, the towns, villages and bazaars, in the European bungalows the keynote was silence."[34] Mulk Raj Anand observed that the "White Sahibs . . . lived and moved and had their being, in a seemingly grim, awe-inspiring silence, only broken now and then by an occasional pink Memsahib's call for the 'Arderly' or the 'Bera.' "[35] Here was one strategy—isolation—for coping with the unfamiliar and intrusive noise of India.

But it was no more possible to avoid hearing India than to avoid seeing it. "I have had the experience of Bombay noises for more than thirty years," wrote a correspondent to the editor of the *Times of India*, "and I despair of finding a quiet place anywhere in this city."[36] Some Britons enjoyed Indian music, but most did not. Indian singing nearly always sounded harsh or discordant to British ears. Sanitation expert Frank Lugard Brayne spent a good deal of time in rural villages, where he and his wife were sometimes treated to song by a children's chorus. "You will find that neither the boys nor the girls can sing a good chorus or indeed sing at all," he wrote. Every piece sounded "mournful," which well reflected their difficult lives, but it meant that "there is no such thing as good hearty singing."[37] Bands might do better, but too often played without proper training, pitch, timing, or feel for the music they frequently adapted from British songbooks. Indian music's two principal forms, Hindustani and Carnatic, both feature *ragas*—musical units, or modes—that differ from European music in scale and tuning. In British Ceylon bands seemed to the authorities to emphasize volume over all else, with tom-tom players "who drum away with all their might" and pipers "blowing, as loudly and discordantly as possible."[38] In Madras, a center of Carnatic music and dance, Julia Charlotte Maitland endured an elderly vina player whose performance seemed to her "miserable, just a mixture of twang and whine, without even a pretence to a tune." Then came girls who danced and sang, "bawling like bad street-singers—a most fearful noise, and no tune." It reminded her of sonic violations in England ("the chimney-sweepers' clatter on May-day would be harmonious in comparison"). "Imagine a succession of unresolved discords, selected at random, and played on twenty or thirty loud instruments," she concluded, "and you will have a fair idea of Hindoo music and its effect on the nerves."[39] Mrs. Robert Moss King had heard European musicians praise Indian music and tried to appreciate it, but soon gave up: it was "the most tuneless, head-splitting, hopeless endless jangle." She found in it "no harmonies, no theme, no tenderness, no meaning."[40] Christmas 1880 in Saharanpur, in North India, brought a quintet that produced "ear-splitting sounds" and "looked much like monkeys of a larger growth escaped from barrel organs," of the sort detested by Londoners when played by immigrants in that city.[41]

British residents found transit points—ports, stations, road junctions—and conveyances especially noisy and generally recoiled from the tumult of the "native places." "Heat noise bustle," recorded a missionary on arriving

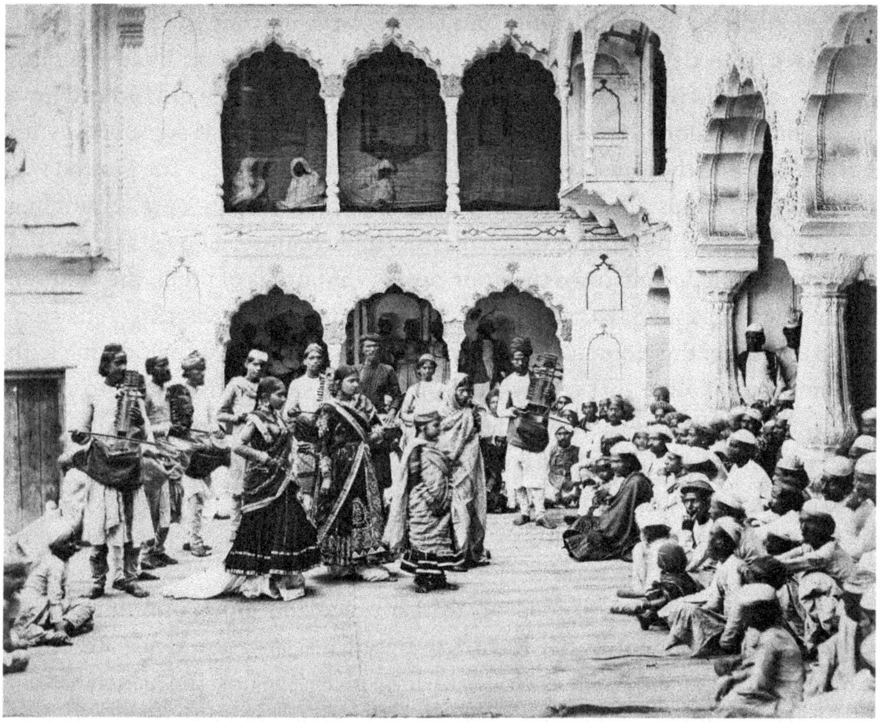

Figure 4.1 A *nautch*—dance and singing—performance at Delhi, 1864. The *nautch* fasincated British observers, though this one has an Indian audience. The dancing carried a whiff of sexuality, but they frequently complained about the music that accompanied it, played here on the *sarangi*. Courtesy of British Library, Asian and African Studies.

in Bombay, the usual port of entry.[42] Evelyn Beeton endured a voyage from Bombay to Karachi, in which the Indian passengers, unused to sea travel, were horribly sick and emitted "dreadful sounds . . . a cross between a lion's roar and the guttural gasps of a person being murdered."[43] "As the ship glided to a stop," recalled Hilda Bourne of her arrival in 1903, "it was a strange and rather bewildering feeling to be surrounded by a screaming mob of Indians trying to sell things."[44] Train stations were hubs of cacophony, as food vendors shouted their wares, families greeted travelers or said their goodbyes, and beggars cried "the thin wail of 'Swami, Swami' " at a pitch that Europeans found piercing and unforgettable.[45] "The noise the natives make at the railway station is positively alarming," wrote a British listener. "It is a suppressed roar, with a sound like a loud angry quack with the squeak taken out, running continuously through it."[46] On the train, passengers jostled for space, their metal tiffin (meal) carriers clanking together over the rattle of wheels against the rails. Viola Bayley recalled the sound of ice melting and draining in tin sinks, and with it the only chance to keep cool during summer in the sweltering passenger cars. At night, bearers made up berths, arriving and leaving with murmured "*salaams*" that expressed both deference and the hope of a tip.[47] Warned off by her English friends, Julia Charlotte Maitland nevertheless ventured to the old fort of Tipoo Sultan, in Bangalore. It was, she wrote, "really '*quite native*.' It is *crammed* with inhabitants, and they bustle and hum like bees in a beehive. . . . The ground was covered with shops all spread out in the dirt; the monkeys were scrambling about in all directions, jumping, chattering, and climbing all over the roofs of the houses, and up and down the door-posts—hundreds of them; the children quarreling, screaming, laughing . . . ; the men smoking, quarreling, chatting, and bargaining; the women covered with jewels, gossiping at their doors, with screams at each other that set my teeth on edge . . . ; and native music to crown the whole. Such confusion was never seen! Landing at Naples is nothing to it!"[48] Part of the problem, Britons thought, may have been the "natives'" habit of wrapping their heads so tightly in their turbans or robes that they could not hear anything, even the shouts of Evelyn Beeton's tonga driver as he tried to warn a group out of the way.[49]

Insects and animals intruded on British peace and quiet, and not only at night. A correspondent in the Rajasthan desert just after the Great Rebellion contended that a "camel's life is a long and loud protest against the load that is put on his back," adding ruefully that he knew "of no sound more sleep-destroying." Then, he continued, there was the trumpeting of elephants, the barking of dogs, the yelling of jackals, and, above all these, the hideous dissonance of the camp, where people spoke over each other in several languages.[50] At a post at Podanur in the inland southeast, Hilda Bourne encountered a coppersmith bird, which got its name from its habit of beating its beak against metal. She fought a headache as the bird's "noise hammered into [her] head," and when her husband, Jim, came home she insisted that he shoot it.[51] Pigs grunted, cows mooed, goats bleated, and working bullocks seemed to moan, as if sounding a dirge, with the effort of turning a water wheel or pulling a plow.[52] Hindu temples were particular sources of aural irritation to the British. Priests clapped and blew horns to waken the god and summoned worshippers with bells, while the faithful talked excitedly as they arrived and departed and chanted once gathered inside the shrine.[53] The conviction that their servants were trying to deceive them came through Britons' ears as well as their eyes. June Norie realized that her cook audibly clicked his toes when he was caught in a lie: "I noticed that when there was a large number of eggs" billed to the household account that "he'd stop suddenly and I'd hear him crack his big toes and I'd know, 'Aha, you've got a guilty conscience over that!'"[54] Jim Bourne died of typhoid in Madras, to which the Bournes had traveled for his treatment. His wife was convinced that the constant noise of the tram bells on the journey from the Tamil hinterland had weakened her husband and bore responsibility for his death.[55]

What tormented British ears most of all was the Indian treatment of language. Britons resented the stubbornness with which (they said) Indians insisted on sticking to their own tongues and dialects and their apparent refusal to learn English. Local languages sounded harsh to western ears, in part, the British claimed, because of their vocabulary rich with "obscenity to an extent almost incredible" to contemplate.[56] Emma Roberts lamented the "shrillness" of the voices of those speaking Hindi; Mrs. King could not sleep through the incessant "chattering of the servants outside, whom we could not contrive to silence."[57] Evelyn Beeton grudgingly learned some Hindi to use with her servants ("it is ugly and there is no literature"), but she also indicated problems with the alternative strategy of demanding that servants use English: "the better a native speaks English the more of a rascal he will be."[58] More than their apparent obstinacy about refusing to learn the language of the conqueror, Indians bemused Britons when they tried dutifully to speak it, for they could not seem to get it right. Mrs. King quoted *Alice in Wonderland*: "This seemed to have no sort of meaning in it, and yet it was certainly English." "That is the essential problem of Bâbu English," she asserted, using the British-English pejorative for an obsequious Bengali bureaucrat. "The words are all good words, but what they mean is what no man can understand."[59] British parents usually sent their young children to Britain for schooling, and one of the main reasons they did so was their fear that the youngsters would otherwise learn to speak English with what Britons contemptuously called a "chi-chi" accent. In India as in England, one's accent mattered as an indication of class and status. It was no good for white children to speak a vulgar form of English in the sing-song cadences of their Indian teachers and schoolmates.[60]

Filipino Soundscapes

In the Philippines, the sharp report of rifle fire was replaced after 1902 by the soundscape of a colony in transition. Americans were immediately struck by the noise of the place: as in India, the cacophony of the city "assailed" the ears of arriving westerners. Teacher Mary Fee took a *carromata*—a horse-drawn cart—from quayside into the heart of Manila. Its "wheels were iron-tired, and jolted. . . . We rattled up the street." They pulled up outside a church just at noon: "Instantly there burst out such a clamor of bells as we had never before heard—big bells and little bells, brass bells and broken bells—and brass bands, lurking in unknown spots seemed to be assisting. I do not know whether the Filipinos were originally fond of noise or whether the Spaniard taught them to be so. At any rate, they both love it equally well now."[61] On a Philippines Commission tour of Luzon in 1902, Edith Moses recorded in a series of letters her impressions of the archipelago's sounds. About to take a siesta in Sablan, she was jarred awake by a band playing "the plaintive strains of 'Just One Girl.'" Next came "a series of dog fights, horses stampeded, Igorrote pow-wows, the squealing of pigs, and the butting of goats, until we were all wide awake." The noise outside abated—at which point Moses's mosquito net collapsed and a cat came into the room, and whenever someone turned over "the whole house creaked and moaned." Three weeks later, the group camped near Itogan. Advised to cover her ears with a towel to prevent moisture or insects from penetrating her ears, Moses found the wrap uncomfortable and discarded it, whereupon her sleep was disrupted. "I never heard so many noises in my life," she complained. "There was a steady crunch, crunch, and the frequent snort of our horses as they cropped the short grass. A thousand insects filled the air with whizz and whirr, making me re-cover my ears precipitately. . . . From far away came the tap of a native drum. A melancholy owl, or night bird, with a hoarse cry, wheeled round and round our mountaintop. Now and again a low guttural sound from the Igorrotes caused me to reflect on the tales I heard of head hunters."[62]

The annoyances and sinister features of Filipino noise did not prevent the American occupiers from listening to it and even trying to understand it. The tours of the islands undertaken by all American governors were exercises in reading landscapes and their inhabitants but also in listening to people and their sonic environments.[63] The Americans heard their subjects out, from Filipino politicians who came to the governor's residence at Malacañan to *presidentes* (mayors) of small towns throughout the archipelago. The Americans were suspicious about what Filipinos told them; the alleged deceitfulness of the insurgents and their leaders during the late insurrection was ascribed by most Americans to a racialized character defect that would not disappear with pacification. Yet Taft himself urged patience. While the Filipino had an "Oriental tendency to speak that which his auditor wished to hear," those "who understood the race" knew that this was less a desire to deceive "than courteous commonplace."[64] Other officials agreed, more or less, though they were not as inclined as Taft to regard the practice with sympathy (and Taft himself was less forgiving in his private correspondence).[65] No one gave up trying to go through the motions, at least, of listening. And there developed a scientific fascination for Filipino hearing practices, including an interest in the physiology of "native" ears. The anatomist and ethnographer Robert Bennett Bean arrived in the Philippines in mid-1907 and immediately began examining Filipinos' ears, in and around Manila and especially at the city's Bilibid prison. Writing in 1909 in a scientific journal, Bean concluded that ear shape had a close relationship to "a physical type of man." The ears of Manilans were much like those of Europeans, while those of most prisoners from outside the city were shaped differently and were "morphologically older."[66] Anthropologist and longtime Philippine Commission member

(a)

(b)

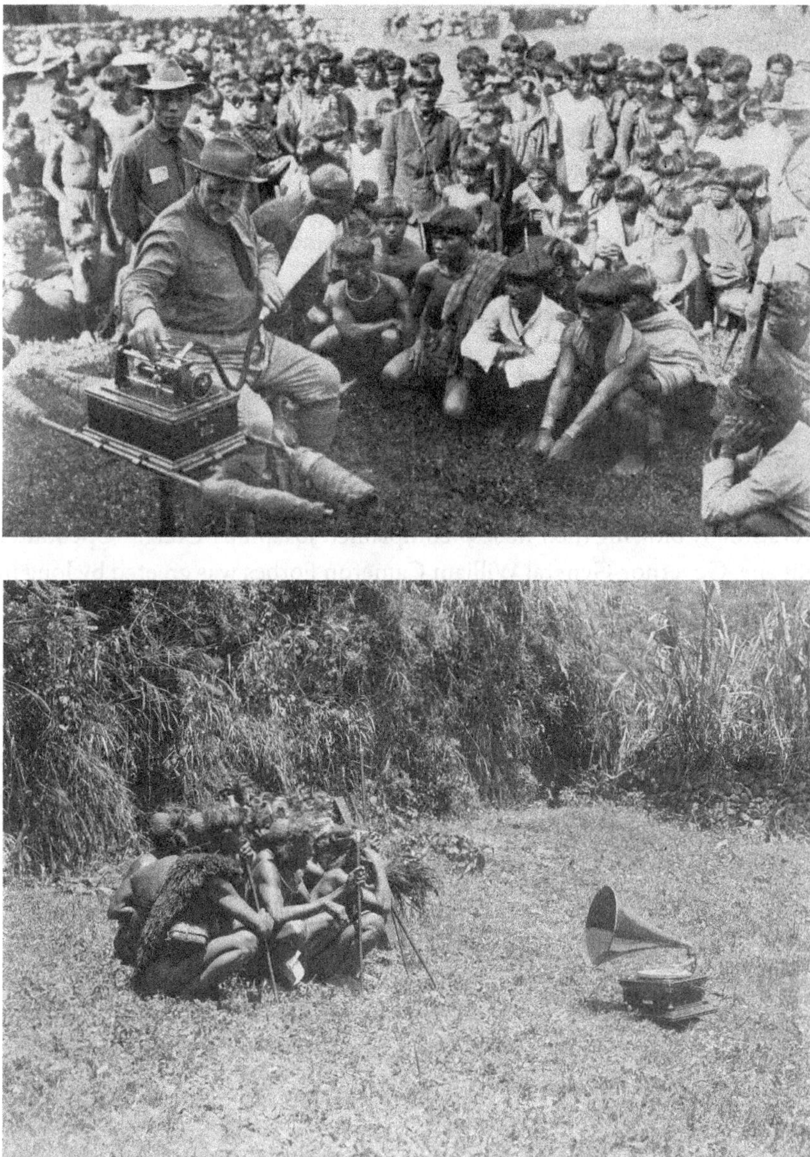

Figures 4.2a and 4.2b Two photographs showing the American hobby of recording Filipino voices and playing them back, which evidently startled and amused the Filipinos. There was a more serious purpose to this practice: Americans used phonograph records and recordings to teach their subjects how to speak proper English, and thus to make them comprehensible. Top: From Dean C. Worcester, *The Philippines Past and Present*, Volume I (New York: The Macmillan Co., 1914), p. 464. Bottom: Courtesy of the Museum of Anthropological Archaeology, University of Michigan.

Dean Worcester liked to "entertain" the upcountry people by recording, then playing back, the voices of their leaders on a Dictaphone.[67]

When they listened Americans invariably heard, as Edith Moses did, the noise of animals and people. John Bancroft Devins found, in a third-class railway car, "a menageries" of noisy beasts, among them a bleating goat, and he heard the "shrill crows" of roosters being transported to and from cockfights.[68] On Mindanao, the grass-walled house of Grace and William Paulding rustled at night with the sounds of scorpions and centipedes.[69] Ruth Hunt's eardrums ached from the "buzzing blare" of locusts. "It is odd to me," she wrote in her diary, "that there are no soft noises here. The birds, locusts, lizards, geckos, cats, dog, and children sound like a shrieking New York tenement."[70] Mainly, though, the people of the Philippines made noise. At work and play they "clatter[ed] and chatter[ed]," for, "like all Orientals," they were unable to interact "without a vast deal of shouting to the other."[71] Babies seemed to cry constantly, and "people are everlastingly blowing their noses," complained Josephine Craig.[72] Upcountry in Silipane, Governor-General William Cameron Forbes was greeted by long lines of people. As he went down the rows shaking hands, "the gongs pealed out" and the Silipanes roared their welcome. "These men just simply yell," Forbes wrote in his journal. "They also have a huh huh huh in unison which a crowd gets yelling; they let it come faster and faster until it all ends in a hurrah. After speeches they all clap, raising their hands and clapping over their heads, the speaker modestly leading both the cheers and clapping."[73] Whenever they hosted Americans in their towns, Filipinos (claimed their visitors) could not refrain from singing and playing instruments at great volume and setting off firecrackers with "the barbarous noise of a salute" even at eight o'clock in the morning.[74]

Many Americans believed that Filipinos were as a people musical, "by nature endowed and by environment encouraged to respond to music and to participate in it," as one listener put it.[75] The Spaniards had brought to the islands the guitar, the harp, and other instruments, with the result that every Filipino town, no matter how small, had an orchestra or a band, and Filipino musicians were much sought after by other East Asian countries. The quality of Filipino musical performance got mixed reviews from the Americans. With cockfighting banned after 1900, some Filipino towns converted their cockpits into theaters that hosted Italian opera.[76] Bishop Charles Henry Brent was once carried across a river by twelve "sweetly" singing Igorots; Helen Taft employed local orchestras in Manila to entertain at official dinner parties; Joseph Stevens listened admiringly to a chorus in Visayan sing American patriotic songs.[77]

Others, however, took a more jaundiced view of the Filipino ear and the effect of Filipino music on the American ear. David P. Barrows, the Superintendent of Education in the Philippines starting in 1903, thought Filipinos clever instrumentalists but incapable of singing well, unlike "the negro or the

Polynesian."[78] Edith Moses would not go even that far. Treated to a performance by a young Filipina on a badly out of tune piano, she was surprised when the Filipinos present and the pianist herself seemed to have no inkling that the sound was discordant, and she found tom-toms and other frequently played instruments "barbaric."[79] William Anderson believed that "the Filipino" loved music but lacked a "sense of interpretation. He has no sentimental feeling in the execution of set music of European composition, and this keeps him from becoming a good instrumentalist"—that is, Filipinos were naturally, emotionally, but not intellectually musical.[80] Again and again, Americans complained that Filipino bands played pieces at inappropriate times. Their favorite tune was "Hot Time in the Old Town Tonight," which they played, grumbled Benjamin Neal, "for weddings, funerals, dances, [and] baptisms." The Filipinos, he suspected, "think it [the] national Air of America."[81] Filipinos were best, Americans decided, at imitating sounds they heard played by accomplished, civilized musicians or more polished performers. Austin Craig taught music at a Filipino elementary school, and had his students sing for visitors. Afterward, while praising the children, several in the audience noted that at the end of each piece, the students had imitated vocally the "whirring" sound of the needle at the end of the record from which they had learned it.[82]

How Subjects Heard

When Britons and Americans said they heard things in India and the Philippines, it is reasonable to take them at their word. What the sounds meant, however, was far less clear. The Anglo-Americans were mapping onto what they heard their own sensibilities, shaped by their perceptions of civilization and its requirement, respectability. When they reacted against noise, they were reflecting attitudes about sound shaped by the sociologies of their metropoles. Loud sounds were dangerous. Cacophony unsettled them. Discordant music and language issued, in their view, from tropical spaces and racially uncouth people who had not yet arrived at an advanced understanding of civilized sonic behavior. Liberal imperialists believed that these places and people could get to civilization with the proper guidance and discipline. Make the streets quieter, insist that men speak truthfully, remove loud animals from human society, train musicians how to choose songs appropriately and how to play them, and, above all, teach spoken English to at least those subjects who seemed in other ways capable of self-control, and India and the Philippines might, someday, be civilized enough to stand on their own.

What Indians and Filipinos made of this logic and of their own soundscapes can be gleaned largely from sources left by Britons and Americans, or written by them since. The westerners found, first, that in both India and the Philippines sonic acknowledgment of rank had meaning, just as it did in the metropoles. Indian princes and Filipino politicians knew, for example, that ceremonial respect for those of the highest status meant saluting them with twenty-one guns. At the Delhi durbar in 1911, the British were willing to greet the Maharajah of Gwalior in this way, offering him "aural recognition of his rank and importance to the Raj."[83] Nearly a quarter century later, American officials in Manila and Washington had a brisk debate over whether to sound twenty-one guns at the inauguration of Manuel Quezon, recently elected president of the new Commonwealth of the Philippines. President Franklin D. Roosevelt at first approved the full salute, but backed down in the face of objections from the American governor in Manila, who insisted that nineteen guns were sufficient for a man of Quezon's position.[84] Second, both Indians and Filipinos remained more committed to oral/aural means of communication than did their more broadly literate and more monolingual rulers. The great Indian epics, among them *The Ramayana*, vary considerably over time because they are "tellings" of stories, passed along orally rather than written down.[85] Herbert Thompson recalled his way of learning about the lives of the Yusufzai people of the Indian northwest. He would ask them to tell him folktales, and he would reciprocate with stories of "the adventures of the wise men of Gotham," in the form of storytelling winning their approval and trust.[86] In early twentieth-century Philippine towns, news of laws and decrees was delivered in the evening not by newspaper but by a town crier, "accompanied by a man with a sepulchral drum."[87] And sounds regarded as rude or simply futile by Britons and Americans were considered vital to health and welfare by Indians and Filipinos. Thompson and his wife burst out laughing when, at a luncheon, a well known local wrestler belched so loudly that "it seemed to roll around the hills and go on and on."[88] In the Philippines, song might have apotropaic qualities. William Freer watched and listened, in sadness and with contempt, as Bicol villagers marched, prayed, and sang—"Perdón, ó Dios mío, Perdón!"—in a desperate effort to prevent a cholera epidemic. When smallpox broke out in Taytay province in the late nineteenth century, healers enjoined the people to go to the river each afternoon and shout at the spirits, "*Apo, dai man cami pagkuhac* (Spirit, please do not get us)."[89]

Most of all, though, Indians and Filipinos used speech, song, and language as subtle modes of resistance to Anglo-Saxon rule, deploying the vernacular when they could to deny their conquerors knowledge of them, and turning English to their own purposes. What Britons and Americans heard as noise could be a strategy.[90] Such may have been the case for the "coolies" employed by the Maude family near Bangalore. The men made up "weird chants" about the Maudes, with the lines of all of them ending with "Ho, Ha." As it happened, the family understood the local language and found the chants "very embarrassing."[91] Disputes over language reached official levels in 1882, when the National Muhammaden Association petitioned the Home Department concerning the substitution of English or the vernacular for Persian as the official language and the decision to write in English the judicial service and bar exams. The Muslims objected that these rules gave advantages to Hindus, who rarely spoke Persian, as they did.[92] Most of all, language became an object of protest and a tool of defiance for Indian nationalists beginning in the late nineteenth century. The poem "Bande Mataram" ("Hail the Mother [India]"), written in 1882 by the Bengali Bankim Chandra Chattopadhyay, was made into a song by Rabindranath Tagore and became an anthem of nationalism: "Who hath said thou art weak in thy lands / When the swords flash out in seventy million hands / And seventy million voices roar / Thy dreadful name from short to shore?" The British banned the singing of the song, but Indians routinely defied them, opening demonstrations with it and, in the northern Madras Presidency in the 1920s requiring its performance by schoolchildren.[93] Anthropologist Bernard Bate has argued that a pivotal moment in nationalist politics came during a massive anti-British rally on Marina Beach, Madras, on April 6, 1919. There, on five stages, leading orators either spoke in Tamil or had their English translated immediately into Tamil, so that the laborers and poor assembled there could understand them. Speakers stood facing the masses directly, and spoke in a familiar "sermonic" style.[94]

Above all, and somewhat by contrast to what Bate heard on Marina Beach, oratory was the means by which Indians at once appropriated "western" oral/aural forms and claimed such discourse as their own. The leading voice of Bengali, and later Indian, nationalism in the late nineteenth and early twentieth centuries was Surendra Nath Banerjea (Surendranath). British educated, Surendranath founded Ripon College in Calcutta and was editor of the paper *Bengalee*, for a time the most influential English-language publication in the country. But his chief skill was speaking, and he used oratory to urge the British to make political reforms and to warn extremists in the nationalist Congress Party against overreach. Liberal journalist Henry Nevinson heard Surendranath speak in English to thousands of young men in Calcutta early in the new century. The content of the speech, wrote Nevinson, was not especially important: "His object was only to sketch out the general programme of the approaching Congress, and to urge all parties to unite for the credit of their country." A simple argument, Nevinson thought, but Surendranath "expounded it with a magnificence of phrase, continuity of expression that held me in wonder. Sentence answered to sentence, period to period, thunder to thunder"—thus did he command a powerful sound of nature. "There was no hesitation, no throwing back," Nevinson went on, "no wandering for ideas or words. Out the great language rolled without a break and without a drop, each syllable in its exact place and order, each sentence following some cadence of its own. . . . It was oratory . . . —such oratory as few living

Englishmen dare venture on for fear of drowning in the gulf of bathos."[95] Yet it was the sort of performance vital to the mobilization of millions who had different languages: whatever Indian objections, the British had given India a potential common tongue. And while not everyone in Surendranath's audience that day understood what they were hearing, they recognized the form and sound of a dazzling oratorical performance, and they responded to it enthusiastically.

With recent experience of resisting outsiders, elite Filipinos also found ways to use language to confound or challenge the occupying Americans. While essentialist caricatures of Filipinos as "theatrical" cannot be credited, there is evidence that Filipinos in the public sphere valued oratory, with all its performative elements. Taft heard from Filipino politicians "a mellifluous flow of words in adoration of liberty," and Nicholas Roosevelt noted "their passion for oratory" which began, he thought, among children, who were "unembarrassed by stage fright" and, like adults, "enjoy[ed] talking for its own sake."[96] A Filipino observed that while the Philippines lacked farmers, it had a glut of lawyers, because "our people love to talk and argue."[97] Americans found here reinforcement for their belief that Filipinos were emotional, and thought their performances reflected their love of show and exaggeration. Much was made of the willingness of Filipino politicians to cry in public. Crying had not worked for Manuel Roxas when he and fellow *ilustrado* Sergio Osmeña lobbied for independence in the United States in 1929, thought Ruth Hunt. "These Filipinos cannot understand our indifference to oratory and tear appeal," she wrote in her Philippines diary. "They both go strong over here."[98]

To some extent, Filipinos adjusted their oral culture to suit American expectations. Accustomed to using the speech of *delicadeza* (delicacy), replete with "euphemisms, circumlocutions, and protective white lies," Filipinos humored American bluntness with the language of blandishment and tactful flattery.[99] More Filipinos learned English, despite reservations that young people were becoming by doing so "unconscious victims of modernity," as the polemicist Teodoro Kalaw put it.[100] Manuel Roxas learned to lower the high pitch of his voice, previously a source of ridicule among American listeners.[101] Gonzalo Cue Malay published a Spanish-language pronunciation guide to English for Filipino speakers: "Du yu spik inglis langüach olredi?" ("Do you speak English language already?"), and "Jaulong jev yu bin jiar in Manila?" ("How long have you been here in Manila?").[102]

More often, though, Filipinos turned their oral culture against their occupiers, confronting them with a nationalist appropriation of their own defense of free speech. Talk was the medium of resistance. The newspapers were full of it: "Talk, talk, talk—they seem made of words," marveled Daniel Williams. "There are a dozen newspapers here, and it seems every Filipino feels it his duty to enlighten the islands with his views."[103] Albert Sonnichsen heard two Filipinas debate independence. The woman supporting US annexation and occupation ("Señorita America") made effective arguments for her position, but these were overwhelmed by "Señorita Filipinas," who spoke "with such force and enthusiasm" that Sonnichsen, despite being held captive by the insurgents, "forgot that I was an American and believed myself a Filipino, to the extent that I almost joined in the burst of applause that followed."[104] On May 14, 1903, a Filipino acting troop performed Aurelio Tolentino's play "Kahapan, Ngayon, at Bukas" ("Yesterday, Today and Tomorrow") at the Liberty Theater in Manila. The play was an indictment of imperialism, and at its climax, one of the characters throws an American flag to the floor and stamps on it. Governor Taft was outraged, and he demanded that Attorney General Lebeus Wilfley prosecute Tolentino under the Sedition Law of 1901. Wilfley was unsure whether the speech in the play violated the law. As for the flag-stamping, his lawyers doubted that the law covered "Pantomimic effect"—that is, if there had been no actual sound of sedition uttered, the office could not proceed. Taft, incredulous, insisted on a broad interpretation of speech, including "everything that occurs in the theater, the expressions of the audience, and what goes on on the stage." Taft's views, predictably, won out: Tolentino was convicted and sent to Bilibid Prison.[105]

Sound Out of Noise?

The British and the Americans hoped to confront noise and substitute for it, or derive from it, civilized sound. Making the nation audible—giving its places and people names one can recognize and pronounce—comes with making it visible. One way to articulate the empire was to rename its geographic and human elements, expecting thereby to make India and the Philippines and their inhabitants sound more familiar. When Sir Herbert Thompson arrived in India in the early 1920s, Lord Willingdon was governor of Madras Presidency. Lord and Lady Willingdon, Thompson recalled, "set their stamp on things Madrassi partly because of a weakness for permitting their name to be used as a label not only on the usual new creations, roads[,] hospitals[,] and schools[,] but also renaming well-known landmarks whose vernacular names enjoyed the sanction of the Presidency's long history."[106] A year after the Great Rebellion, the Deputy Secretary to the Government of Bangalore argued that the British needed a "systematic way of representing native names in the English character." Existing practice was baffling, leading to "a great and increasing evil" as officials tried to keep track of Indians involved in government proceedings.[107] The British did undertake to know their subjects by appropriating their speech. After 1858 British authors and compilers of census reports, reference works on caste, and land revenue documents increasingly incorporated into their texts oral Indian proverbs, chosen to reflect the behavior of the compliant and uncooperative alike. The selected proverbs reified newly rigid representations of caste, and reflected the interests of Indian elites. The voices of the "authentic" Indians were recontextualized in official documents "to create the illusion" of consent to British policy.[108] Within two decades of their arrival in the Philippines, Americans had christened Taft Avenue and Ike Beck had built a thriving market called the American Bazaar that sold Kellogg's Corn Flakes, among other things.[109] As if anticipating American wishes, and doubtless to convince the Americans of their loyalty and admiration, Filipinos began baptizing their children with American names and Anglicizing their Spanish names. Pedro became Pete; Beatriz, Betty; Maria, Mary; Juan, Johnny.[110]

Another possible way to alter a soundscape was to add bells to it. The sound of bells communicated to residents quickly and equally. Town or church bells defined space, extending authority as far they could be heard and demarcating the limits of the polity: those within their earshot were part of the community they inscribed, those who could not hear them fell outside its ambit. Bells summoned people to church, announced elections and deaths, drove off demons and witches, broke up dark clouds, and invited in angels.[111] But they could go too far, be too loud, or be rung at inconvenient times. Bells were less welcome in cities than in villages, in part because urban dwellers stayed up later than townsfolk, more because their sounding was increasingly associated with the masses—the early morning churchgoers and people who started work before dawn and used public bells to mark their days. Complaining about noise from bells was increasingly common among urban "elites, who were intent on imposing their fastidious tastes and reducing noises to some sort of harmonious order against 'rough music,' charivaris, and rackets, which all served to define the people." It was no accident, according to one author, that the Chinese used bells as torture devices.[112]

Anglican missionaries in nineteenth-century India welcomed the bells of churches and their congregants, or "hearers," numbered at nearly twenty thousand by 1850.[113] On the whole, though, the British seem generally to have regarded bells in India as sources of noise. The *Times of London* correspondent at the Delhi durbar in 1903 heard the jangle of bells hung from the backs of elephants bearing the princes to their audience with Viceroy Curzon, but thought them the soundtrack to "a barbaric display."[114] Mainly bells were associated with the constant distressing noise of Hindu temples, all of which had at least one large bell to summon worshippers. Arriving for an inspection of a village in the Deccan plateau, the Bombay Deputy Surgeon-General T. G. Hewlett encountered in a small shrine a *pujari* (priest) "ringing a series of bells which are suspended from the roof by brass chains, whilst he mutters his mantras."[115] The sound of bells thus defined the boundaries of a superstitious, premodern community; there was neither enough of a state nor of an Anglican presence in India to wrest control of the bells' sonic meaning from the Hindu majority. Using bells to wring sound from noise seemed hopeless to the British in India.[116]

The situation in the Philippines was different. The islands had a recognizable sonic culture of bells put in place by the Spanish friars. A "glad ringing of the bells" greeted the dawn of Easter morning, and bells heralding at the start of Lent, baptisms, weddings, and funerals sounded familiar to American ears.[117] The problem was the same one that deafened urban Americans at home: the abuse of bells. The Balangiga affair during the Filipino insurgency had given grim indications of this. On the night of September 27, 1901, a group of Filipino fighters slipped into the town of Balangiga, Samar, then occupied by Company C of the US Ninth Infantry. Some of the fighters were dressed as women, and the actual women arriving along with them carried small coffins, which they claimed held child victims of cholera but in fact concealed bolos—the weapons of choice for the insurgents. The next morning was Sunday, so the Filipinos signaled their attack by having children ring vigorously the bells in the church belfry. "What happened was indescribable," recalled Eugenio Diaz, who was present. "The ringing of the bells, the general shouting of the words of 'courage, brother, advance,' was heard everywhere; a noise horrible, imposing, sad and hair-raising, which excited the patriotic blood of the rebels; the disorder and confusion among the American soldiers, who, disorganized and horrified, fled in every direction."[118] Fifty-nine members of Company C were killed and twenty-three were wounded by the bolomen.[119]

Such sonic deception persisted, claimed the Americans, after the conflict had ended. On Taft's order, Victor Heiser, the director of health, investigated the silencing of church bells on Batangas. He discovered that the local authorities, who had been ringing bells each time someone died of cholera, had decided that the people panicked when they heard the ringing and so had stopped. Heiser insisted that they resume, thus lifting the people's mood and enabling the secretion of strong "gastric juices" that he claimed would help protect people from the disease.[120] The bigger issue was Filipino enthusiasm for sounding bells too loudly and too often. Ralph Buckland complained of "the dreadful clanging of the dozen or so of discordant bells . . . in the belfry" of a nearby church, and Daniel Williams was dismayed by the "pound[ing]" of bells in Manila during the nine days surrounding Christmas, beginning at five in the morning and so disrupting his sleep.[121] An American soldier threatened to shoot two young boys who kept trying to ring the bells of their village church. Lieutenant Laurence Halstead put a stop to the threats, but only after hearing with sympathy the soldier's objections: "Those damn kids are ringing them damn bells at all hours of the day and it jest has got on my nerves."[122]

Common to India and the Philippines, if improbably, were brass bands. These had European origins, British in the first case, Spanish in the second. In India the British heard Hindu *ragas*, which most deprecated, but also Mughal public performances featuring the energetic playing of drums and blowing on horns and conches.[123] British military bands toured parts of India, including the band of the Royal Scots with the Prince of Wales in 1872 and of the XIIth Hussars, which arrived in Lucknow in 1874 and stayed in India for twelve years.[124] These bands and others incorporated Indian musicians into their ranks, and when sepoys mustered out they formed bands of their own in cities and small towns. Brass instruments were at a surplus in Britain, and unlike strings or reeds they were mostly impervious to "extremities of humidity or temperature."[125] British civil servants recalled that as they toured their districts in the early twentieth century, they were greeted by the local bands nearly everywhere.[126] At a festival in the Northwest Frontier Provinces, Sir Fraser Noble heard pipe bands, and a Sikh regimental group, "magnificent . . . in their colourful uniforms." His own contribution was patronage of the Adolescent Convicts' Pipe Band from the nearby jail at Haripur.[127]

Views differed as to the quality of the bands. There was some admiration for the music they produced, though any success was generally ascribed to the military training or British leadership of the bandsmen. British observers often made fun of the bands, leaving no doubt that the musicians' output remained for them

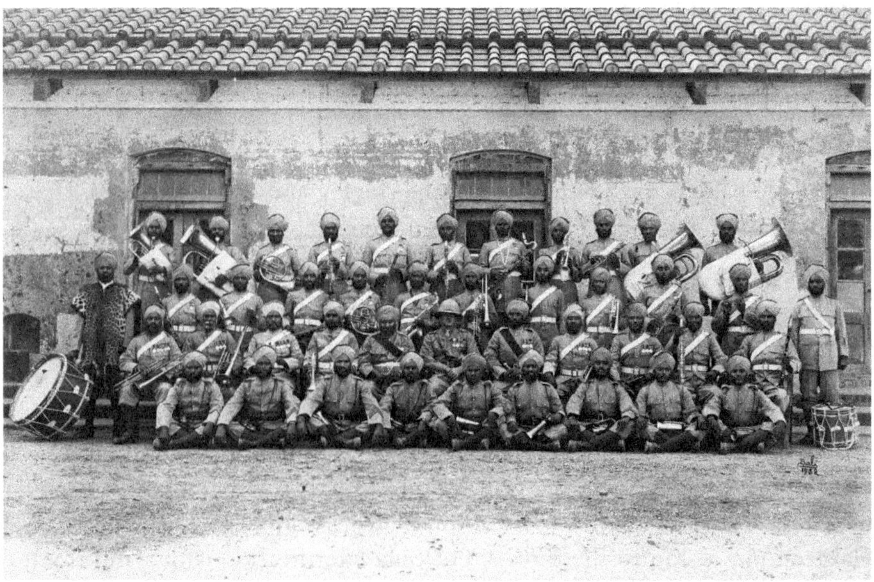

Figure 4.3 A Sikh brass band, 1932. British officers regarded military bands as opportunities to impose sonic and somatic discipline on "native" troops. Note the British conductor (in pith helmet) seated in the middle of the second row. Courtesy of British Library, Asian and African Studies.

noise, not sound. Song selection was not always appropriate, as when Douglas Gordon heard the Madras Carnatic Infantry Band strike up "Yes, We Have No Bananas" at the funeral of a prominent Madrasi.[128] In Goa, a band playing "The Colonel Bogey March" woke Anne Bremner at five in the morning, and "each bandsman played the tune to his own time and his own idea of music."[129] Hilda Bourne thought the band she heard play in late 1913 made "a funny noise with all their different instruments."[130]

The British hoped for improvement. Most of all, they sought to impose on Indians and their other subjects a sonic (and somatic) discipline by organizing them into marching ranks and teaching them how to play on key and strictly in time—4/4 if they were playing a march. Missionaries and, later, British conductors wished to rid their colonial charges of bad musical habits, including the pursuit of different tempos in the same song, the "sudden passions of African drumming," and the "wild screeches at irregular intervals" of choruses.[131] The British did not invent band music in India, but they attempted to impose their soundscapes on existing ones, shaping longstanding practices with the orderliness of their sartorial tastes (thus the uniforms) and sonic preferences. As two music historians have put it, "The brass band was a small-scale metaphor for the colonial process itself—a single foreign bandmaster exerting authority over numerous native bandsmen who were expected to abandon their traditional ways of making music in favour of more 'civilized' European ways."[132]

Every Philippine town had a brass band or small orchestra. The musician's vocation was often handed down from father to son, as were instruments. Like the British, the Spaniards created regimental bands, and the Americans inherited these in 1898, along with more casual village groups and a handful of drummers and trumpeters recruited from Aguinaldo's army as it surrendered over time. The bands performed at every civic and religious function, including welcoming visitors, births, weddings, and deaths.[133] In 1913, military bands from the towns of Bani and Agno were used to drive out locusts that threatened the local crops.[134] Americans praised the energy with which Filipinos played, their apparent feel for the music, and frequently the way in which they picked up songs by ear. Whatever they possessed by way of emotional connection to music, though, they lacked in terms of a disciplined, orderly approach to the score. They could not read music, nor could they follow rhythmic convention. The Igorots would not be cured of "beating drums and gongs in seemingly chaotic fashion," and three tribal "fanatics" in Jolo, who "ran amuck" and tried to attack the band, were prevented from doing so only by the heroic action of the bass drummer and tuba player who blocked the way with their instruments. But the majority of Tagalo bandsmen might be taught to temper their inherent musicality and produce a fair version of a John Philip Sousa march, and to play songs appropriate to occasions, rather than blaring "Hot Time in the Old Town

Tonight" at funerals.[135] "The Filipinos as a people are extremely musical," wrote Helen Taft, "but in the early days of the American occupation a vast majority of the musicians were the rankest amateurs who played 'by ear' only. . . . They did not know the words, or the 'sentiment' of the songs; they knew only the tunes, and these they played at all times, for occasions either solemn or gay."[136] They *felt* the music, but they did not understand it—they were emotional Asians.[137]

To American ears, lack of musical knowledge brought many Filipino bands to grief. Two bands greeted William Cameron Forbes at Morong in 1904 and began playing the "Star-Spangled Banner" simultaneously. "They played badly, I think purposely," he recorded in his diary, "and one got through before the other and struck up another bit of music," a piece that Forbes later learned was a revolutionary song. Forbes rode forward on horseback, stopped the bands, and scolded the provincial governor, Lopez Santos, for the disrespectful performance. Forbes would later call the governor and the bands' conductors on the carpet in Manila for a further dressing down. "I shall permit no lack of courtesy to the American flag nor the national music," he wrote.[138] Similar performances received Helen Taft (1901) and Governor Theodore Roosevelt Jr. (1932), who heard the anthem played "so haltingly and so slowly that time and again we think they are stuck."[139] Amused, distressed, but not discouraged, the Americans, like the British, used the bands to discipline Filipino musicians with the ultimate goal of civilizing them.[140] Governor Taft encouraged the creation and support of the

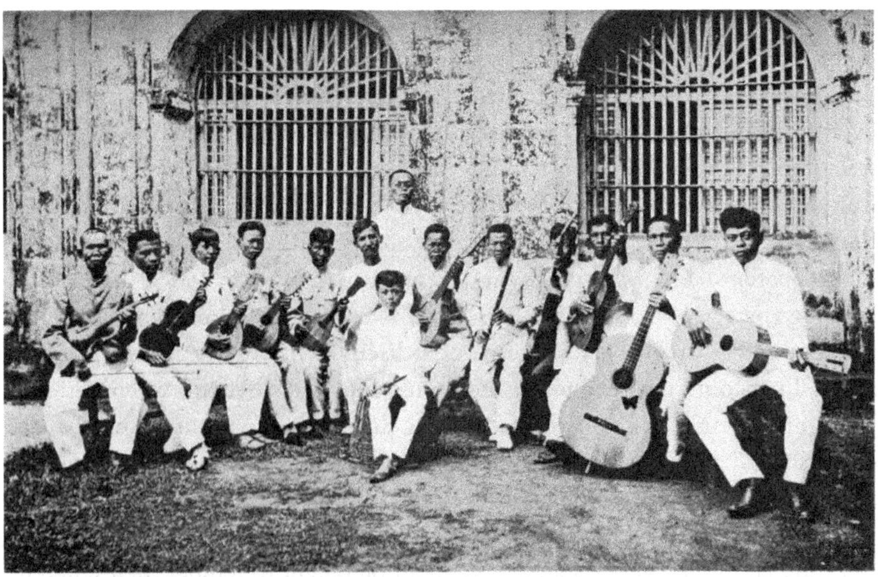

Figure 4.4 A leper orchestra, San Lazaro Leper Hospital, Philippines. Courtesy of British Library, Asian and African Studies.

Rizal Orchestra in Manila—"an excellent company of musicians that would do credit to any city in America," he wrote in 1902—and a decade later the Manila Symphony Orchestra played a western classical repertoire under the baton of Vincenzo Gambardella.[141] And the primary school curriculum written by the Americans included considerable scope for learning and performing American songs.[142]

Noise Abatement and Teaching Spoken English

Britons and Americans regarded schools as the most suitable places for imposing sonic discipline on their domestic lower classes, immigrant children, and imperial subjects alike. Every school, wrote the ethnologist Michael Haberlandt in 1900, ought to teach an eleventh commandment: "Thou shalt not make noise."[143] Noise was to be replaced with the sound of English speech, properly modulated and accented. To learn to speak English was a vital part of becoming civilized. And, significantly, it made subjects comprehensible to their rulers—vital to those with recent memories of rebellion.

This did not mean, in India at least, the abandonment of local languages. British Orientalists admired Sanskrit and eagerly absorbed the classic texts in which it was written.[144] Vernaculars were retained for the training of Indian health care providers, for example.[145] Advice manuals written for Britons going to Indian recommended learning some words of the local language, or else servants and merchants would keep secrets, spread scurrilous gossip, and take advantage of sahibs and memsahibs. Well before 1857, British officials who wished to move up the civil service bureaucracy were required to be proficient in one of their province's Indian tongues.[146] Their fear was falling into "helpless and dependent thralldom" to an Indian assistant or being treated with scorn by a servant.[147] Starting in 1889, Queen Victoria employed the former Indian clerk Abdul Karim to teach her Hindi so that she might speak to her servants.[148] "The first duty of a mistress is, of course, to be able to give intelligible orders to her servants," wrote Flora Annie Steel and Grace Gardiner in their popular guide. "Therefore, it is necessary that she learn how to speak Hindustani. No sane Englishwoman would dream of living, say, for twenty years, in Germany, Italy, or France, without making the *attempt*, at any rate, to learn the language."[149] The India Civil Service considered this a matter of honor; Iris Portal's father told her that if as an educated woman, she could not "speak the language of a man who is illiterate" she was not "fit to employ him."[150] The language they meant to learn was hardly classical Sanskrit, but rather a serviceable street Hindi, Tamil, or Punjabi that reflected the social positions of speaker and listener. John Gilchrist, an army surgeon, published a Hindi phrase book that limited itself to essentials.

Among these expressions were "'Row fast, pull away, don't be lazy'; 'Hand me my toothbrush and powder'; 'Brush the curtains well that no mosquitoes may remain'; and 'What! Has no one yet told you that bearer is in our tongue a very low word like slave or drudge.'"[151] Sanskrit or Hindi words had already made their way into British lexicons. The first volume of *A New English Dictionary on Historical Principles*, published in 1888 and part of the project that would be renamed the *Oxford English Dictionary*, contained the words *achar* (pickle), *brinjal* (eggplant), *banian* (trader), and *budgerow* (barge).[152]

The effort to learn to speak Indian languages was not without its hazards. Speaking like a "native" could bring with it the kind of degradation that contact with polluted Others might cause through touching them or ingesting their unfamiliar food. The possibility of sonic damage to British children was particularly alarming. In contrast to Steel and Gardiner, for instance, Edmund C. P. Hull, in his book *The European in India; or, Anglo-India's Vade Mecum* (1871), warned that use of the vernacular threatened innocent children, as "the language of the vulgar in India is corrupt, and interspersed with obscenity to an extent almost incredible." Worse, learning to speak in Indian cadences could distort the accent of a child's spoken English. The result was "chi chi" (or "du du") English, much dreaded by British parents. It was best, Hull concluded, to keep respectable white children away from spoken Indian languages, thus "totally in ignorance of so muddy a stream."[153]

So it was for Indian children to learn English. Hearing a group of them "bawling their hearts out" as they did lessons in their own languages was proof enough, said Britons, of Indians' need for sonic discipline.[154] Thomas Macaulay's *Minute on Education* (1835) urged the creation of English medium schools throughout India, in order to build an English-speaking class "who may be interpreters between us and the millions whom we govern—a class of persons Indian in colour and blood, but English in tastes, in opinions, in morals, and in intellect."[155] The English Education Act, through which English supplanted Persian as the official language, was adopted that same year.[156] Thereafter local languages did not disappear from schools, but those teaching in English were more likely to receive government funding, the three universities at Bombay, Madras, and Calcutta (founded in 1857) were English medium, and considerable effort went into attracting the right sort of children, men, and eventually women to their halls. The founding of the Doon School for boys in Dehradun (1935) was the belated culmination of this effort. "It is a big experiment, this idea of an Indian public-school," Gerald Hare wrote to its head, Jack Gibson, "but it is obviously an essential part of the still larger and bolder experiment which we are carrying out in India trying to graft an English outlook onto the Indian mind."[157]

As inspector of schools in the Punjab in the early 1930s, W. A. Barnes witnessed the progress of the "experiment," mainly with frustration over the

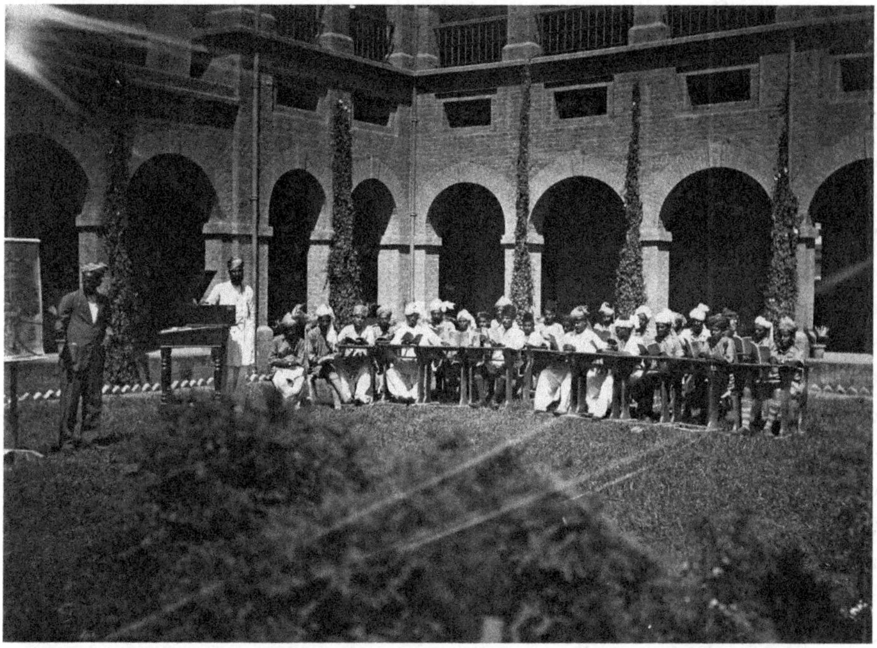

Figure 4.5 Like the Americans, the British used recordings to teach some of their subjects English. The audience here is a group of elite schoolboys. Courtesy of the American Historical Collection, Rizal Library, Ateneo de Manila University.

inadequacy of its execution. Nearly every school he visited was, according to his diary, staffed by lazy incompetents, including Qasim Shah, headmaster and "a thorough liar," and those at the Government Manual School, scene of "a lot of worthless tamashery [troublemaking]." Barnes was most unhappy with the students' phonetic failings that prevented them from speaking clear English. Part of the problem, he thought, was the persistence of instruction in languages beside English. At Raikot, he found "a terrible waste . . . Arabic, Persian, Hindi, Punjabi, Sanskrit, all taught!" He complained of the frequent misuse of English, as when Indians greeted each other with "Good morning" at all hours of the day: "The expression good-morning is only used amongst educated English-speaking people when they meet before twelve o'clock noon or, at the latest before one o'clock in the afternoon." In notes to himself, Barnes jotted five "Reasons for learning English," pointing out that the language was the medium of instruction not only in Anglo-Saxon homelands but India, Hawaii, and the Philippines, that it was the surest "way to power and wealth," and that the language offered "national salvation" through a peerless combination of "democracy education business invention religion." Above all, it was vital that Indian children learn to speak properly, with clear diction and without a "chi chi" accent. The curriculum Barnes enforced included lessons on phonetics which emphasized "the importance of attending to pronunciation from the very first," especially with boys, who were prone to resist imitating the "right" sounds coming from the teacher.[158] Boys were also potential soldiers, so it was imperative that their future British officers be able to understand their speech, lest they plot rebellion once more. Even girls, considered better candidates for learning English, struggled to read it; Nora Scott heard a young woman read "*This is a cat*" in a "slow, child-like way."[159]

Like the British in India, the Americans encountered a welter of tongues in the Philippines and heard cacophony in Filipino schools. Most Filipinos spoke local languages; only a small number spoke Spanish.[160] Education under the Spaniards took place in the vernacular and was done orally. Americans commented in amazement about the noise emanating from school rooms, discordant in substance and tone. These were, wrote Emily Conger, "like pandemonium let loose; all the pupils studying together, making a deafening, rasping noise."[161] On his first day teaching in the Philippines, one American recalled: "I went across the plaza and found two one-story buildings of stone with an American flag floating over one, and noise which resembled the din of a boiler factory issuing from it. The noise was the vociferous outcry of one hundred and eighty-nine Filipino youths engaged in study or at least in a high, throaty clamor, over and over again, of their assigned lessons."[162] In fairness, admitted David Barrows, director of the Education Bureau, noise from outside the school required teachers and pupils to raise their volume: in Manila schools were frequently repurposed family homes, close to the street and with windows that opened to "the noise of traffic and travel. Carromatas and carabao carts rumble past, street hawkers shout their cries, and all the sounds of a quarreling, jostling, idle population burst into the rooms."[163] American educators would nevertheless demand of their pupils proper auditory deportment, including "ears free from discharge" and "a voice of pleasing quality."[164]

English instruction in the Philippines "became the wedge that separated the Filipinos from their past and later was to separate educated Filipinos from the masses of their countrymen," according to historian Renato Constantino.[165] The US military made efforts during the insurrection to build and staff schools, believing, as Brig. General Robert P. Hughes put it, that "half of our difficulties would disappear if our men could communicate directly with whom they are dealing." Brig. General Samuel B. M. Young established over two hundred schools in Ilocanos, stocked them with teachers, and even provided them with an English-Ilocano primer.[166] In April 1900, President McKinley charged the Taft Commission to build more schools in order to "fit the people for the duties of citizenship and for the ordinary duties of the civilized community."[167] By the following January, the Commission had created the Bureau of Public Education and made English the national language of instruction. That summer, five hundred American teachers arrived in Manila and, following a few weeks' acclimation and a brief training, were dispersed across the archipelago with the mission to teach Filipino children how to read, write, practice good hygienic habits, exercise domestic skills—and, above all, to speak English correctly. "It is very important that English be taught in all the schools, in order that the next generation shall have a common medium of communication," wrote Taft. "A knowledge of English, and a consequent familiarity with American literature and American newspapers, will furnish the people a means of understanding American civilization and American institutions, and will greatly assist in teaching them self-government on Anglo-Saxon lines."[168] Filipinos would use English to talk to each other, and understanding them, the American authorities could better rule them.

An absence of textbooks, blackboards, and even pencils and paper plagued American teachers, as it had Spanish ones, but it meant that oral instruction was the only alternative.[169] In spite of the clamor it produced, the emphasis on speaking Filipinos had grown used to under Spain's control could be turned by the Americans to purposes that fit with their aspirations, for hearing and speaking were, they concluded, the best ways for "imitative" Filipinos to learn English. Verbal economy was part of an oral education that had as its goal the civilization of young Filipinos. "The child is trained [in school] to be regular and punctual, and to restrain his desire to talk and whisper—in these things gaining self-control day by day," observed a writer for the journal *Philippine Teacher*. "The essence of moral behavior is self-control."[170] Patriotism—to the Philippines as a subject of the United States—was taught through song, and on the assumption that Filipinos were naturally musical, had good ears, and could not resist performing. Teachers formed choruses and glee clubs, and put into the repertoire "Our Philippines," sung to the tune of "My Country 'Tis of Thee" (or "God Save the Queen"), with new lyrics: "Long live the Philippines / Adorned with noble scenes / By patriot sons. / We hail the glorious day / When all the people pay / True homage to thy sway / Our Philippines."[171] Oral, hands-on instruction worked well for vocational training, whose advocates included Fred Atkinson, the first superintendent of schools, and Taft, who appointed him and directed him to visit Hampton, Carlisle, and Tuskegee Institutes, in all of which young men of color were trained to use their hands, before he left the United States to take up his post.[172]

Education Director David Barrows resisted the emphasis on teaching trades. Doing so would, he argued, reduce the time available for instruction in "letters," chiefly English. Civilizing the Philippines depended on the extension of literacy throughout the population. "In civilized communities an illiterate class suffers a grievous handicap in the social competition," he wrote. "Civilized communities are civilized because they are literate."[173] It was vital to make English more accessible to the people, and the best way to do this was to make it easier to identify English vocabulary, thus enabling Filipinos to read and speak with greater facility. Spelling should be simplified. And more Spanish and Tagalog words should be incorporated into English speech, among them "banca," "tuba," "bolo," and "nipa" (but not "chowchow," which was "a little beyond the limit").[174] On the whole, Barrows got his way. Schools emphasized oral recitation and presentation, and hearing and speaking English. While teachers tried to curb the "hubbub" inspired by Spanish methods, they worked to modulate rather than silence their students, understanding, as teacher Ralph Buckland put it, that "memorization is aided by vocalization." In his classroom, "the mouths were made to do most of the work."[175]

These lessons were codified in the *Survey of the Educational System of the Philippine Islands* (1925), undertaken on behalf of the US government by a group of American and Filipino educators. "The learning of a foreign language proceeds by imitation," the survey found. "If Filipino children are to succeed in mastering the language, an accurate model of speech must be set, and systematic ear training in discrimination of the spoken language must be given." Unhappily, half of Filipino children were already nine years old when they started school, by which age they had learned "a totally different set of vocal habits" than those needed to speak English. "Whereas English is a highly staccato and accented language," the authors explained, with "stress being continually employed in conveying the refined shades of meaning," the various Filipino languages were "dominated by a singing unstressed monotone." Filipino teachers, who had by the mid-1920s largely supplanted the Americans, struggled to hear and pronounce English. Thus, the teaching of English must be done using phonograph records made by native speakers. This was, the authors admitted, a "makeshift solution," and one dependent on the availability of working machines for playing the records. Still, since Filipino children were said to be naturally good at imitation, it followed that they should hear and follow English that was properly pronounced.[176]

The curriculum subsequently developed by officials—*Course of Study in Phonics for Primary Grades*—did not fully adopt the recorded method of teaching, but rather continued to place faith in teachers to learn phonics and to impress their students with its importance. The book was clear that "ear training should precede eye training," and that it "should be continued after eye training has begun." Filipinos, teachers and pupils alike, had difficulty pronouncing the letters f, j, and z, short u and a, and ch and sh. They also tended to introduce initial "s" words with a short e, as in "es-school." The *Course* urged teachers to eliminate these errors. Students could learn z's if they "buzz[ed] like bees"; m and oo would come if they mooed like cows. The curriculum included many rhymes and songs, mostly familiar American ones, but sometimes with modifications designed to help the children articulate them. For example, there was this exchange between "Luis" and his father: " 'Hurrah for the old, old flag!' said Luis. 'Hurrah for Jose Rizal!' said his father." The nursery rhyme "Juan Be Nimble" was chanted by hundreds of schoolchildren.[177]

It was an ambitious undertaking. Yet even Barrows, who hoped that English would become lingua franca throughout the islands, uniting all Filipinos, was realistic in his expectations. The "old dialects" would "persist," he told the Senate Insular Affairs Committee in 1902. But he thought it was "possible, in a very few years, to raise up an educated class . . . who will understand English, understand ourselves, [and] will know something of English literature."[178] Such a class would appreciate American efforts to reform Filipino society and government because it would share a sonic environment with the Americans. Its members would be respectfully quiet, appreciate sound not noise, and speak good English. If and when that occurred, they might be ready to rule themselves.

The British heirs of Thomas Macaulay sensed this happening in India too, but were less easily reconciled to it. Some admitted that a certain class of Indians, particularly those educated in Britain and those who lived or traveled there, had "outlook[s] on life and mental processes that appear to be . . . European." And, "in India too you meet the highly educated Indian who speaks your language perfectly yet uses its words in a totally different sense. And when such an Indian startles you by remarking, for example, that it is a great pity that the proper enunciation of mantrams (religious spells) is a lost art, which if revived might give mankind great power over the elements, then you are tempted to go to the opposite extreme and ask whether we have really influenced Indian thought at all."[179] In 1858, the Governor-General Lord Ellenborough had had a conversation with the Calcutta businessman Dwarkaneth Tagore concerning Macaulay's plan to give Indians an English education. "You know," said Ellenborough, "if these gentlemen succeed in educating the natives of India to the utmost of their utmost desire, we should not remain in the country for three months." "Not three weeks," replied Tagore.[180] The founding of the Indian Congress Party, and the movement for independence, in Tagore's Bengal, was less than three decades away.

5

Sanitizing

The Campaigns Against Odor

> For people could close their eyes to greatness, to horrors, to beauty, and their ears to melodies or deceiving words. But they could not escape scent. For scent was the brother of breath. Together with breath it entered human beings, who could not defend themselves against it, not if they wanted to live. And scent entered into their very core, went directly to their hearts, and decided for good and all between affection and contempt, disgust and lust, love and hate. He who ruled scent ruled the hearts of men.
>
> —Patrick Süskind, *Perfume: The Story of a Murderer* (1986)

> Smells have no place in the constitutive triad of civilization: hygiene, order, and beauty. In the empire of hygiene and order, odor will always be suspect.
>
> —Dominique Laporte, *History of Shit* (2000)

> Smells are surer than sights and sounds to make your heart-strings crack.
>
> —Rudyard Kipling, "Lichtenberg" (1916)

Smell is at once the most evanescent and enduring of the five senses. Odors are volatile and fleeting, carried on the breeze, encountered with an unexpected inhalation, then gone again. They are difficult to retain. An odor can only be described in its own terms. Fish smell like . . . fish; the odor of roses resembles only itself. Yet odors are penetrating and powerful. They inspire emotion, entering areas of the brain unmediated by intellectual process. They are the most likely of the senses to trigger memories. And odors have long served to distinguish the fresh and familiar from the putrid and disgusting, Selves from Others, who is civilized from who is not. "Odors," writes the novelist Patrick Süskind, "have a power of persuasion stronger than that of words, appearances, emotions, or will. The persuasive power of an odor cannot be fended off, it enters into us like breath into our lungs, it fills us up, imbues us totally. There is no remedy for it."[1]

Britons and Americans claimed that uncivilized people stank: of their strange strong food and drink, of the sweat that clung to their bodies or clothes, of excrement, of death. The civilized did not stink. Their bodies smelled clean. Their breath did not reek. Their public spaces were odorless or pleasant-smelling. The scent of their animals was contained, their refuse was buried or moved far away, and the stench of human waste was sent underground, where it would not offend refined nostrils. Making Indians and Filipinos mannerly, and therefore civilized, remained one of empire's central and most audacious missions, and critically important to it was deodorizing their bodies and their environments.

As is true of all senses, there is a biological and a cultural basis for odor. Smells have chemical form: odor-producing molecules arrive with the intake of breath on the nerve endings of the nostrils, and the information they contain is instantly conveyed from olfactory receptors to those sites of the brain related to emotion and memory.[2] Most smells also have complicated meanings, which have shifted over time and depend on place. Humans have long distinguished between the civilized and the primitive on the basis of smell, the aesthetic and moral evaluation of which is learned through acculturation. The Romans found the scent of barbarians disgusting. Christians claimed to give off the odor of sanctity (and knew the devil because he stank); the Hindu *Kama Sutra* insisted that beauty had less to do with appearance than with the right sort of smell; the Muslim tellers and authors of *The Arabian Nights* had it that Europeans ate "evil-smelling, putrescent things, such as rotten cheeses and game which they hang up," that they never washed, and that they drank "yellow liquid with foam on top . . . which is either fermented urine or something worse."[3] As Norbert Elias has argued, the European sense of what stank changed with the Enlightenment, with its new definition of what was mannerly and therefore what it meant to be civilized.[4] People suspected of bad behavior were called "stinkers," "stinkoes," or "stinkpots."[5] But even in the late nineteenth century, there was no consensus about what smelled good or bad. British and American soldiers who went to fight the wars of empire might know the odors of excrement and death. Yet the smell of incense in India or coconut shampoo in the Philippines usually revolted them. Their body odor, redolent of the foods they ate and their sweat, disgusted their hosts.[6] Odor was and is evaluated in the nostrils of the smeller.

Post-Enlightenment writers claimed that rural or primitive people relied on their senses of smell, touch, and taste to know their environments, to gauge the health or illness of human bodies and the fitness of the land for cultivating. Over time hearing rose in importance as information was distributed aurally, then print replaced speech as the chief medium of knowledge circulation, elevating vision over what were now regarded as "the lower senses."[7] Acuity of touch, the willingness to eat the seemingly inedible, and the frequent urge to smell things were reserved for those who lacked sensory refinement. "Civilization evidently despises odor and will oust it with increasing ferocity" over time, writes historian Jonathan Reinarz.[8] To smell, in ways both active and passive, was to be uncivilized. Unrefined people sniffed the air too searchingly and too well: by the nineteenth century, "smell was the sense of madness and savagery."[9] The broad noses of Africans and African Americans suggested to Anglo-Americans an atavistic olfactory skill. Yet these nasal endowments did not, evidently, prevent so-called primitives from smelling terrible themselves. "Groups considered 'other' are generally considered malodorous, and good smells (or no odor at all) are believed to characterize the critic's own social group," writes scholar Jim Drobnick.[10]

Among the senses, smell had a vitally important role to play in the British and American empires of bodies. Nasal encounters with Others were immediate. British travelers in the nineteenth century often claimed to smell India even before they saw it, as they approached by ship. They came to know India's odor as extraordinary, a smell "difficult to pinpoint, partly the populace, partly the different vegetation, partly the very rapid fall of dusk and the cooling off which leads to a most lovely scent just after sundown."[11] "The smell was the first thing they noticed," according to Margaret MacMillan. "Even before they landed, a whiff of India was borne out to them on the breeze."[12] It was "un-nameable . . . a queer intangible drift never experienced before."[13] "I remember," recalled Major T. E. Browsdon, "one of the ship's officers telling me that if they arrived off a port in the East at night or early morning . . . he could tell where they were without looking out at the port hole, which port it was, as they all had their characteristic smells."[14] "Has any one thoroughly investigated the Big Calcutta Stink?" wondered Rudyard Kipling. "There is only one. Benares is fouler in point of concentrated, pent-up muck, and there are local stenches in Peshawur which are stronger than the B. C. S.; but, for diffused, soul-sickening expansiveness, the reek of Calcutta beats both Benares and Peshawur. . . . It is faint, it is sickly, it is indescribable . . . And there is no escape from it. It blows across the *maidan*; it comes in gusts into the corridors of the Great Eastern Hotel . . . ; it pours out of by-streets with sickening intensity, and the breeze of the morning is laden with it."[15] Americans in the Philippines, for their part, smelled uncleaned horse stables, festering canals (*esteros*), unfamiliar foods frying in the bazaar, copra (dried coconut) and coconut oil, and human and animal excrement.[16] Most Britons and Americans in their Asian possessions believed they were inhaling smells fundamentally different from those they knew at home, the tropical temperatures and moisture, distinctive plants and animals, and dangerous new diseases producing peculiar and noxious smells.[17] Stench was intensified by the presence of crowds that jostled in the sunbaked streets of Calcutta and Manila—as in southern American cities, and elsewhere in Britain's empire.[18] Strong odors registered to Anglo-Americans as exotic, threatening, and repulsive.[19]

Britons and Americans who arrived in Asia were well aware of—indeed, were frequently part of—campaigns in their metropoles to clean things up for the benefit of the senses. Victorian British and Progressive American cities were sites of reformist campaigns to render them more legible, quieter, less congested, and free of stench. City planners imagined an end to slums, with their twisting lanes that concealed disease and misconduct and defied efforts by authorities to sanitize them. Like their campaigns to limit noise, reformers undertook vigorously to eliminate bad smells, associated particularly with the working classes.[20] Hector Gavin surveyed the Bethnal Green neighborhood in London. His 1848 report castigated the authorities for allowing the horrors of insanitation and odor to reside among the poor. At Digby Street and Globe Road, Gavin found the corpse of a man named Baker that "formed a receptacle for every kind of manure." Alongside "this table mountain of manure, extensive and deep lakes of putrefying *night soil* are dammed up with the more solid dung, and refuse, forming together, mountain and lake, a scene of the most disgusting character. . . . The decomposing organic particles which are ever being set free from this putrescent mass, are wafted by each wind that blows, over a population to whom they bring disease and death." At Gibralter Walk: "The odour of these streets is *always* most offensive and disgusting. Near the southern end of this filthy walk are two gully-holes, which constantly emit the most abominable stenches, and give rise to fever in the neighbourhood." Gavin had no doubt that the odors of the place sickened and killed its residents.[21] Forty years later, police reporter Jacob Riis began to capture visually the lives of poverty he witnessed in New York City's immigrant neighborhoods using a camera and new techniques of photographic lighting, and resulting in his chronicle *How the Other Half Lives*. While the book is rightly remembered for its pictures, Riis was led to his subjects by the smells of their surroundings. In the tenements downtown he found hallway sinks shared by the tenants, "poisoned alike by their summer stenches," further tainted "with the smell of boiling cabbage, of rags and uncleanliness all about." The poorest Italian worked in sanitation if he worked at all, and he might well make his home in the garbage dump, "in the filthy burrows where he works by day, sleeping and eating his meals . . . on the edge of slimy depths and amid surroundings full of unutterable horror." "The filth and stench were unbearable," even to the police who routinely raided the Lower East Side's "stale-beer dives." From Chinatown wafted the odor of the opium pipe; Jewish homes and shops produced the pungent smells of cabbage, onions, and frying fish. Common to all tenements, regardless of the ethnicity of their residents, was the single air shaft that belied its name by "letting out foul stenches from below."[22]

By the time Riis undertook his research, efforts to displace, reduce, conceal, or eliminate bad smells were underway in Britain and the United States. These included removing garbage from city streets, moving or closing slaughterhouses, tanneries, and fertilizer plants, endorsing personal cleanliness through bathing or the masking of body odor (deodorant was introduced in the United States in 1888), paving streets to prevent noxious fumes from rising from the soil to assail the nostrils, and building underground sewer systems that would sweep wastes away, out of sight and scent, as far as possible from respectable human habitation.[23] Such campaigns could not be confined to the metropoles. Reformers believed that the blessings of public health and sanitation should be extended not only to their own poorest citizens but equally to the downtrodden men and women of their empires. In tropical lands where people were said to live close to savage nature, men and women evidently had little control of their bodies. Ruled by instinct and emotion, they lacked civic responsibility and thus the ability to form and maintain governments. Self-control might be taught to some of them by imperial agents who could master the environment and the bodies they found in it, and if achieved would be reflected in the decency and mannerly practices of the "natives" henceforth.[24]

What emerges from the writings of Britons and Americans in Asia was anxiety about their safety in a tropical environment. Strong odor frightened them perhaps most of all. Their efforts to promote hygiene, end public defecation, and build sewers and latrines and compel their use, were undertaken not just with a feeling of certainty that "sanitation *was* civilization," as Florence Nightingale put it, but out of fear that they would otherwise be sickened and perhaps killed by the odors of the tropics.[25] The olfactory biopolitics of empire were especially powerful because they concerned "fundamental, existential questions about the survival of bodies understood to be out of place, in physically and morally hazardous locations."[26] More than any other sense, smell registered these dangers.

The Anglo-Americans asserted that strong, unpleasant odors and a penchant for sniffing others too brazenly marked the bodies and practices of the uncivilized. Post-Enlightenment westerners used smell to make distinctions among ethnic, national, and religious groups. Among those said by the "civilized" to stink at various times were Finns, Eskimos, Cossacks, Jews, "the filthy Hottentot," and the "Boche." The French were alleged to cover their foul body odor with excessive perfume or cologne; the French scientist Pierre Cabanis claimed that the "stale" smell of the English lingered in their bedrooms for years.[27] Women were associated with the production of strong sexual or menstrual odors, and were said to be uniquely able to "sniff things out" with their superior sense of smell.[28] Those in cities insisted that rural-dwellers had both keener senses of smell and stronger body and social odors; on farms, in the countryside, deep in the mountains or jungles, people were supposedly less likely to wash themselves, and they lived close to animals and reeked of their bodily emanations, including their manure.[29] Smells denoted class: excrement clung to the poor and the working classes, as did many forms of body odor now judged offensive to the civilized nose. The poor were called "the great unwashed." The stalls of the butcher and the fishmonger reeked of the remnants of their trade. "Greasy and fetid sweat" glistened on the skin of workers; their clothes, unwashed for days, gave off a sharp smell that staggered anyone respectable within olfactory range, and their own sense of smell, dulled by lives of sense-numbing exertion, concealed from them their odor or left them indifferent to it.[30] "I do not blame the working man because he stinks, but stink he does," wrote novelist Somerset Maugham. "It makes social intercourse difficult to persons of sensitive nostril. The matutinal tub divides the classes more effectually than birth, wealth, or education."[31]

Above all, smell was used to divide the world according to the construct of race. Race was the servant of imperial domination and an embodied imaginary constituted by all five senses. As whites conceived it, race involved perceptions of skin color and texture, hair texture, the form of the skull and physiognomy and the size of the lips and nose—and the supposedly repugnant odor of dark-skinned bodies. Anglo-Americans were disturbed by the alleged insistence of the "uncivilized" on sniffing the bodies of others and by the shape and condition of their noses. "The nose is the most prominent and noticeable feature of the face," asserted a late nineteenth-century American etiquette manual. "It should never be fondled before company, or, in fact, touched at any time, unless absolutely necessary. The nose, like all other organs, augments in size by frequent handling, so we recommend every person to keep his own fingers, as well as those of his friends or enemies away from it."[32] More distressing to whites was the sharply unpleasant body odor that allegedly characterized people with dark skins, particularly Africans and African Americans. "In the torrid zone," wrote a French commentator early in the nineteenth century, "the Negroes' sweat always has such an evil-smelling odor that it is hard to stay near them for a few minutes."[33] White Americans in the antebellum south were convinced that their difference from black slaves was corporeal and indicated by odor—so powerful that it was, said an observer, "absolutely capable of being *weighed* and *seen* as well as *tasted* and *smelt*."[34] German evolutionary theorist Carl Vogt declared in 1865 that "the specific odor of the Negro remains the same whatever attention he pays to cleanliness and whatever food he takes. It belongs to the species as must does the musk deer that produces it."[35] Twentieth-century white Americans attributed to blacks a "hircine" (goatish) smell that could not be washed away.[36]

To some extent, such racialized olfactory stereotypes clung to Indians and Filipinos as well. In the Indian hill station Simla, Margery Hall panicked at "the strong smells of the strange people," and once posted to remote Rajasthan she routinely doused her bed pillows with cologne, which "help[ed] a little to dim the stink" that pervaded the small settlement there.[37] Dead animals, especially cattle, seemed to be ubiquitous in India, polluting local water supplies with a "sickening" stench.[38] In Peshawar, magistrate Herbert Thompson struggled with a persistently "smelly" courtroom.[39] Writer W. H. Hudson told a story of a British army doctor who instructed his Indian servant to enter the doctor's church each Sunday and tell him, in front of the congregants, that he had an "urgent case" to attend to, in this way raising the Briton's status with his peers and releasing him from the sermon. One evening the doctor agreed to attend a meeting of Indians on the outskirts of town. It was a hot night, and the doctor was quickly overwhelmed by the stench. He ran from the room, took several deep breaths, and said: "'What a relief to get out! In another ten minutes I should have collapsed. The smell!' To which his servant replied: 'Ah, Sahib, *now* you will understand what I suffer every Sunday when I have to go right to the middle of the church to call you out!'"[40] "Critical Americans speak of a 'Filipino smell,'" wrote John Bancroft Devins, and Lieutenant Lee McCoy, stationed in Manila, told his hometown newspaper that "the natives are a repulsive lot smelling of cocoanut oil. . . . They nearly all smoke and chew betel nut."[41] Josephine Craig thought the capital had "a decidedly brown smell."[42] In northern Luzon, Ruth Hunt observed: "The smells are pretty bad, and the sewers are all open and covered with a filthy green slime."[43] Those who traveled to India and then to the archipelago found similar the odors of the streets, markets, and waterways.[44]

There is an important qualification to be made here. Race was a protean concept, and like the empires with which it kept company it evolved over time. Most Britons and Americans declined to attribute the odors of Indians and Filipinos to something inherent in them. In contrast to Anglo-American characterizations of black people, Asians were thought to fashion rather than generate bodily their stenches, and thus could reduce (if not fully eliminate) them. Members of a Spiti family in the Punjab were "very smelly" because they bathed infrequently, the village of Trichalur in South India reeked with the odor of the fetid Hindu temple well, and the stench of burial grounds, in which bodies had been too shallowly buried, was emitted by "putrefaction" that expelled into the air "unpleasant" and "death dealing gases."[45] A British resident explained: "Many of the natives are addicted to practices which make them anything but agreeable *compagnons de voyage* in close quarters. In the first place, they lubricate the body with oil, sometimes cocoanut, but often castor or margosa oil; the two latter kinds having a most foetid and, to a European, a most disgusting and nauseating smell. Secondly, being often fat, the natives perspire very freely, which they can hardly be blamed for, but which intensifies the effect of the anointment."[46] The British complained also about the Indian food and body odors of asafetida, garlic, turmeric, garlic, and "curry stuff."[47] In the Philippines, Americans, like Lee McCoy and Ruth Hunt, objected to the smells of coconut oil and tobacco smoke and sewers, and as well of stuffy interior spaces in which families nursed their sick, bad breath, and garbage.[48] In all of these cases, according to the British and Americans, Asians could lessen the offensive odors. They could wash (with far less coconut oil), lose weight, clean up their water and their roadways, open windows, bury their garbage, build sewers and latrines, and dispose more thoroughly of the dead. All of these things they could, or the best among them could, in theory, be taught or helped to do. Make Asian bodies smell fresh, not stale or sharp. Eliminate the stink from their breath. Render their public spaces odorless or pleasant-smelling. Send human waste underground, where it would not offend civilized nostrils. In short, deodorize or reodorize the Other and he begins to become civilized.

Odor and Disease

Foul odors remained in the late nineteenth and early twentieth centuries associated not only with supposed racial inferiority but also with contagious diseases that were themselves said to be a product of dark-skinned bodies and the places they lived. Stench was alleged to be common to racial Others and the causes of the illnesses they harbored, particularly in the tropics. Bad smells were not, by this logic, merely unpleasant: they could be fatal.

Dark-skinned residents of the tropics held no monopoly on illnesses, but they were usually blamed for having started them. Asian diseases had apparently traveled west on fomites, objects retaining the smells, and thus the corrupt essences, of those who fashioned or handled them. Europeans used *parfumoirs,* wooden chests with chafing dishes filled with pellets that smelled pleasant when burned, to fumigate mail arrived "from the contaminating Orient."[49] The British in 1858, and to some extent the Americans even forty years later, regarded bad smells as possible indicators of miasmas, poisonous exhalations of the soil and water that caused disease. The British sanitary reformer Edwin Chadwick famously observed in 1846: "All smell is, if it be intense, immediate acute disease; and eventually we may say that . . . all smell is disease."[50] Plague was long ascribed to the putrefaction of dead or dying bodies, and London's mid-nineteenth-century "disease mist" reputedly produced cholera, smallpox, measles, and whooping cough.[51] "Beneficial odors are sweet and fragrant; hurtful vapors are offensive and unpleasant," claimed *The Saturday Evening Post,* and in the 1870s, American scientists blamed typhus on foul odors from sewers or exhalations from the tenements of the immigrant poor.[52] Objects imported to the United States, especially hides, coffee, and rags, might contain "foul or contaminated air," indicated by their smell—the residue of damp or rot—and carrying the prospect of infection.[53] Diseases themselves exuded particular odors. Tuberculosis smelled of stale beer, yellow fever of butchered meat, the breath of diabetics of acetone.[54] The judgment of odor was not merely aesthetic.

In June 1858, as the British were ending the Great Rebellion in India, a terrible odor rose from the River Thames, left low after a long dry spell. The *Journal of Public Health and Sanitary Review* recorded tales "of men struck down with the stench, and of all kinds of fatal diseases, upspringing from the river's banks." Workers tried to suppress the smell, and its presumed malignant effect, by dumping quantities of lime into the river, and covering the windows of Parliament with sheets soaked in chloride of lime. When these efforts failed, the members fled Westminster; Benjamin Disraeli, the leader of the Commons, held a handkerchief to his nose as he left, declaring the Thames a "Stygian Pool." Aboard a hospital ship docked in the river, a sailor named Richard Billingsley felt nauseated and "complained of a general debility" while suffering from diarrhea. A surgeon diagnosed him with cholera, "as he said he could not get the stench off his lungs." When Billingsley died, the surgeon, coroner, and a jury at the inquest agreed "that the deceased died from the effects of an attack of Asian cholera, brought on by inhaling the noxious vapour of the Thames." For years Londoners had channeled their excrement directly into the Thames. Now, at Disraeli's insistence, Parliament empowered the Metropolitan Board of Works to build an enormous sewer project that would carry wastes miles downriver, where they would presumably be washed away to the sea. As the *Times* observed, "the stench of June . . . did for the sanitary administration of the metropolis what the Bengal mutinies did for the administration of India." The London sewer system, designed by Sir Joseph Bazalgette, consisting of eighty-three miles of water mains fed by hundreds of miles of tributaries, was finished in 1875.[55]

The miasma theory that odors themselves caused disease began to weaken in Europe and America in the 1880s. The discoveries of Robert Koch and Louis Pasteur implicated bacteria in several illnesses, including cholera, and suggested their role in causing many more. When Paris underwent its own "Great Stink" in 1880, the first reaction of officials and ordinary citizens was, as in London, to attribute illnesses that followed in its wake to stench. Yet studies done in Pasteur's city in the aftermath of the Stink suggested caution. In the aggregate, their conclusion was that "some—but not all—odors are hazardous to human health." The sanitarian Paul Brouardel modified Chadwick's earlier formulation: "not everything that stinks kills, and not everything that kills stinks." What evolved thereafter was an effort to reconcile the evidence absorbed by the public nose with the incontestable truths revealed by the scientist's microscope. Scientists concluded that bacteria imparted stench to air and water. It might be that an unseen pathogen rather than a bad smell made people sick, but if the two were so closely associated the agent of cause seemed functionally no more significant than that which made it manifest to the nostrils. Foul odors continued to have their own pathology; that which stank *might* kill, and "could not be bacteriologically innocent."[56] Even as the germ theory made its way fitfully to Britain and the

United States, miasmas remained suspect, and strong smells in both places continued to engender suspicion and fear, a threat to civilized men and women.[57]

In the wars of empire and after, Britons and Americans in their Asian possessions believed they were experiencing smells fundamentally different from those they knew at home, even if their supposed pathogenic effects were in some cases the same. The odors of their tropical empires had a pervasiveness and an intensity that both attracted and (more often) repelled the Anglo-Americans. Thus, the sweet and evocative smells of India: sandalwood and aloewood; fragrant tea and pungent chilies; spices, including cumin, turmeric, ginger, and cloves; jasmine and the pine scent of the hill stations; incense; attar of roses.[58] And the noxious ones: "the smell of fresh blood pouring down the streets of Delhi, the sweetish odor of human flesh decayed"; in Sind an "ammoniac odor which more or less grips you by the throat"; in Goa the odor of drying fish; the reek of ubiquitous Hindu temple wells ("a stench pervades the whole place of an intensity not to be described"); the bearers of *doolies,* rough carriages used to convey Europeans up mountain paths, who smelled of "rank" tobacco and dirty clothes and were "redolent of saturated humanity and *ghee*"; the stench of domestic servants—"the awful smell of my bearer as he entered my room," wrote Evelyn Beeton; an overall "decay of urine and spices"; foul food that "tasted of the smell of the natives."[59] Americans in the Philippines acknowledged that the people they encountered frequently bathed, and the smell of pine in the hill station Baguio invigorated those who spent the hot weather there.[60] But there was also the "decayed or dirty food" too often sold in the markets; excessive use of "oils or pomades" with their "distinct odor which is most offensive to people with good taste"; the "musty" smell of cockroaches; the animal smells in village homes in which pigs rooted through garbage under permeable bamboo floors.[61] Upcountry, Dr. Victor Heiser witnessed an Igorot funeral practice: "The feasting mourners would squat in the house of the deceased, and custom demanded that the corpse be there with them, propped up in a rude chair with a smoke fire going under him to keep him. I have known these affairs to last six months, and in that warm climate the corpse, even in its smoked condition, was likely to become rather high."[62] In Manila, recalled Florence Horn, "the heat, the streets crowded with human beings, and the horses combine to produce a smell that is overpowering: the heavy, gamy smell of human perspiration, the smell of urine, equine and human."[63] Even when they used a pleasant-smelling substance, Indians and Filipinos were said to overdo it, as if compensating for foul odors. At parties, Indian women splashed scent on the handkerchiefs of their British guests, garlanded them to the point of suffocation with jasmine, poured liquid sandalwood into their hands, or, according to Fanny Parks, "sprinkled us most copiously with rose water."[64] On the hot afternoon of a Philippines commission session in Ilagan, several Filipinas poured full bottles of perfume on Governor

Taft and his party, making "the recipients smell," according to one of them, "like a wrecked drug store."[65]

Indian and Filipino insistence on maintaining proximity to animals seemed to British and American sanitary reformers evidence of olfactory barbarism. Foul-smelling livestock surely carried diseases, and their odor corrupted the atmosphere of houses in, near, or under which they lived. Britons were nauseated by the presence of pigs (which when dead and smelling "unbelievably awful" neither Muslims nor Hindus would touch), camels ("their smell . . . is powerful exceedingly"), and, in Lady Reynolds's case, a pair of reeking live tigers held in chains by servants while she and her husband stood uneasily next to them for a photograph.[66] Animals in Philippine villages must not be kept under houses, instructed the Americans, lest their wastes "poison the air" above them.[67] Westerners in both India and the Philippines were fascinated and repelled by civets, wild cats bearing anal sacs filled with a greasy, foul-smelling secretion that nevertheless, when diluted and mixed with other scents, became something of a rage among European perfumers by the nineteenth century. (Often compared to musk, it acted as a fixative to hold the scent longer on the skin.) South Indians collected the scent of civet by gathering twigs or logs onto which the cats discharged it, harvested it, then used it to anoint their kings and the images of gods in Hindu temples.[68] Dean Worcester, the US commissioner who spent many years studying people and animals in the Philippines, was given in the summer of 1899 a "fine lot of civet cats," presumably dead, for his experiments. His work was frequently interrupted by a garrulous Spanish friar. Worcester contrived to use the cat to ward off this nuisance. One day, just as the friar arrived, Worcester sliced open the civet's odor sac, and within seconds "the defunct cat was 'doing itself proud,'" filling the room with its stench. The padre tried smoking, but it was not enough. "In another moment my visitor's eyes suddenly filled with tears," Worcester wrote. "Dropping his cigarette, he covered his mouth and nose with a handkerchief and rushed from the room," and he did not return.[69]

Above all, in both India and the Philippines, Britons and Americans recoiled at the odor of excrement, especially human waste. Excrement was a pollutant of all the senses, inverting the body by turning what was inside out and thus violating its boundaries.[70] Its presence in public indicated to Anglo-Americans a widespread lack of self-control, an indifference to hygiene, and a profound failure to act with the sort of bodily discipline required of civilized men and women. It was not just the odor that disgusted them—no one wished to see excrement, nor touch it. But the smell was worst: feces (and urine) stank.[71] In India, women especially used cow dung for fuel or building material and, despite its smell and other polluting qualities, showed no hesitation in handling it. Such activity "degrades the women" and "makes them filthy," wrote the sanitation specialist F. L. Brayne.[72] Cesspools and open trenches of cities ran with a "black semi-liquid deposit" that reeked of decay, while in villages, according to a British sanitary official, "even the cleanest privy emits an offensive odour, and all such smells near a house are unwholesome"—the odors from the public latrine were "perfectly indescribable, and make me feel quite sick."[73] Indian *ayahs* (nannies) had to be trained not to leave soiled diapers unwashed in the bathroom for more than a day.[74] Aden, on the Arabian peninsula but part of the Bombay Presidency, was plagued with excrement-laden sanitation carts that passed near middle-class homes on their way to discharge their contents in the Arabian Sea, bringing tears to the eyes of residents and leaving behind a "vile stench."[75] In the Rajasthani outpost of Jacobabad, Margery Hall "followed [her] nose" to the servants' lavatory. The toilet, a wooden box open to the roof, "had not been emptied in many moons, and it was overflowing all over the little room it was housed in. Not only that, but it was all walking, huge maggots covering the whole area. The stench was unbelievable and the whole pot seethed and bubbled with life. I fled, retching and sweating, down the blazing hot path to the house."[76] In the Philippines, residents squatted everywhere, without regard, the Americans said, for propriety or their proximity to the gaze of others or sources of food and water.[77] The Philippines Bureau of Education instructed Filipinos with latrines to dump

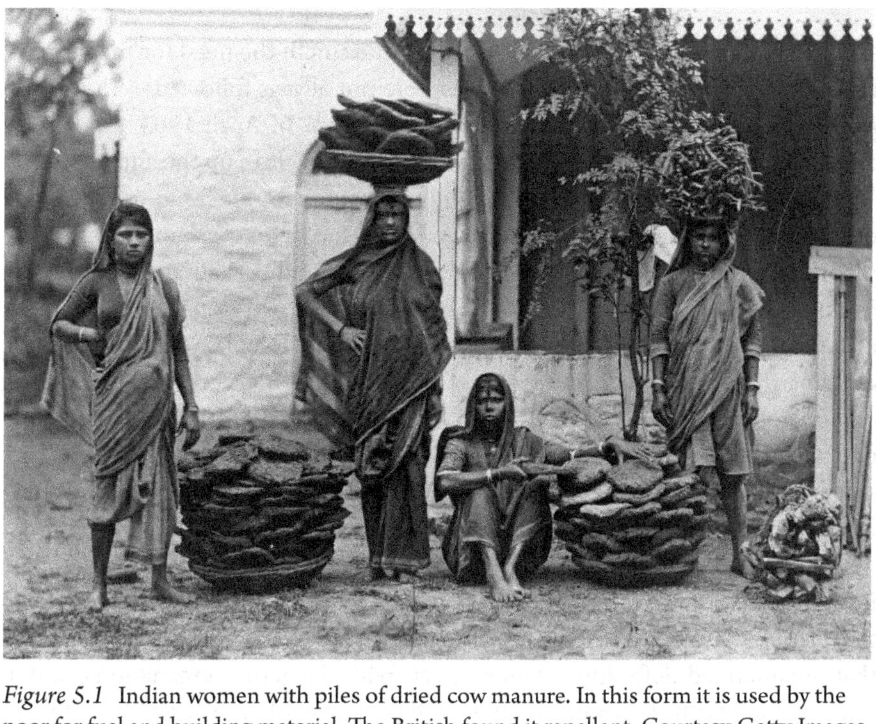

Figure 5.1 Indian women with piles of dried cow manure. In this form it is used by the poor for fuel and building material. The British found it repellent. Courtesy Getty Images.

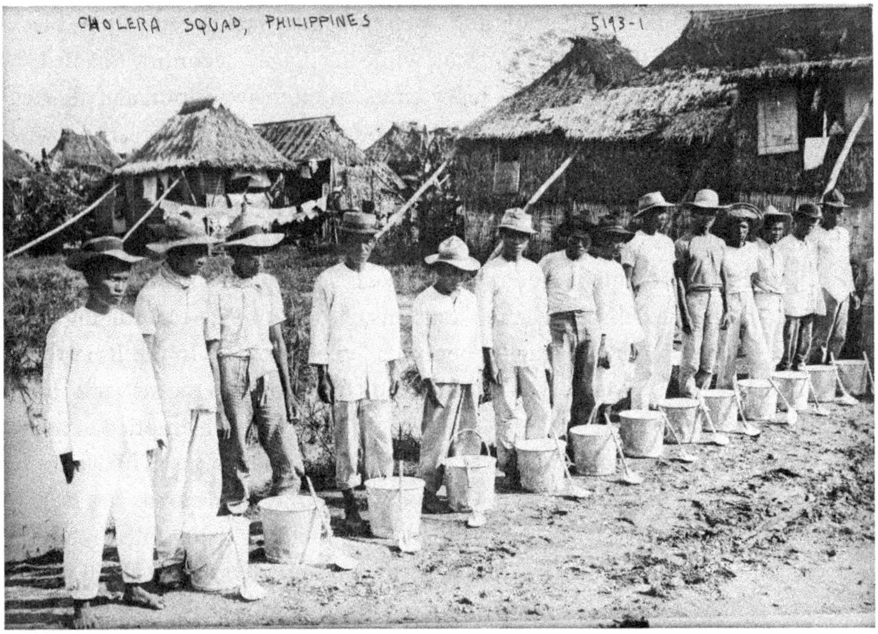

Figure 5.2 A pail brigade prepares to attack cholera during an epidemic in Manila. Courtesy of Library of Congress, Prints and Photographs Division, LC-DIG-ggbain-30474.

sand into them every day in order to absorb the smell; the need for the instruction was evidence that such procedures were not always followed.[78] The *esteros* of Manila carried wastes openly to the Pasig River. In April 1903, an editorialist for the *Manila Times* pleaded with authorities to clean up the *esteros,* whose "heavy foulness can be not only smelt but almost felt for blocks away." It was an odor "quite enough to knock you down."[79] So, too, with carabao urine, which reportedly inspired the only sanitary law Grace Paulding had ever heard of in Cebu: the driver of a carabao-drawn cart was obliged to prevent his animal from urinating in the street, either by "twist[ing] his tail violently" or, if that failed, catching the urine in a chamber pot and disposing of it accordingly.[80] "Calls of nature are attended to wherever . . . it is the most convenient—indoors or out of doors," wrote George Telfer to his wife, Lottie. "Capt. Prescott has been on smelling detail among the monasteries near us. He is a very robust man, but he has to excuse himself from the balance of the party now and then—to vomit."[81]

And excrement was dangerous. Adherents to the miasma theory continued to hold that the odor of feces could itself be fatal to those who inhaled it. In 1896, the Deputy Surgeon-General in India, T. G. Hewlett, admonished villagers that uncontained defecation "taints the air with dangerous emanations, and it fouls the soil with dangerous matter."[82] Imperial health and sanitation officers increasingly came to recognize that smelling excrement, unwholesome as it might be, did not actually kill people. But even if the smell of shit was not dangerous, it remained an indicator of morbific (disease-causing) substances close by. Any sort of contact with wastes could be fatal. Ingesting the bacteria they carried almost certainly would be. In 1912, the Philippines Bureau of Health cautioned that human wastes "are more dangerous than arsenic or strychnine" because "dysentery, typhoid fever, cholera, and kindred diseases are conveyed to the person, regardless of whether he be a king or peasant, with minute organisms that, probably, have passed through the bowels of another person."[83] And the odor of excrement was offensive to civilized noses. It must be masked, altered, or—best of all—sent underground, out of sight and smell.

Cholera in particular was the disease caused by excrement out of place, one of the most dangerous illnesses encountered in India and the Philippines. The foul odor of feces was invariably present where the cholera vibrio, or bacterium, bred, and so stink drew the attention of the offended nose to what was threatening but unseen. In the summer of 1854, cholera raged through the Soho neighborhood in London, ultimately claiming at least six hundred lives. Doubting that the disease was caused by miasmas, as most scientists then believed, physician John Snow focused his investigations on a water pump on Broad Street. He went door to door, finding gruesome evidence of the epidemic, and mapping the houses wherein residents had fallen ill. In this way he demonstrated that all those affected by the disease had drunk infected water drawn from the Broad Street pump, and that those in the area who had taken water elsewhere—or, in the case of a group of brewery workers, drunk only beer—had not been afflicted. Local authorities removed the handle from the implicated pump, and the disease tapered off. Thirty years later, Robert Koch would identify the bacterium *vibrio cholera* as the source of the disease.[84]

Snow had traced cholera to India (it was known in full as "Asiatic cholera"), and as sanitary conditions improved in Europe epidemics were far more frequent in Asian countries. That the water in London had been fouled by feces was Snow's conclusion, but not everyone was convinced or certain of the disease vector, and for many years after the Soho epidemic argument continued concerning cholera's etiology. In 1868, the sanitary commissioner of India's North-West Provinces blamed an outbreak in part on "air . . . tainted by fermenting or decomposing animal excrement."[85] As late as 1894 Indian Army medical regulations advised "troops when attacked by cholera to march at right angles to the wind," and into the third decade of the twentieth century some scientists believed that the humidity in the air played an independent role in spreading the disease. Two severe outbreaks of cholera raged in Chittagong in 1897. The civil surgeon blamed the first on low and dirty water tanks resulting from drought, the second on debris blown into the tanks by a cyclone and "the use of excessive quantities of bad-smelling fish" during a food shortage in the city.[86] All of these hypotheses were remnants of the miasma theory.[87] Many Britons wore "cholera belts," webbed straps cinched tight around the waist, which were said to prevent the body from "cooling" and thus becoming receptive to the cholera germ.[88]

Whatever else they suspected as a cause of the disease, the British understood that the use of water polluted with human waste was extremely dangerous. It was also ubiquitous in India, where tanks or cisterns, open to street and sky, provided villages with drinking water, and where rivers were nearly always used for bathing, doing laundry, dumping garbage and human and animal wastes, as well as supplying water for consumption. One official noted the definition of an Indian village made by a government report: "a collection of insanitary huts situated on a dunghill."[89] Another described the scene in Indian towns of all sizes: "The conditions of life and the general sanitary arrangements, or want of sanitary arrangements, in village and town alike were such as to give a fine field for epidemic disease and an excessive mortality. The village tank was too often mere sewage, abounding in life. Every shower washed surface filth into it, every dust shower carried some more; clothes and cooking utensils left their modicum of dirt; as the dry season lasted it grew lower and dirtier. When it appeared in a city like Calcutta it was a mere pool of fermenting sewage, the common cloaca of neighbourhood, where the wretched denizens of the huts that crowd its banks might be seen bathing, washing their cooking pots and garments, and filling drinking pots with a fetid liquid about the colour of London porter."[90] Most dangerous were the gatherings of devout Hindus at the great fairs (*kumbhs*), which brought thousands of pilgrims to sites along the River Ganges to worship, bathe, wash clothes, and commit the ashes of dead relatives to its sacred water. *Kumbhs* were implicated in cholera epidemics in 1875–1877 and 1891–1892. The celebrants not only drank directly from the river, but also filled bottles with river water and took them home to those unable to make the pilgrimage.[91] Authorities struggled to gain some measure of control over these festivals. In 1893, bacteriologist Waldemar Haffkine successfully tested in Bengal a vaccination for cholera, but it was hard to persuade Indians to submit to it, in good part because inoculation had gone wrong in the villages before, and it was not always possible to deliver hygienically the vaccine and syringes.[92]

On one matter there was agreement: cholera was a terrible way to die. Accounts emphasized the panic that came with the realization that one had the disease. Those afflicted suffer from rampant "rice water" diarrhea, which quickly dehydrates them. As one doctor described it, the patient " 'tosses about continually, and evinces the utmost distress.' His skin turned cold and corpse-like, the pulse grew sluggish and breathing labored; his voice became 'feeble, sepulchral, and unnatural.' "[93] Irene Bose left an account of a cholera attack in the village of Loni. She deplored the fatalism of the villagers, who (she said)

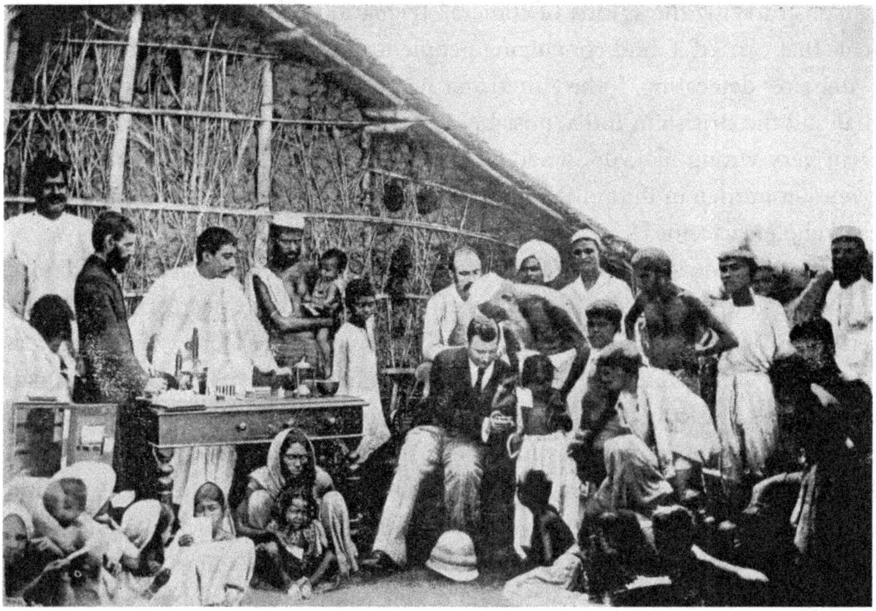

Figure 5.3 Waldemar Haffkine, assisted by the British Health Officer in Calcutta and several Indian doctors, inoculates a child against cholera, 1894. Not all patients were as cooperative as this one seems to be. Wellcome Collection. CC BY 4.0.

offered futile offerings to the gods and were otherwise inclined to accept their fate. That changed, she said, when children caught the disease: "Parbati, age ten, as graceful and vivid as a hibiscus flower, died of it in terror calling to us for help. Two small sisters came down with it screaming." The epidemic abated when at last the village leaders begged Bose and her colleagues for help, and isolation and hydration of victims commenced.[94]

So too did cholera prove devastating in the Philippines. The disease was soberingly familiar to Filipinos: an epidemic had killed an estimated ten percent of the population of Manila in 1882. The Spanish board of health believed that cholera was caused by miasmas and recommended that people protect themselves with smudge pots burning lemongrass and tar and by putting camphorated quills in their mouths.[95] Corpses piled up too quickly to be buried; the stench was reportedly "so dreadful that one could hardly go through it."[96] After 1898 American health officials followed European findings on the cause of the disease, and in general they got it right, though many of them, like Britons in India, continued to wear cholera belts.[97] By 1908, at least, doctors and sanitationists agreed that cholera was carried by Robert Koch's "pathogenic bacteria," that it was found in the sewer system of Manila "either in its fluid contents or in vermin," and that if water supplies could be kept free of cholera, preventing an epidemic still depended on policing the "improperly cared for stools of the persons carrying the spirilla of cholera," trying to eradicate flies and other animals that carried it, and convincing people to wash their hands with soap and water after defecating.[98] The Americans had even less success with vaccination than did the British in India, possibly because an experiment with vaccination went very wrong in 1906, when an American doctor accidentally inoculated twenty-four men in Bilibid Prison with a virulent strain of plague serum rather than cholera vaccine.[99]

Cholera made its presence felt in a fast-moving epidemic that struck Manila, then surged upcountry, in the spring of 1902. Officials suspected that the bacterium arrived on fresh vegetables from Canton or Hong Kong, where growers used night soil as fertilizer, but it was more likely conveyed through a human carrier who had contact with someone from China.[100] The timing of the epidemic was fortuitous but may have been significant: the American military effort against the Philippine insurgency transitioned into a militarized health and sanitation campaign undertaken by Dean Worcester, Dr. Louis Maus, and others in response to the crisis. "It was, in a sense, the old war in a new, more complex setting," writes historian Reynaldo Ileto; one cannot miss the militant rhetoric of Worcester's account of the epidemic, nor his use of the US army to secure the city's water supply against Filipinos who would, however inadvertently, pollute it.[101] When Worcester discovered that the first cases of cholera were concentrated in Farola, a poor neighborhood of nipa huts and warehouses built on the mudflats along the Pasig, he at first quarantined the place, then removed 1,200 of its residents to a detention camp at San Lazaro, after which he ordered the burning of its huts and disinfection of its "more substantial buildings." (The scent of burning nipa huts filled the air in every town where cholera was suspected or found.)[102] Alongside the detention camp were two hospitals, a morgue, and a crematorium, though most Filipinos were horrified at the thought of immolating their dead. Those in the camp lived in tents and were separated from the outside world by barbed wire. If the sick were discovered in private houses, they were removed to the hospital while their families were left behind, a policy that defied the Filipino practice of nursing family members at home.[103] "Four times out of five this was the last they ever saw of their loved ones until shortly they received a curt notice to come to the hospital and claim their dead," recalled Health Commissioner Victor Heiser.[104] Worcester closed all the wells, destroyed the Chinese vegetables, and made provision for the distribution of more distilled water throughout the city.[105] To the despair of health authorities, Americans seemed to think that drinking alcohol would prevent their getting the disease, "and many lives were sacrificed through this erroneous idea."[106] The epidemic finally ran its course in early 1904. The death toll was 109,461 in the archipelago, with 4,386 of the victims in Manila.[107]

Deodorizing and Detoxifying the Empire

Efforts to control bad smells and cholera were thus largely one and the same for sanitary reformers in Great Britain and the United States and in their nations' imperial possessions. Cholera germs accompanied stink; identify and eliminate the odor and the disease would abate, even in the absence of visual identification of the implicated bacteria. Elites needed protection from pathogens and the poor required cleaning up at home, and so did the civilizing mission demand attention to the comparable classes abroad, in India and the Philippines. It would be difficult work, given the supposed cultural and racial limitations of those who were the targets of sanitationists' and physicians' hygienic plans, and as the Asians' seemingly passive response to controlling cholera demonstrated. Many Britons doubted that the vast majority of Indians were interested in sanitation; as a sanitary commissioner wrote in 1868, "It seems to be a hopeless task to attempt by means of legislation to force on so large a population occupying so vast a continent reforms which involve . . . a radical change in their everyday habits and customs to which they cling with a reverential persistence partaking largely of superstition."[108] American officials claimed to know all too well how hard it was to get immigrants to clean themselves up and pointed to New York's Chinatown for evidence of the distinctive, unwholesome, and intractable smell of Asians.[109] Yet decency required sanitation and hygiene, as did the safety of their own citizens and control of people who would not control themselves. In the end, Americans professed confidence that they could deodorize and cleanse the Philippines. "It remained for us to prove that the thing could be done," wrote Isabel Anderson, who visited the islands in 1915, "that a tropical country could be made sanitary and hygienic for all inhabitants, whether they were white or brown or yellow, and whether they wanted it made so or not."[110]

Despite the exertions of Progressives, American cities lagged behind London in building sewage systems. Washington, DC had some eighty miles of sewer pipe by the time Joseph Bazalgette's project was finished on the Thames in 1875, but many of its neighborhoods remained unserved, connections were incomplete, and maintenance was poor. The Chicago River was an open sewer to Lake Michigan, polluting Chicago's water supply. Milwaukee stank of horse manure and dead animals and lacked the water needed to flush its sewers, and Baltimore's wastes simmered in the harbor as sewerage commissions and politicians squabbled over building plans; the city did not have a complete, enclosed sewer system until 1915.[111] "A person who knowingly takes into his mouth the excrement of another human being is certainly defective," wrote the sanitary engineer George Johnson in 1916. "A community having a public water supply known to be contaminated by the sewage of other cities, and using it without even attempting its purification, is certainly a victim of defective civilization."[112] He could have been describing either the United States or its most recent Asian possession.

None of their shortcomings at home prevented the British in India and the Americans in the Philippines from waxing sanctimonious about the lack of sewers in their colonies and the need for their installation. In India, British officials' concern began with the destructive effect of poor sanitation on their army in the aftermath of the Great Rebellion, but efforts to manage sewage soon spread. An 1882 government study recommended as a first measure "the cleansing and safe removal and disposal of house sewage."[113] The Bombay Presidency adopted in 1888 a Municipal Act that defined a "nuisance" broadly as "a thing which causes, or is likely to cause injury, danger, annoyance, or offence to the sense of sight, smelling, or hearing," and prohibited its commission, but enforcing the law was an uphill fight: nearly two decades later, citizens of the city still complained bitterly about the "horrible stench" from drains and the "foul and putrid smell" at railroad crossings.[114] Towns developed their own methods for dealing with the sewage problem—or not. The Viceroy, Lord Dufferin, toured the Calcutta slums in 1888. It proved, "from a sanitary and olfactory point of view, a terrible morning walk" through the capital city. With "handkerchief to nose," he transited a "labyrinth of dark and stuffy gutters" and "hideous, squalid narrow lanes, where an odour reigns supreme, with rancid ghee for its basis," a stench at once "indescribable, omnipresent, overwhelming."[115] Belgaum was considered a model of sanitary innovation, but there remained in 1919 a "striking smell" issuing from the city's public drains, next to which vendors at the bazaar spread their wares on the open ground.[116] Poona dumped its wastes from "foul-smelling" open receptacles into a small stream, polluting the local river; Muzaffarpur, in Bengal, replaced trenching not with sewers but with a septic system; Madras chose increasingly to bury its wastes with soil or sand; and on a tea plantation high in the Annamalai mountains, James L. H. Williams conceded that latrines smelled far worse than open air toilets exposed to the hot South Indian sun—though he would later have workers build deep latrine pits, called "Long Drops," adjacent to the plantings, covered by shelters and disinfected by sweepers each day.[117] Even the hill stations were afflicted by bad odors: in Ootacamund in 1868, the Madras sanitary commissioner detected " 'a general foecal taint to the atmosphere' due to defecation in the surrounding undergrowth" by servants of the Europeans who visited there.[118]

India's rural villages were the despair of officials. Appalled by the stench of feces and the sight and smell of pigs and cows feasting on fresh excrement, T. G. Hewlett offered precise instructions for the building and maintenance of latrines. They must be located "at least 250 yards" from the edge of the village and have "separate areas for men and women." Residents caught relieving themselves within the boundaries of the village "shall be dealt with." Each user of the latrine must rake or kick dirt "over what has come from him," while low-caste sweepers were to clean the privies and police the village for filth left by scofflaws. In the latrines there were to be stone footrests, an "iron receptacle" with two chambers, "the upper one of which retains the night soil, and is perforated to allow of the ablution-water and urine flowing into the lower chamber," and a floor of asphalt or brick to allow for thorough cleaning.[119] Civil Servant F. L. Brayne spent years in the Punjab and in Gurgaon district, near Delhi, visiting villages and exhorting their residents to clean things up. "When you lose your way in Gurgaon district you find your way by your nose," he advised. "The greater the stink the nearer the village." There were "FOUR THINGS" villagers must do if they "wish to be regarded as civilised human beings: (1) Dig pits and clean the villages. (2) Stop making *upla* [cow dung cakes]. (3) Open windows in your houses. (4) Treat girls equally with boys and send them to school together." The first three of these of course concerned smell, and lessons learned by both girls and boys were meant to reinforce hygienic habits at home. Brayne was struck by the relative lack of manure used as fertilizer and the abundance of it strewn about the village or stuck to its children. In *Village Uplift in India,* Brayne imagined himself approaching a Gurgaon village sometime in the future: "By th[at] time we had reached the village, and I at once detected something radically different from my idea of a village. There was no smell, no filth, no dust, no rubbish, no dung cakes, no manure heaps. I said, 'What have you done with the dear old village smells, and the dung-cakes and everything?' But no one seemed to understand me, and I had to explain. Then they told me that everyone keeps his cattle on his farm now-a-days, where he had his manure pit, and a large number of the farmers live on their farms. 'We don't huddle together in crowded villages like our ancestors used to. The village streets have long since been paved out of the profits of our banks, latrines were built and water-taps were put up to be fed from the tank at the top of the village.' "[120]

"The centres of population as first known to me presented an appearance of much neglect," wrote the sanitary commissioner of Allahabad, Charles Planck, in 1881. A city of around a hundred thousand people, Allahabad was not just a visual but an olfactory affront to Planck's sensibilities. Local authorities "gave little thought to sanitary conditions," though they admitted that when they entered certain parts of the city they smoked a cigar or scattered "an occasional pinch of powdered camphor as a defence against the prevailing unwholesome atmosphere." Planck tried to persuade them that unsanitary conditions, indicated by the awful stench, were "the true death penalty" of the city. He built public latrines and encouraged the use of latrines at home, but the success of his plans depended on the citizens' willingness to use the toilets and keep them clean. Earth had to be spread over the contents of the public latrines after use, and their contents had to be removed as promptly as possible. Planck encountered considerable obstacles to his plans. For a time, the authorities used urine to water Alfred Park, but that spread enteric fever and smelled foul. Indoor ("cupboard") latrines were built and opened with a shutter to the street; their contents were dumped into a short trench that emptied into a pit or a larger open sewer. The city's main sewerage channel carried wastes from the railway station across the city to flow into the Jumna River. Planck described the sewer system as "a noisome ditch everywhere, with crawling fetid contents." Sanitary success in Allahabad was, in short, elusive.[121]

Delhi, the old Mughal capital, was roughly four times the size of Allahabad. Its sewer system, completed in 1873, proved inadequate, inasmuch as it relied on open trenches and basins, the sluice water for which was unavailable and "which accordingly," complained a newspaper editorialist, "are always full of exceedingly foul smells." The lanes of the city "are too narrow and lined with open privies." In 1888 the Viceroy, Lord Dufferin, launched an inquiry into the sanitation problem. A Delhi official responded that, "to the masses of the people, sanitation is foolishness," but he held out some hope that the "better class of Indians" might be persuaded to observe its basic rules and serve as an example to the others. With manual labor more abundant than water, the city resigned itself to a system whereby residents threw garbage out of doors or windows and evacuated night soil via pit toilets into holding receptacles along the streets. These were then collected and taken by bullock carts to a landfill on the outskirts of the city. The carters, men of the lowest caste, were presumed impervious to stench, but the stink caused protests as their carts transited neighborhoods, and as the city's population grew it impinged on the landfills. Under pressure from British residents, whose homes and clubs were in the summer months downwind of the Malkaganj landfill, the Delhi Municipal Corporation opened new dump sites south of the walled city, near the "native enclave." (The Indian representative on the Commission asked the medical authorities to "devise some medicine that every citizen should be made to eat so that he loses his sense of smell.") New technologies of disposal, including the development of digestive sludge tanks, allowed the construction of treatment plants, around which authorities planted aromatic bushes in vain hope of masking ambient odors, and the advent of a "Refuse Train" in the 1930s replaced remaining dumps near the city. By that time, Delhi's British Health Officer had proposed that "as many houses of a good class as possible" receive the water necessary to connect them directly to the sewers. This reinforced the British view that the better sorts of Indians might be made mannerly.[122]

The Americans encountered a similar situation in the Philippines, especially in villages and towns outside Manila. Work here was influenced by their experience of sanitation in Cuba and Puerto Rico. The Americans' first concern was to protect themselves from harm caused by slovenly hygiene, and as long as soldiers were in garrison their health was as good as that of men in the United States, or so the authorities proclaimed. Official travelers resorted to carrying and preparing their own food to avoid cholera, even at risk of offending hosts who planned lavish banquets in their honor.[123] But American sanitation practices took hold slowly otherwise. "The Filipino people," wrote Dr. Thomas Marshall, "should be taught that . . . promiscuous defecation is dangerous and should be discontinued."[124] According to a scientific report, in one provincial capital of eight to ten thousand people, the river served "as a sewer and water supply, as a universal bath-tub for people and animals, and as a wash tub for the clothing" of town residents. Along the streets visitors encountered a variety of animals including pigs, "many of them with decorations of human faeces on their heads and backs, foraging for garbage or the droppings from passing horses and carabaos." Markets were open to the dusty air, and flies swarmed over the sweets and raw meats, while dogs and cats tracked through fruits and vegetables arrayed on the ground. "Defecation is performed in public at all times upon the streets and river banks," and what latrines the locals had were "of the pig-flushing variety."[125] Close inspection of 1,300 houses in the town of Taytay in 1909 revealed that nearly half had no provision for the disposal of excrement. About a quarter had outhouses a few meters from the house, in which seatless privies opened directly to the ground. While the space under the floor was enclosed, it always featured a hole large enough to admit a pig, which scavenged in the pit. Otherwise, residents in their homes defecated into pots emptied randomly outside each morning, urinated through the kitchen floor, or, if they lived "near the edge of town, they go into the nearest clump of bushes," the women squatting with their skirts arrayed about them in "as wide a circle as possible," while the men "simply go up and face the nearest bush, tree, or wall."[126]

Things were somewhat different in Manila. The Spaniards had built an underground sewer system there during the 1850s, but it lacked sufficient connection to individual toilets and the water needed to flush the wastes.[127] Most Manilans, especially the poor, deposited their wastes in the *esteros* in the hope that they would then flow to the Pasig and out to sea. What happened instead was that low tide drew everything in the canals through Manila's business district, "attended by all its disagreeable odors and unhealthful emanations."[128] "When the tide is out the black mud is tinged green with a disgusting slime," the *Manila Times* reported, "and the stench is horrible."[129] Americans quickly began to import home water filters and, like wealthy Manilans, sought out bottled water.[130] When Governor Taft arrived in Manila in 1900, he immediately wrote to a friend in Coronado, California, to inquire what the town did with

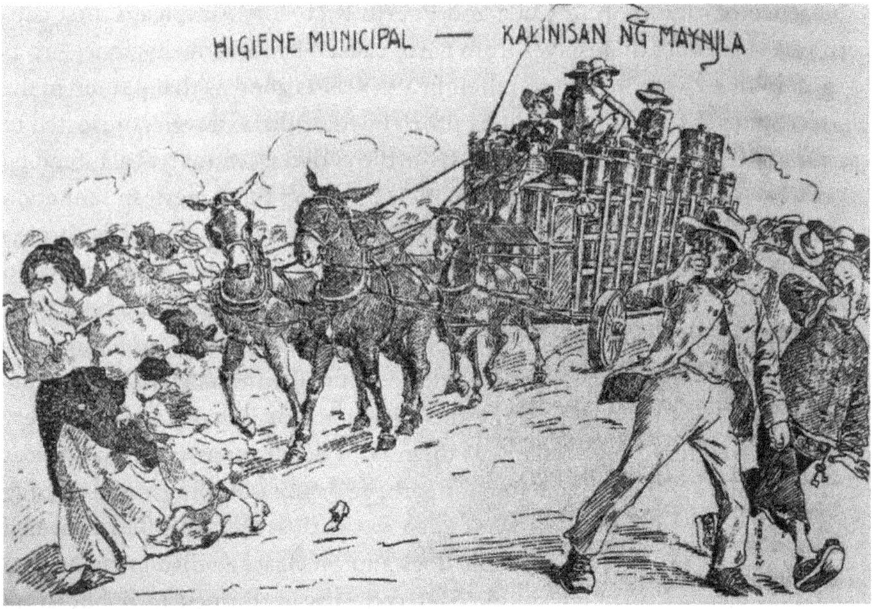

Figure 5.4 In the absence of sewers, human waste was carted through the city streets to the river or dumps on the outskirts. Here, a respectable-looking crowd flees the stench of a fully loaded wagon. The caption reads "Municipal Hygiene—Hygiene of the Man." Digitized by Dennis Villegas, http://pilipinokomiks.blogspot.com/2005/10/.

its sewage, hoping to create in Manila a system "by which the tide should carry it away" to the sea.[131] Two years later, Congress approved and the president signed a bill to provide funds to build sewers in Manila, but progress thereafter was slow.[132] In August 1903 the *Manila Times* complained that "the same old wooden pipes or boxes partially carry the sewage to the sluggish esteros, where it festers and pollutes the air that must be breathed by the city's population. . . . The noisome odor from any estero in this city should be ample warning that this sewerage cannot be exposed to the rays of a tropical sun without endangering everybody who comes within the range of the atmosphere vitiated by such agency."[133]

Dr. Victor G. Heiser, originally Manila's Chief Quarantine Officer and then the nation's Health Commissioner, was confident that he could "sanitate" Manila and the countryside beyond, and transform Filipinos from "the weak and feeble race we have found them into the strong, healthy and enduring people they may yet become." Heiser understood the connection between untreated human waste and cholera, and he was determined to build enclosed sewers to prevent further outbreaks of the disease.[134] Although Manila opened a new sewer system in May 1908, the system remained imperfect, and Heiser was still complaining about limited sewer hookups in his annual report four years later.[135]

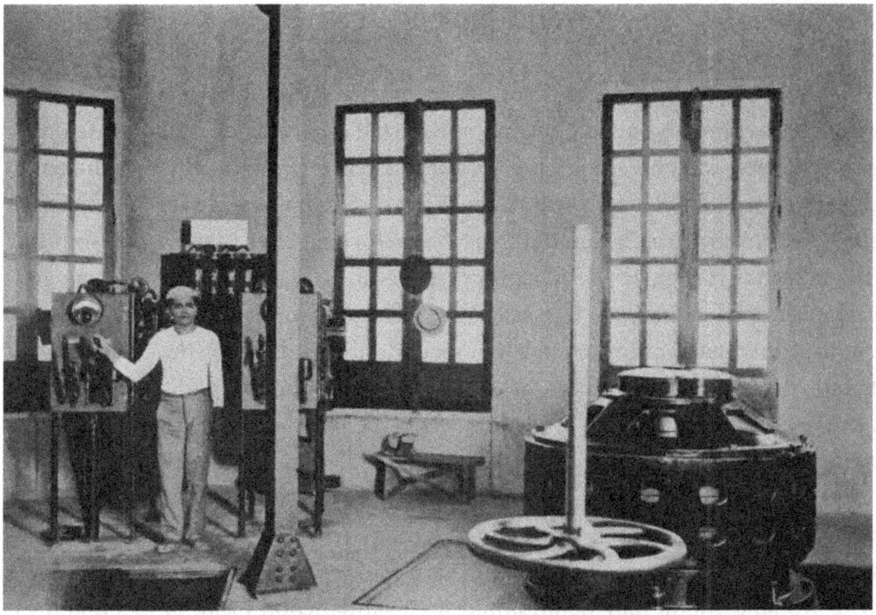

Figure 5.5 In contrast to the previous image, here is what the Americans hoped to do throughout the Philippines. This is a photograph of the Central Pumping Station at Tondo Beach, Manila. The interior of the facility is orderly and sparkling clean, even including the worker's shirt. Courtesy of the American Historical Collection, Rizal Library, Ateneo de Manila University.

Outside Manila, as Heiser and others studied toileting practices, they also collected thousands of fecal samples; in 1916, a sanitary commission found intestinal parasites in 98.7 percent of the 1,036 people it examined in Pasay.[136] Heiser worked with engineers to design toilets that contained bacteria and suppressed odor, assuming villagers used them properly. The Antipolo toilet, named for a city east of Manila, was introduced in the 1910s. It was a pit toilet with a drop of at least five feet, tightly covered (ideally, the lid closed automatically after use), secured against pigs, and vented above the roofline of the structure that held it.[137] Heiser expressed satisfaction with Antipolos in 1929, though he noted that they were said to "smell badly."[138] Two years later, Heiser wrote in his diary that engineers were experimenting with latrines bored directly into rock. He inspected several of them and "found none of them creating any nuisance or giving off odors," and was amused to see villagers building their own structures over them, providing "an outlet for the repressed artistic inclinations of the people."[139] By the 1930s, the government claimed to have built more than a hundred thousand latrines, and rural public health expenditures continued to increase dramatically. "The privy," concludes historian Warwick Anderson, "was nowhere more firmly affixed to the nation."[140]

The Subject Nose

Thus did Britons in India and Americans in the Philippines recoil against the odors of the land and people that no one foisted on them, represent those odors as uncivilized and dangerous, and set out to alter or eliminate them in the name of sanitation, health, and good taste. What did Indians and Filipinos think of the smells of their rulers and of the new olfactory regimes they tried to impose? The evidence is slight, but a few observations are possible. First, smell is in general important to Indians. Classical Sanskrit texts emphasize, for example, the connections between odor and memory, desire, and loss. The *Dharmaśāstra* (ninth century) characterizes as "stinking" the odors of garlic, onions, and human excrement, and the epic *Mahabharata* describes nine basic odors of the earth, among them "sweet" and "pungent." Stench denotes the "ritually impure," according to historian James McHugh, including carrion and the birds and animals that eat it. Children made ill by demons reek of blood, urine, or animal fat. Good smells are used in the performance of religious ritual; gods, and those who worship them, may be anointed with sandalwood paste or civet, and incense is generally present at the heart of Hindu shrines. And Hindus believe that the sense of déjà vu is triggered by scent. Odors allow those who smell them "to locate odorants in more complex schemes for classifying the world: divine and social hierarchies, cooling and heating, pure and impure, and so on."[141]

The Ongee people of India's Andaman Islands find their identity in their smell and the difference between it and that of others. When an Ongee wishes to refer to herself, she touches the tip of her nose, and when Ongee greet each other they ask, "How is your nose?" Ongee help those feeling " 'heavy' with odor" sniff some of it away; if one is, on the other hand, low on odor, an interlocutor will gently blow on him. Not just Ongee but many Indians prefer sniffing the head of a child returned from travel to hugging or kissing. This is consistent with a passage from the *Vedas*: "I will smell thee on the head; that is the greatest sign of tender love."[142]

The extent to which these practices persisted and retained meaning into the nineteenth and twentieth centuries, thus affecting colonial relations, is difficult to say. The English army doctor's servant for a time endured in silence the olfactory torments of entering a crowded British church on hot Sunday mornings. An East India Company factory was prevented from locating close to a mosque in Gujarat because, as a company official admitted, it "offended the moores [Muslims] especially our people pissing rudely and doing other filthiness against the walls," and Muslims in Aden objected to the carnal smell of smoke from nearby incinerators.[143] Auspicious occasions like weddings prompted the distribution to guests of silk handkerchiefs scented with sandalwood.[144]

Odor was, or became, an issue of class or caste, in which Indians who sought entrée into British society tried to demonstrate their own olfactory respectability and therefore their contempt for the insanitary habits of their less exalted countryfolk. In the early nineteenth century Sake Deen Mahomed, a former soldier from Patna, established the Indian Vapour Baths and Shampooing Establishment in the seaside town of Brighton. He persuaded Britons that a steam bath, followed by massage, would relax muscles because the waters were permeated with "sweet-smelling" herbs brought from India. Like British sanitation experts in Indian villages, Thakore Saheb walked through a London neighborhood near the Thames in 1883, and recoiled at the filth he saw and smelled there.[145] George Orwell's novel *Burmese Days* imagines the Indian doctor Veraswami complaining to a British friend about his South Asian patients: "As the last patient disappeared the doctor sank into his chair, fanning his face with the prescription-pad. 'Ach, this heat! Some mornings I think that never will I get the smell of garlic out of my nose! It iss [*sic*] amazing to me how their very blood becomes impregnated with it. Are you not suffocated, Mr. Flory? You English have the sense of smell almost too highly developed. What torments you must all suffer in our filthy East!' 'Abandon your noses, all ye who enter here, what? They might well write that up over the Suez Canal.' "[146] Proverbs collected by British officials seeking an "authentic" voice suggested olfactory sensitivity. "A low caste man is like a musk-rat," went one. "If you smell him you remember it."[147]

For the Philippines, the evidence concerning smell is skimpier. The nineteenth-century French visitor Jean Mallat claimed that Filipinos boasted of their keen sense of smell, and found servants who said they could recognize an employer's newly laundered shirts by their distinctive odor and men and women who asked for a shirt from their lover, to be exchanged for another when the first had lost its scent.[148] In the Danasalan market, an American observed a Filipina sniffing a number of frying hotcakes before deciding which one to buy, it having "passe[d] the censorship of her olfactory nerves."[149] Carabao reportedly disliked the odor of Americans.[150] "Filipinos," writes historian Ambeth Ocampo, "venture on a typology based on smell: Indians approximate spicy curry, Americans are supposed to reek of beef, Thais exude the aroma of patis (fish sauce), and so on. But ask Filipinos to describe the typical Filipino scent and they will reply that we don't smell because we bathe every day."[151] It is possible to imagine the Filipino reaction to the widespread use by Americans of cologne, to Americans' body odor, their canned imported food, the "beery" smell of Manila's commercial Escolta after 1898, and chemicals, including carbolic acid, used frequently by the Americans to disinfect houses, boats, and hospitals.[152] And there is this: in late 1934, Rep. Vicente Rama launched a broadside against the last American governor, Frank Murphy, excoriating him for his unwillingness to approve laws sent to him by the Philippines legislature demanding immediate independence. Rama charged Murphy with false piety, with being a "devil" in a "monk's robe" seeking to gull the people. But Murphy could not escape his true nature; he was betrayed by "the smell of the vestry cockroach about him."[153]

6

Touching, Feeling, and Healing

Hapticity and the Hazards of Contact

> The experience of India was . . . perceived to be written on the Anglo-Indian physique, from the boils, mosquito bites and the altered composition of the fibres and tissues of the body, to the colonists' characteristic clothing and confident demeanour.
>
> —E. M. Collingham, *Imperial Bodies* (2001)

> It is often forgotten that in the name of public health the state is licensed to palpate, handle, bruise, test, and mobilize individuals, especially with those deemed dangerous, marginal, or needy.
>
> —Warwick Anderson, *Haunted by Empire* (2006)

Imagine the body moved to a new and wholly different place, from a damp, cool environment of light-skinned people staying more or less in line on the street or pavement as they rode or walked, to a warm, humid land where animals joined dark-complexioned humans in a jostling scrum. Where sudden encounters with alien bodies happened with some frequency. Where insects collided with skin, rain poured down like a waterfall, and the surface of the earth was broken and irregular, causing walkers to stumble and riders in conveyances constantly to bounce. And where, most of all, the body came in contact with other bodies suspected of carrying sickness that seemingly could be transmitted through the merest brush of skin. India and the Philippines were for their British and American interlopers empires of profound physical and psychological anxiety, and nothing made empire's agents more anxious than the fear that their bodily boundaries might be trespassed, and thus violated, by the bodies of those they had come to rule.

Hapticity is the pauper and king of the senses. It is generally relegated to realm of the lower senses, beneath even smell and taste. Connected not to one organ or feature but to a network of nerve endings, touch lacks specificity or distinctiveness. Touch and feel tell the body nothing about objects at a distance, and the information they provide—is the surface rough or smooth, hot or cold?—seems trivial when compared to inputs received through eyes, ears, noses, and tongues. Yet while seeing is believing, as the saying goes in full, "touching is the truth."[1] Touch, argues scholar Yi-Fu Tuan, "is the sense least susceptible to deception"; direct haptic contact, the temperature, resistance, or pliability of an object, "is our final guarantee of the real."[2] Touch was of great importance in medieval Europe, where families shared a bed for warmth. The feel of one's clothing signified standing: the roughness of the cloth worn by peasants indicated their alleged coarseness, while the silk that enveloped the skin of the wealthy suggested their refinement and delicacy. By the mid-nineteenth century Europeans and Americans were washing their bodies more frequently, mostly to smooth their skins. The routine touching of others' bodies was viewed with suspicion, suggesting dangerous intimacy, effeminacy, or the felt necessity of crowding together, skin to skin—a sign of poverty or depravity. The growing denigration of touch, accompanied by the elevation of sight and hearing, could not reduce its apparent power to do harm; touch retained a fearful power. The treatment and condition of the skin, its texture, permeability, sensitivity, and exposure, said a good deal about the level of civilization of its inhabitant. No respectable people would allow their skin to stay rough or dirty, to be encased in clothing that might abrade or irritate or overheat. Those who allowed such abuses of their skin, or whose skins permitted such abuses, were members of "primitive races." And, as germ theory gradually took hold in the late nineteenth and early twentieth centuries, a terrible reality became clear: touching the wrong thing or a diseased person could sicken or kill.[3]

The metaphors used to describe empire were frequently haptic. India and the Philippines were held, grasped, and gripped, and their people, Anglo-Americans claimed, clung to their masters with a tenacity that revealed their gratitude for a civilized presence—but that could also weaken the connection. Viceroy Lord Curzon insisted that "every nerve a man may strain, every energy he may put forward cannot be devoted to a nobler purpose than keeping tight the cords that hold India to ourselves."[4] For the viceregal councilor Sir Bampfylde Fuller the lessons of such physical dependency were otherwise: "India enfeebles white races that cling to her breasts," he warned.[5] Corruption at all levels, from venal government officials to servants skimming a few pice or pesos from the household budget, was known as "the squeeze" and considered common practice in India and the Philippines.[6] Filipinos were to be "led by the hand" by the Americans out of the uncivilized darkness, or, more ambitiously, "lifted from the slough of ignorance and filth in which they have wallowed for centuries."[7] In places where the economic "field" was difficult to keep "smooth" for the "merchants who played ball," where poverty and sloth too often remained "untouched," and where colonists and "natives" alike had a tendency to lose their "hold on religion and morality," it was imperative for the agents of empire to stay in touch, maintain their grip, and hold tightly to their colonies and their elusive and dangerous yet physically dependent residents.[8]

The skin offered some protection against bodily violation, but it was no armor. It could be burned by wind and sun, stung by insects, made to smart by a blow, made to bleed with a prick or stab or shot. Worst of all, it could be penetrated or breeched by an organism held in the alien body of an Asian and too small to be noticed until its pathogenic effects became manifest in the unwitting western victim. For this reason, Britons and Americans sought to remove themselves as far as possible from contact with Indians and Filipinos.

Yet the Anglo-Americans, Victorians and Progressives, would not be content with haptic withdrawal. They had come to civilize their subjects, and having moved to make them legible, audible, and less odorous, their mission became the supremely important one of smoothing and healing their land and curing and preventing disease. The British and Americans were in the first instance concerned with their own safety, with policing their own bodily membranes against disruption or encroachment. But this determination was never wholly distinct from their desire to cleanse, soften, purify, and heal the terrain and bodies of others, as a way to protect themselves and as a way to do good in the empire, thereby fulfilling their philanthropic mission.

The Haptic Menace of Nature

Anglo-Americans arriving in their Asian colonies noticed at once the inhospitability of the land itself. Surfaces were torn and rough. When it was dry, dust rose from roads and pathways; when it rained, the same thoroughfares turned into quagmires of mud. Steep mountains defied efforts to move quickly over the terrain, while travelers stuck fast in swamps or sank helplessly into a muck of rotting vegetation. The land shook with volcanoes and earthquakes. At Naini Tal, India, in late September 1880—the morning after census takers had counted the town's population—an earthquake cast the public library into a lake, buried a hotel, destroyed scores of houses, and killed hundreds.[9] In January 1911, Luzon's Taal volcano erupted with "the loudest noise in the world," after which "the ground shook and the earth opened," killing at least 1,340.[10] The Americans found most of the buildings in the archipelago rickety and poorly maintained, and attributed this in part to the unstable "climatological and telluric conditions of the country."[11]

The British dreaded to travel across India. "The jungle was silent and savage," wrote a correspondent. "If one of those brutal little bushes but caught a hold of you, how he tore and scratched and bled you." Roads were cratered, pitted, and strewn with rocks, and the means of transport were ill-suited to them.[12] Travelers walked, rode horses, elephants, and camels, sat in carts and carriages of various constructions, and were borne by coolies in sedan chairs ("these fellows shook me to pieces," lamented Juxon Jones; "I did little else but vomit the whole way from Sirsa to Hansir").[13] "Travel was glamorous only from a distance," Margaret MacMillan has written. "The reality, for all the privilege, was generally slow, dirty, uncomfortable, and sometimes dangerous." Riders "bounced and rattled from side to side in anything from a bullock-drawn cart to a horse-drawn carriage."[14] Perhaps the land itself could be healed, as if it were a body. Lord Dalhousie, who served as Governor General just before the Great Rebellion, attempted to put in place an ambitious program of public works, including road improvements, bridge and canal building, and the construction of railroads.[15] Some progress was made. Near the civil lines of several towns prisoners were employed to repair roads, and in Ahmedabad in the early 1880s women dispensed water from enormous "water-skins" to reduce dust and keep surfaces smooth.[16] Railroad mileage would treble in the last two decades of the nineteenth century, and passengers would praise the trains for their relative comfort and efficiency.[17]

On the whole, however, progress on transport was maddeningly slow and seemed to Britons evidence of the intractability of the Indian landscape. From Mowana in 1878, Mrs. Robert Moss King reported: "In camp again. The roads worse than ever—unmetalled and nothing but rows of deep ruts. It is impossible to drive a pair [of horses], so we put in one horse and go about five miles an hour; we were obliged to get five or six coolies to push in several places where there were deep sand-drifts over the road."[18] Thousands of miles south, the tea planter J. L. H. Williams recalled that the roads in rural Travancore "were very poor, bad and holey surfaces and dusty with volumes of white dust." It took many hours to go from the nearest town to his settlement, though the distance was only twenty miles.[19] The arrival of automobiles did not necessarily make things easier. "Mum, you'd scream if you could see some of the obstacles the poor old car has to tackle," Carol Hyde wrote her mother in England. "We always have to carry a pick axe with us, and quite often the two servants have to use it on the hard clay to level up the ruts two or three feet deep. Sometimes we cross rivers that go along dips in the road, and we have to pick our way over boulders to reach the water, struggle through mud and stones and goodness knows what to get to the other side, then up an unbelievable slope to reach the level again!"[20] Jack Gibson's short ride over "the most awful roads" resulted in a dismembered front bumper and the car grounded out with its exhaust pipe under water.[21] Even the Delhi to Rajasthan train seemed no match for the land it bisected, "jolting," plunging down declines, and hopping on its imperfect rails.[22]

In the Philippines, the conveyance of choice for Americans and middle-class Filipinos was the *carromata,* a horse-drawn wooden cart with bare iron wheels. "There may be vehicles which jar one more than a carromata," wrote

John Bancroft Devins, "but they have not come under this writer's observation."[23] As in India, roads in the Philippines in the later nineteenth century were narrow, mostly unpaved, and barely maintained. In 1898, the American Consul in Manila lamented that the miserable condition of the islands' roads illustrated the indifference to progress of both Spaniards and Filipinos. There was hardly a roadway anywhere that allowed the easy passage of a cart or carriage, which meant that almost all commercial traffic went by water.[24] The cobbled streets of Manila made the jolting worse, such that ambulances had to slow down in order to avoid further injury to their passengers.[25] Governor Taft arrived in the Philippines in June 1900 determined to address the situation. The first act approved by the Philippines Commission was a million dollar appropriation for building and improving roads.[26] Taft and others planned to modernize the islands with infrastructure. "Roads are the great civilizers if history is any guide," asserted Bishop Charles Henry Brent.[27]

Problems arose almost immediately. Washington stinted with money, and officials in Manila found that the needs for ongoing pacification, sanitation, and public health, among others, competed with roads for resources. But nature proved the most serious obstacle. The weather conspired against the modernizers: typhoon rains washed away road beds, the heat caused asphalt and tar to melt, and steep mountains and ravines challenged engineers and increased costs. Maintenance was a nearly constant task.[28] "I traveled yesterday over a road in Cavite province which was supposed to be kept in repair in which I stuck in the mud five times and nearly lost two horses," complained David Barrows, the islands' education director, in mid-1909.[29] Taft contemplated railroads, eying the British example in India, but found it hard to persuade investors to build beyond the environs of Manila.[30] Members of the government who liked to retreat to the cool hill station at Baguio were disappointed for years by the failure of efforts to construct either road or railway through the hard country that separated it from Manila, a distance of less than 130 miles.[31]

As Governor beginning in 1909, William Cameron Forbes made road building his chief task. Forbes substituted concrete or macadam for asphalt as a building material, and he assembled corps of Filipino *camineros* (road laborers) to maintain the roads, assigning each man a kilometer and supplying him with a cart or bamboo box filled with stone, a shovel, and instructions to repair any holes that appeared.[32] Forbes contrasted the well-built and maintained roads he demanded with those that had thus far escaped his notice, or were under the authority of an indifferent local official, or from which the *camineros* had fled. "The difference between American and native administration is nowhere more evident than on the roads," he wrote. "In the center of towns, where the municipal *presidentes* are supposed to maintain the roads, and where they are most used, there were puddles and holes, no ditches, and generally a mess. We had to slow

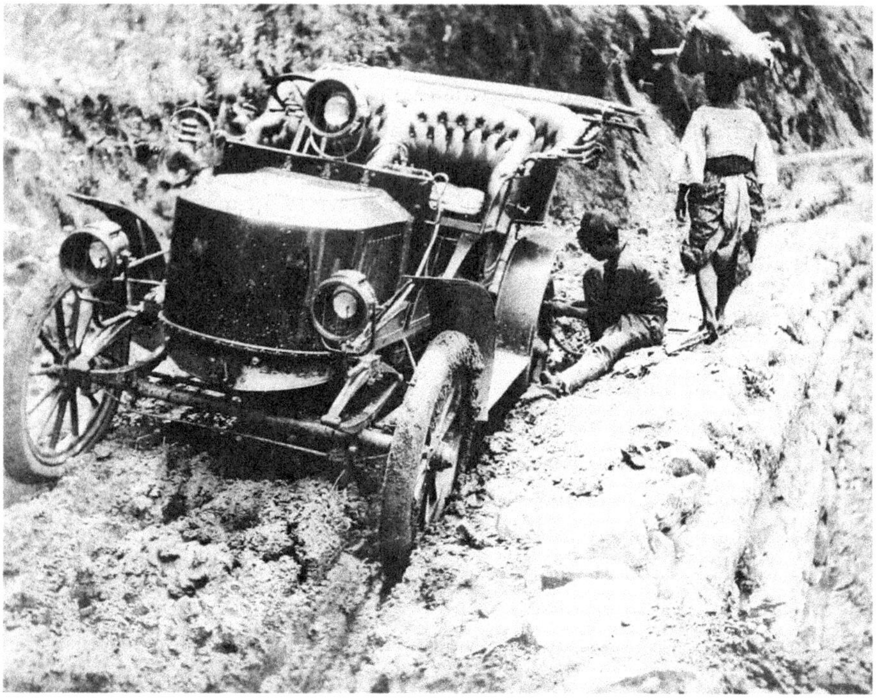

Figure 6.1 Stuck in the muddy ruts of the Benguet Road, the final leg of the journey from Manila to the hill station of Baguio. Courtesy of the American Historical Collection, Rizal Library, Ateneo de Manila University.

up and still got jolted to the sky. Upon reaching the outskirts of town, the fair, white-crowned, and ditched road would begin . . . and jolting and jarring ceased, and the world flew or flowed by."[33] Forbes insisted that officials accompany him as he drove over provincial roads, calling their attention to every bump.[34] Road mileage in the archipelago grew quickly under Forbes's leadership.[35] "It was the keenest satisfaction to me," Forbes wrote in his journal, "one of the pleasantest things that I can remember having happened to me, to have seen this policy beginning to take form and bear fruit. It worked wonders for the people and justified itself many times over."[36]

If the surface of the land could in theory be smoothed and healed, it was harder to reform the air that surrounded residents of India and the Philippines. In the cities, on the plains, in swamps and jungles, transplanted Anglo-Americans complained constantly about the heat. The sun seemed to strike them physically. "When you walk out of the customs shed into the sun of India it hits you like a blow, and it continues to do that all through the years you're in India," recalled a Briton. "Every time you walk out of doors during the middle of the day you feel as if you've been hit by something."[37] An American doctor questioned by the

First Philippines Commission about the effects of the sun acknowledged that it was "always dangerous," and that during his time in the islands he had "felt it very much."[38] The heat in both countries exhausted visitors. Maria Jane Jewsbury arrived in Bombay, "alias biscuit-over, alias brick-kiln, alias burning Babel alias Pandemonium, alias everything hot, horrid, glaring barren, dissonant, and detestable"; John Scott wished "to take off one's skin, and sit in one's bones"; and Fanny Parks confessed: "this heavy, unnatural atmosphere overpowers me. . . . The air is so oppressive, it appears full of dust, so white, so hot!"[39] Experts believed that women and children were especially susceptible to injury from the heat. One insisted that European women in a hot climate were "peculiarly liable to menstrual derangement and uterine disease," while another advised women with "uterine disorders" or who were "anaemic or sallow" not to go to India at all.[40] British children born in India were sent to live with relatives in England, partly because the heat was said to cause them to "deteriorate physically and morally" and made them likely to grow up "slight, weedy, and delicate" and unable to tell right from wrong, "deceitful and vain, indisposed to study, and to a great extent unfitted to do so."[41] In the Philippines, Americans found the heat unyielding for days on end.[42] And the humidity was remorseless, the air absent "any crispness" and "lack[ing] tone and brace."[43] Shirts stuck to backs, postage stamps to each other, leather and cloth grew moldy and sour.[44] "Never have I seen a man suffer more than Mr. Taft at Ilagan," wrote Dean Worcester of the Philippine Commission's 1901 tour of the Cagayan Valley. "The air was suffocating. My bed was in a corner. I dragged it out between a window and a door and threw both wide open. Still I could not sleep. Slipping off my pajamas, I seated myself on the broad window sill. The heat was intolerable. I poured water over myself and resumed my seat by the window. . . . I sat there until morning, as I could not endure the heat lying down."[45]

The atmosphere was not merely uncomfortable but dangerous, or so the Anglo-Americans believed. Whites claimed to be debilitated by the tropical climate. They feared that the heat and humidity abetted sickening miasmas that rose from the ground. James Johnson blamed "vegeto-animal miasmata" for the "foetid exhalations" that afflicted Europeans with fevers and other "malignant diseases," while James Ranald Martin, in his *Notes on the Medical Topography of Calcutta,* found the land itself "most deadly," the source of miasmas "summoned up by tropical humidity and a powerful sun, wafted along on insalubrious winds, or rising up in invisible clouds" from the rotting Indian earth.[46] The Philippines Commission concluded that the heat "interferes with the process of digestion," leading inevitably to diarrhea. "People who have lived here a long time gradually grow pale," the Commission explained, evidently without reference to the millions of Filipinos.[47] Testifying before Congress concerned about reports of American military atrocities in the islands, General Arthur MacArthur, who commanded US forces there 1900–1902, seemed to blame the climate for any soldierly indiscretions:

> Under the influence of the far-eastern sun the heated imagination had a boundless scope for indulgence of the boldest assumptions. Discrimination and sound judgment were taxed to the limit in order to reach anything like a conservative conception of the situation, which was filled with paradoxical suggestions and apparently hopeless conclusions. Visible indications manifested themselves which were incongruous with each other and irreconcilable with facts regarded of reliable record and which generally accepted as the bases of important deductions in the premises.[48]

Britons and Americans did what they could to combat the exhausting climate. The British used large fans (*punkahs*), *khus khus tatties*, which were bundles of grass fixed to the outside of windows and kept wet to cool incoming breezes, and thermantidotes, boxes with treadle fans enclosed with moistened *tatties*. All of these devices relied for their use on coolie laborers, who had to keep fans moving manually and water the *tatties* day and night.[49] Taft installed electric fans in his house in Manila, but these were subject to the vagaries of the city's power supply.[50] It would be decades before air conditioning arrived in India or the Philippines.[51]

If the air in most of India and the Philippines felt hot, still, and heavy with moisture, it was nevertheless hectic with flying, buzzing insects. Locusts filled the air, swarmed heedless into faces, and destroyed wheat and rice crops and their seed.[52] Moths "flew in to commit suicide against one's lamps"; scorpions and centipedes sheltered in shoes and delivered painful stings or bites. There were flies of many types, including biting sandflies and flies drawn perversely to eyes, and beetles that "banged into everything, until some heavy collision deposited them on the floor, normally upside down with their legs waving helplessly in the air"—and "squash[ing] them left a horrid stain" and "a very nasty smell."[53] Ants delivered burning bites and chewed through paper, wood, plaster, even tin cans.[54] Herbert Thompson hung his mackintosh on a peg in a whitewashed wall. When he retrieved it a few minutes later, he found that white ants had eaten away the lining.[55] There were cockroaches, grasshoppers, wasps, termites that silently bored into wood, causing furniture to collapse unexpectedly under those sitting on it, and ubiquitous fleas.[56] Most dangerous were the mosquitoes, whose bite was by the beginning of the twentieth century implicated in malaria. There were few window screens in India or the Philippines, and mosquitoes dismayed residents with their ability to resist insecticides and penetrate the netting that Britons and Americans erected over their beds.[57]

Other animals brought their own haptic annoyances and dangers. Carol Hyde's tent was invaded one night by frogs, one of which jumped into her pajama pants and left her queasy.[58] All mammals were susceptible to rabies, though the wild dogs in Indian and Filipino villages were most often infected. Britons still could not always resist them; Jackie Smyth admitted that she lost four dogs to rabies, and worried with each death that she had been licked by one of them.[59] Snakes alarmed westerners. Not all were poisonous—at Grace Paulding's house in the Luzon countryside a king snake living between the sail cloth ceiling and the thatched roof kept the rat population down—but the kraits, coral snakes, and especially cobras created a good deal of anxiety in both places.[60] Kipling's story "Rikki-Tikki-Tavi" captured this fear: "Then inch by inch out of the grass rise up the head and spread hood of Nag, the big black cobra, and he was five feet long from tongue to tail. . . . He looked at Rikki-tikki with the wicked snake's eyes that never change their expression, whatever the snake may be thinking of."[61]

The Hygienic Self, the Pathological Other

Neither Britons nor Americans ever absolved the tropics for their discomforts and their illnesses. The terrain of their Asian colonies defied costly and strenuous efforts to heal it. Miasmas, exaggerated by the hot, wet climate, remained suspect in disease. There would always be insects and other irritating (or worse) fauna. But increasingly, as the twentieth century dawned on empires in sensory flux, westerners more and more assigned responsibility for the threats to their bodies to Indians and Filipinos and the invisible menace they carried. Physical contact with primitive people transmitted sickness; actually touching them threatened trespass of civilized bodily membranes. The germ theory shaped this perception, as did the related ascription of pollution to racial Others.[62] The British and Americans sought in the first place to remove themselves as far as possible from contact with their subjects, having decided that Indian and Filipino bodies, more than "miasmatic fluxes," were the true repositories of disease.[63] The touch of the Other was defiling. It demanded disinfection.[64]

The rising fear of touching unclean subjects accompanied growing alarm concerning crowds. Conservatives had long mistrusted mobs, but by the end of the nineteenth century they were joined by progressives on both sides of the Atlantic, who worried not solely about the political power of the masses but who also preferred not to rub against them, or who were suspicious of excessive physical contact. French sociologist Gustave Le Bon published *The Crowd: A Study of the Popular Mind* in 1895. "Civilisations as yet have only been created and directed by a small intellectual aristocracy, never by crowds," he wrote. "Crowds are only powerful for destruction. Their rule is always tantamount to a barbarian phase"—a judgment that echoed the views of imperialists.[65] In late nineteenth-century Britain and the United States, middle-class whites found in crowds, undifferentiated as they were by race and class, the source of their dread of pollution and miscegenation.[66] Imperial behavior in India and the Philippines reflected these concerns. Bernard Cohn has observed that the British in India tended to survey their colony "from above and at a distance"—astride a horse or an elephant, from a carriage or a railway car. "They were uncomfortable in the narrow confines of a city street, a bazaar, a *mela* [fair]—anywhere they were surrounded by their Indian subjects."[67] Following the 1919 police massacre of hundreds of Indians gathered in a public garden in Amritsar, the word "crowd" appeared 280 times in the 175-page self-exculpatory British report on the incident.[68] Assigned to the first Philippine Commission, Daniel Williams was buffeted by the traffic, pedestrian and vehicular, in the streets of Manila, which remained always "in a state of constant turmoil and congestion."[69]

The subjects in these haptic exchanges had the curious advantage of relative invulnerability: unlike their refined conquerors, Indians and Filipinos were alleged to have coarse, tough skins, and were therefore imagined to be impervious to the kinds of physical insult that threatened Caucasians. Whites had long believed that dark skin was thicker and coarser than theirs. This was a myth with several sources, including the alleged nonchalance with which African Americans took beatings, the apparent ability of dark-skinned people to manage life under a tropical sun, and even the supposed "nervelessness" of the Chinese, extended to other Asians, regarded altogether an unfeeling race.[70] "So very long it took me to shake off my . . . assumptions that the lower classes and the coloured races didn't 'feel' things the same way, having simple nervous systems, like lobsters," recalled Iris Macfarlane.[71] Most Indians slept on some version of a *charpoy*, a wooden frame interlaced with slats or crosshatched with rough fabric and perhaps a thin mattress. Britons complained about having to use these "hard wooden beds . . . with a thin and ancient mattress, through which the wooden frame showed like the ribs of an old cab-horse."[72] Indian skin seem unaffected by proximity to coarse fabrics that would have chafed Britons, and the near-nudity of Indian manual laborers was startling in the way it exposed workers to the harsh elements, evidently without harming them.[73] Most of all, the insensitivity of Indian skin suggested an indifference to civilized forms of discipline and the futility of getting soldiers and servants to do one's reasonable bidding in the absence of physical punishment. The stories are depressingly similar: Flora Annie Steel, using a whip, "belaboured" a male servant "with it till I nearly dropped, he shrieking in terror that a female demon had got him"; high-caste men whom the British took pains to punish in public "where their shame would be seen by all," including the local prostitutes; village "agitators" given six blows each on their bottoms, then left in an agony that puzzled D. H. Biscoe until he learned that "the stripes were inflicted with the branches of a certain tree which, the recipients believed, rendered a man impotent."[74] Evelyn Beeton recalled with apparent satisfaction that her two riding whips "returned to England bent and broken," the result of her having "hit these lazy beggars"—her servants—"as though they were dogs."[75] Reformers had tried in the mid-nineteenth century to outlaw whipping in India, but the practice was still commonly used decades later.[76]

Americans in the Philippines also ascribed haptic insensitivity to their subjects. The "natives" slept on bamboo platforms, suffered pillows "stuffed with sawdust or something equally hard," and tolerated nights of sleeping on beds without mattresses, frames made of rattan with a sheet thrown over, or "just an arrangement of ropes and quilts folded over it and not too heavy ones, either," explained Grace Paulding. "You were lucky if you didn't wake up in the morning with a pattern pretty well printed on your body."[77] The president of the Pneumatic Mattress and Cushion Company tried to sell Governor Taft inflatable "Air Beds" for the soldiers, for "sleeping on damp ground has ended many a soldier's career."[78] Like Indians, Filipinos wore clothing the appearance of which abraded American sensibilities. Taft politely rebuffed a request from the wife of Henry Cabot Lodge for some *piña* cloth to make a dress; it was, the governor wrote, "like a coat of armor" and unsuitable for clothing an American.[79] Other fabric was "starched with rice and stands out rigidly" against the skin, or made from the maguey cactus, and John Clifford Brown saw a Filipino wearing a suit of bamboo.[80] Filipino hygiene experts warned against the practice of applying to the skin of babies heated coconut shells or leeches, said to prevent convulsions, and advised instead daily ice rubs and massage.[81] Like their British counterparts, Americans beat their servants for seeming "impertinent."[82]

In February 1906, a group of American scientists working for the Philippines Government Bureau of Science published the first issue of *The Philippine Journal of Science*, meant to provide a forum for their research on tropical health and medicine. One of the subjects of greatest interest to journal authors was the effect of the tropical climate on whites, and the apparently greater facility with which darker-skinned people functioned in it. Studies ruled out the popular claim that brunettes fared better than blonds in the tropics.[83] An experiment by Hans Aron found that while brown skin heated more quickly than white, it also began to sweat earlier, cooling the skin with perspiration. It may have been that the color of the skin itself made the difference, though Aron also considered the possibility that "the negro has larger and better developed sweat glands than the white man." Whatever the cause, wrote Aron, "it seems to me that the brown man is superior to the white in this economy of sweating."[84] That opaque skin helped people endure the heat of the tropics indicated a particular kind of superiority, but also confirmed the imperviousness of their bodies to physical and moral refinement and haptic sensitivity.

The chief physical distinction whites made between themselves and those with dark skins was that between the clean and dirty body. William Cohen has defined filth as "a term of condemnation, which instantly repudiates a threatening thing, person or idea by ascribing alterity to it. . . . That which is filthy is so fundamentally alien that it must be rejected; labeling something filthy is a viscerally powerful way of excluding it."[85] Britons and Americans claimed to be clean, while Indian and Filipino "natives" were inhumanly filthy. While Indians and Filipinos, the Anglo-Americans admitted, seemed to bathe more often than their conquerors, their bathwater—often a river or a village tank—was itself unsanitary, as anyone could smell. The "natives" had no soap or used the wrong sort. Even if bodies were clean, the clothes that covered them were not. Above all, the habits of Indians and Filipinos were filthy. It did no good, westerners claimed, to bathe, then consort with animals, defecate in the open and fail to clean oneself or the site immediately after, handle garbage and scatter it, eat with one's fingers on poorly washed dishes, smother the body with strong scent, linger near the sick and the dead, and even touch cow dung or night soil. No amount of bathing compensated for the primitive social practices of millennia. The dirt people generated and with which they lived polluted them, and rendered them physical threats to the Britons and Americans who ruled them.

Whites had long regarded as defiling the touch of a person with dark skin. It was as if the darkness itself carried filth, or concealed it. Even dark skin might be cleaned. Soap, which was adopted for hygienic (rather than merely olfactory) reasons as part of Anglo-American bathing practices only in the last third of the nineteenth century, quickly became an object of fetish in the empire.[86] Advertisements for Pears' soap promised those with dark skins that they could wash off "the very stigma of racial and class degeneration," though the agents of empire were less sure of this.[87] Monica Clough, whose family lived in Madras State, recalled her mother's obsession with cleanliness: "contacts with Indian children were forbidden, and Indian food and water." "Don't touch it, it's come from the bazaar," was her refrain, and she, like most *memsahibs,* insisted on washing nearly everything in potassium permanganate. Clough suspected that her mother's hygienic fears were rooted in "racial hostility."[88] When Maria Jones sent her daughter Minnie to school in Simla, she warned her against contact with Indians and even Eurasians who worked there: "Don't kiss Miss Byrne or let her kiss you. . . . I would just as soon you kissed the Mehta"—the sweeper, lowest on the ladder of caste.[89] In the United States, racism was grounded in anxieties about "mixing" and pollution taboos. With respect to the Philippines, an 1898 cartoon, titled "Cares of a Growing Family," depicted President William McKinley looking vexed as he contemplated sullen and dark-skinned representatives of Puerto

Rico, Cuba, and the Philippines while seated on a box marked "Soap: Have You Tried It?"[90] Soon after arriving in the archipelago, Bishop Brent ordered a case of soap to treat the "skin troubles" of the rural people.[91]

In so many ways, insisted the Anglo-Americans, Indians and Filipinos were anathema to civilized touch. Robert Minturn recoiled at rubbing up against "oily, black bodies" in Bombay harbor.[92] Britons coming to India were cautioned to avoid unnecessary contact with the inhabitants. One should "never shake hands with an Indian," insiders advised, "because you never know where his hand has been."[93] Britons watched, appalled, as an Indian servant used his fingers to put ice in drinks or held a mixing bowl between his feet while he "mixed a cake with his hands. I was assured that he had washed them with soap," wrote Irene Bose, but "with a dark skin it was impossible to tell."[94] Margery Hall was frequently traumatized by the behavior of her servants in remote Jacobabad. She discovered that the family driver, who had put her children on his knee while he drove, had syphilis, and later learned that her cook had been entertaining a

(a)

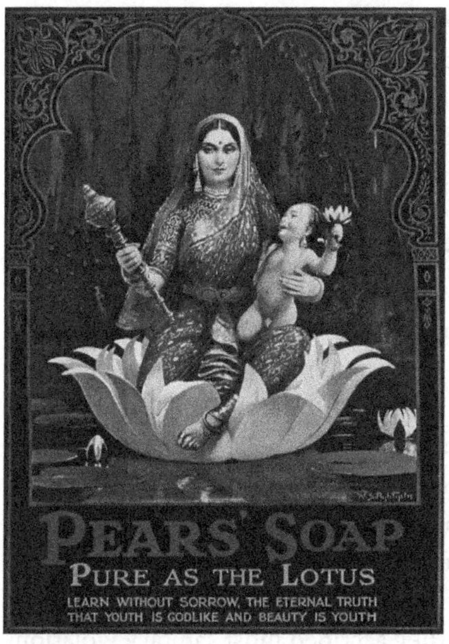
PEARS' SOAP
PURE AS THE LOTUS
LEARN WITHOUT SORROW, THE ETERNAL TRUTH
THAT YOUTH IS GODLIKE AND BEAUTY IS YOUTH

(b)

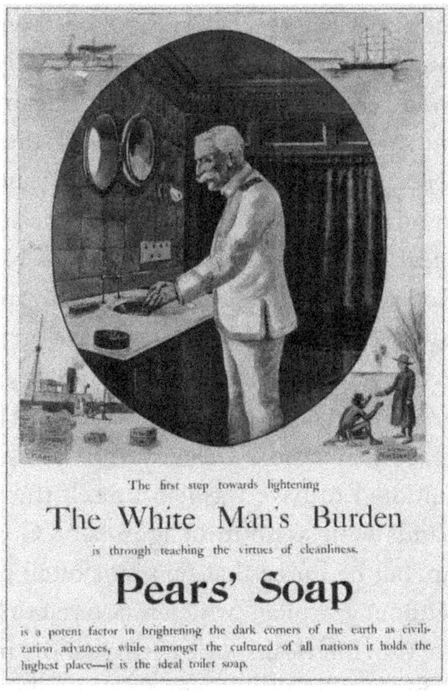
The first step towards lightening
The White Man's Burden
is through teaching the virtues of cleanliness.
Pears' Soap
is a potent factor in brightening the dark corners of the earth as civilization advances, while amongst the cultured of all nations it holds the highest place—it is the ideal toilet soap.

Figures 6.2a and 6.2b Two images praising the benefits of Pears' Soap. The first shows the goddess Lakshmi, seated on a lotus, holding her very white baby, presumably purified with soap. The second is of a white-clad Admiral Dewey washing with Pears, thus "lightening the White Man's Burden" even in "the dark corners of the earth as civilization advances." A missionary gives a bar to a loincloth-clad "native." Top: Courtesy Alamy Images. Bottom: Wikimedia Commons.

"bazaar prostitute" in the house. She directed the servants to "take the bed to pieces. Boil it and the webbing in Phenyl Water. Burn the mattress. Wash all my possessions in disinfectant. Wash out the room with Phenyl."[95] When the Prince and Princess of Wales toured India in 1905, the government distributed a series of sanitary guidelines to those whose districts would host them. It was imperative to keep them away from sites of epidemic disease, to ensure that the houses they stayed in and their surroundings were "in a thoroughly sanitary condition," and that at assemblies, the dozens of members of princely entourages "be medically inspected every day."[96]

The American regime regarded Filipinos in much the same way: the men, women, and children of the archipelago were filthy. "One glance," wrote Emily Conger, "and there was a wild desire to take those dirty, almost nude creatures in hand and, holding them at arm's length, dip them into some cleansing caldron."[97] Robert Carter ranted in a letter to his father: "All natives are a walking bunch of sores, small pox, and leprosy. . . . The majority of the niggers have sores on their legs and feet. . . . I hate the sight of niggers and, although they are always bathing and are cleanly as people as far as washing goes, in other ways they are filthy. I avoid them like the plague."[98] "And oh! They are so dirty," complained the American teacher Harry Cole from Leyte. "Of course, they have not been taught any better, and so they can hardly be blamed, and yet I do not believe they would care to exert themselves to clean up. . . . Their habits are frightful."[99] Just as Indian servants touched food with their hands and feet, so did Filipino orange sellers placed their hot feet on the fruit to cool.[100] For years before they arrived in numbers in the Philippines, American men had shaken hands, a sign of respect, equality, and masculinity. On New Year's Day 1907, President Theodore Roosevelt would shake hands with over eight thousand people. (Secretly he hated it: "What a lot of bugs I have on my hands, and how dirty, filthy I am!")[101] While handshaking would become a common greeting in the islands, it was at first undertaken with some reluctance or confusion on the part of the Filipinos. Francis Harrison, the governor of the Philippines from 1913 to 1921, was rumored to have washed himself thoroughly with carbolic soap after shaking hands with a group of Igorots.[102] Governor Forbes apparently did not wash up, but he noted that Filipinos often proffered their left hands and "touch[ed] without grasping," which registered to him as unmanly.[103]

The Americans were perhaps more optimistic than the British that their Asian subjects might be taught cleaner habits. They ascribed most sanitary violations to the lower classes and rural people, which meant that a lack of hygiene was not inherent in the race as a whole. The Annual Report of the Bureau of Public Health for 1903–1904 admitted that many Filipinos possessed "insanitary habits which are the result of their oriental customs" and their ignorance of the causes of disease, and while it conceded that "racial habits and customs which have prevailed through centuries cannot be changed in a few years," it was "possible to improve them" over time.[104] Victor Heiser titled chapter 6 of his autobiography "Washing Up the Orient," and his text indicated that he thought he had to some extent succeeded in doing so in the Philippines. "We applied water, soap, and disinfectant rigorously," he wrote. "Whenever a ship came in from Hongkong or Amoy, the crews, many of whom had loathsome skin diseases due to filth, were scrubbed, sometimes forcibly." Filipinos refused to boil their water and insisted on dipping coconut halves into a common jar. High infant mortality resulted from violent or unsanitary delivery practices: when a baby got stuck, men tied a rope around the birth mother's waist and pulled, and midwives dressed umbilical cords with manure, killing many babies with tetanus. Heiser was fond of such horror stories, but he refused to believe that "the Oriental could not be sanitated." He issued instructions for the Manila food market, requiring that all entrants wash their hands in a barrel of mercury bichloride, providing forks to the butchers, and prohibiting the sale of "low-growing vegetables," which he believed were polluted with night soil. His "Knife and Fork" societies taught children table manners. And he presided over a public health program that included latrine-building, vaccination against disease, and, most ambitiously, a campaign to "collect" and quarantine the country's lepers.[105]

Heiser pursued his sanitation efforts through the schools. Authorities resolved to teach children hygienic practices and hoped that the lessons would go home to families, who were otherwise difficult to reach. Children were taught to eat with utensils, to brush their teeth, and not to touch animals immediately before eating. And they were to take care of their skin. It was important to bathe frequently, nude and with soap and if possible warm water. Each person should have a towel, washcloth, and "toilet articles" of their own. According to a popular textbook, "clothes should be clean. . . . We should not sleep in our underclothes or the clothes we have worn during the day, but change to night clothes. It is equally uncleanly to wear sleeping pajamas and nightgowns during the daytime."[106] Edward J. Murphy, the Superintendent of Education at Bagombong, managed some modest success in convincing local boys to bathe more often, despite the local custom not to do so between rice planting and harvesting. He wrote to David Barrows, "now they get off the biggest layers before they come to pay their respects."[107]

All the while, the British and the Americans policed their own delicate skins, evidently vulnerable to the menacing tropics. They donned hats and smoked glasses or goggles to avoid the damaging effects of the sun.[108] Men wore wool or silk hats on formal occasions, though they complained about the heaviness of both in the heat. Over time they reverted in large part to linen suits, always white.[109] And they were greatly concerned with their underwear, the cloth membrane they wore against skin that they sought to protect from their tropical clothing and the environment.[110] Linen underwear had become popular in Europe during the nineteenth century, but James Johnson advised against wearing it in India, recommending instead cotton, which "conducts more slowly the *excess* of external heat *to* our bodies."[111] British women were to buy their undergarments at home, as Indian versions were poorly made. The best fabric for them, according to Flora Annie Steel and Grace Gardiner, was silk or cotton blended with silk, and no woman should wear more than one undergarment, for piling them on "keeps in perspiration and conduces fatally to prickly heat."[112] Anne Wilson recommended "4 pair of medium fine drawers, 4 pair of medium thick merino knee drawers" (presumably for the hill stations), and "12 pair of white calico knee drawers," while some doctors insisted that flannel, despite its weight, absorbed perspiration better than other fabrics and was therefore preferable to them.[113]

William Howard Taft, who at well over three hundred pounds weighed more than twice the average American man, found his skin constantly irritated by the climate and the need to dress formally for official business. Six months after arriving in Manila, he ordered from a department store in his hometown of Cincinnati "a dozen suits of undershirts and drawers of very thin French balbriggan; size No. 50 for the drawers and 48 for the undershirts, 'short and stout.'" (He would order more drawers a year and a half later, remarkably requesting a larger size.)[114] Balbriggan was made in the eponymous Irish town, famous for its undergarments. Originally balbriggan drawers were made of wool, but by 1900 dress reform advocates were urging men to reject woolens, suspected of "clogging the pores of the skin, which was 'thus rendered incapable of performing'" its function as a "vomitory of impurities."[115] Taft asked for drawers made from woven Egyptian cotton, "soft finished" and with sateen waist bands and buttons made of pearl. *Vogue* magazine proclaimed in 1903 that these new "open mesh" underpants were "among the most healthful and sanitary of all kinds."[116] Others made do with less sophisticated underwear. Too often, wrote George Telfer, it "sticks to you and tears when you take it off," and while captured Spanish underclothing was reasonably well made it was, in Telfer's case, much too small.[117]

Medicalized Empires: Campaigns Against Illness and Disease

Liberal empire was a medical enterprise, the urgency of which was intensified by a mix of confidence and anxiety: confidence that grew from the presumed racial superiority and requirements of mission and reform harbored by

Anglo-Americans, anxiety borne of their tenuous presence in dangerous tropical lands, with their threatening nature, their reckless and ignorant and sickly people. Both feelings resided in the haptic. It was possible, westerners believed, to tame (though not master) nature through physical contact, by building straight flat roads and railroads, and by using technologies of touch—fans, mosquito nets, proper clothing—to mitigate the effects of climate. Physical contact might be made less dangerous by avoiding others, or otherwise by persuading subjects to keep themselves clean, to respect modern hygienic practice, to allow their tactile examination by medical practitioners, and to accept injections through the skin for infectious tropical diseases, thereby protecting their rulers and themselves. The diseased Other would be cured by the healing touch of the white, generally male, westerner, or by his colonial representative. Never mind that many of the diseases—smallpox, measles, syphilis—were brought to Asians by Europeans and North Americans; never mind that expanding trade networks and road building projects had by the nineteenth century spread disease vectors, among them fleas and lice, to areas previously free of epidemic scale disease. For Florence Nightingale, providing health care to Indians was "a noble task," a necessary act of civilization.[118] In the Philippines, wrote Victor Heiser, health authorities were "presented with a medical situation of unparalleled gravity; an entire nation had to be rehabilitated."[119] Confidently, anxiously, the Anglo-Americans moved to civilize and rehabilitate the dangerous bodies of their subjects.

They felt increasingly that they knew what they were facing. Norway's Armaeur Hansen found the leprosy bacterium in 1873; the German Robert Koch implicated bacteria in anthrax, tuberculosis, and cholera (the last while he was in India) during the 1880s; and Robert Ross, who was born in India and did much of his work there, discovered the malaria parasite in the gut of mosquitoes in the late 1890s. Even so, tropical medicine was recognized in Britain only in 1899, with the creation of schools dedicated to its study in London and Liverpool, and seven years later the US Army created the Board for the Study of Tropical Diseases as They Exist in the Philippine Islands.[120] Scientists and health workers clung to other theories, especially those blaming miasmas for illness, and as late as the 1920s British epidemiologist Sir Leonard Rogers persisted in finding correlations between rainfall and the incidence of leprosy and smallpox.[121] Local medical practices were largely dismissed by the British who, according to David Arnold, "mocked what they saw as the fatalism, superstition and barbarity of indigenous response to disease," though by the late nineteenth century they were encouraging the devolution of medical practice to Indian states and even smaller polities—something the Americans resisted in the Philippines.[122]

Isolation, Enclosure, Protection

Concerned most of all about their own health, Britons in the aftermath of the Great Rebellion and Americans arriving in the Philippines after 1898 tried so far as possible to distance themselves from physical contact with their subjects.[123] They closed their bodies against India and Indians, the Philippines and Filipinos. British military cantonments were self-contained communities, with their own sanitary facilities and markets and located well outside of Indian towns.[124] The bungalows designed for British residents stood back from the road, featured a monitored gate, a long drive up to the house, and a verandah to which most Indian visitors were restricted.[125] In the hot season, officers, officials, and their families retreated to hill stations in India's mountains. Simla, Mt. Abu, Darjeeling, Ootacamund, and Kodaikanal were havens for those, recalled a surgeon in Madras, "who are simply exhausted in mind and body from prolonged exposure to a high temperature in the low country, and who need rest from work and a cooler air to breathe."[126] The stations offered the company of other Britons and the relative absence of Indians. Britons also wrapped their bodies against the elements, hoping to tighten or thicken the barrier against hazard. Fearing the jolting of Indian roads and other shocks to their backs, the rays of the sun, or the presence of hidden microbes, British women dressed in layers of clothing, including corsets, and adopted cork "spine-protectors," worn under clothes from neck to mid-back, and flannel cummerbunds.[127] They hunched in armchairs over dinner, their "crinolines and petticoats" held snugly against them, as if to keep out the malignant air.[128] To their sun *topis* and goggles women and men added "cholera belts"; problems with one's bowels were frequently attributed to the failure to wear one of these.[129] All of these protections were meant to isolate or envelop the British in ways that would insulate them against undesirable contact.

The Americans, at times consciously following the British example, tried many of the same strategies for keeping themselves aloof from Filipinos. They kept to themselves in military camps and their homes, permitting Filipinos to enter their lines or residences only with permission and after inspection. Governor Taft summoned Daniel Burnham, the architect of the National Mall in Washington, to build a new Manila, and Burnham designed large plazas, parks, and wide avenues for human traffic, the better to prevent unwanted jostling with Filipinos.[130] Burnham also designed the American hill station at Baguio. Modeled deliberately on the British stations in India, Baguio offered relief from the heat of Manila, and American officials used it often, with some of them building bungalow-style houses there.[131] "I cannot say too much about the climate, surroundings, and beauty" of Baguio, Taft wrote to Henry Cabot Lodge. "It is the solution of the problem of retaining Americans in the service out here permanently." Manila had "a somber hue," but "with the opportunity to come up here for two or three months, or four months, in the year, a great change will be worked."[132] Dean Worcester, among the first Americans to explore Baguio, noted British statistics showing a decreased mortality rate for invalid troops allowed to recover in the hills.[133] British *topis* failed to catch on: the Americans substituted for them felt hats with sweat bands.[134] The Americans took readily to "stomach bandages," alleged to prevent cramps, vomiting, and diarrhea; Benjamin Neal reported that a fellow teacher had left his off one night and as a result was "taken sick in school" with dysentery.[135]

None of these strategies for isolation and enclosure worked. It was impossible to live in India and the Philippines and avoid contact with their environments and inhabitants. Verandahs notwithstanding, houses in the tropics were built on open plans to take best advantage of incoming breezes. This made privacy inside them problematic. Servants showed up constantly to touch their employers in bedrooms and bathrooms: the sahib needed dressing, the American commissioner required attendance in his bath. Servants

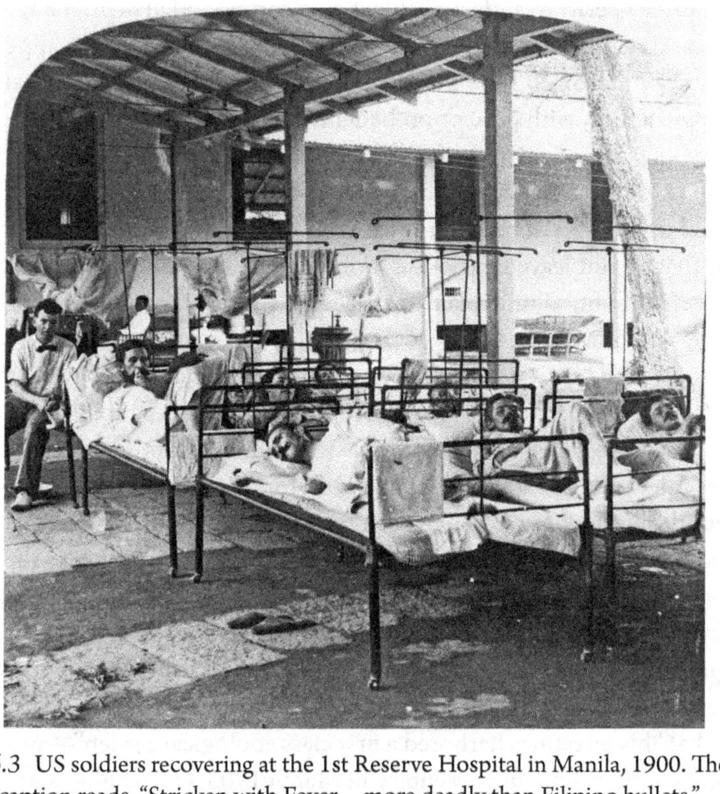

Figure 6.3 US soldiers recovering at the 1st Reserve Hospital in Manila, 1900. The original caption reads, "Stricken with Fever—more deadly than Filipino bullets." Courtesy of Library of Congress, Prints and Photographs Division.

generally disliked the relative cool of the hills, but the Anglo-Americans could not do without them there; the hill stations were shared, however grudgingly, with brown men and women.[136] As Iris Macfarlane observed, the British brought their values with them to India and "wore them as a protection like solar topees and veils, against the threatening hordes of the brown, the pagan, and the ignorant poor." They—and the same could be said of Americans in the Philippines—were "walled in, physically and mentally."[137] Or so they hoped. But they knew otherwise.

Diseases of the Skin

Deadly disease was the gravest threat to the imperialists, but it occurred far less frequently than ordinary afflictions of the skin. *Dhobi* itch, the scourge of soldiers, afflicted civilians too. The humidity caused prickly heat—"little pimples rising over every inch of the body so that you couldn't put a pin between a pimple"—which proved very hard to cure.[138] "The sensations arising from prickly heat are perfectly indescribable; being compounded of prickling, itching, tingling, and many other feelings, for which I have no appropriate appellation," wrote James Johnson. "I have tried lime juice, hair powder, and a variety of external applications, with little or no benefit."[139] People complained of bed bugs, boils, eczema, impetigo, and lice.[140] They dreaded small cuts or sores, which could quickly turn septic.[141] In the summer of 1901, Taft reported that he had been "laid up for a week with a tropical sore" on his big toe, and the doctor had insisted that he not leave the house. "Sores of that kind in this climate it is well to be careful about," Taft explained, "because they occasionally lead to blood-poisoning and other difficulties."[142]

Worse awaited him. That fall, Taft developed an ischiorectal abscess, the "poisoning from which," wrote his personal secretary, "spread so rapidly as to require surgery to remove gangrenous flesh." For twenty-four hours doctors were unsure whether Taft would live, according to his wife, for "the abscess was of long growth, the wound [incision] had to be made a terrible one, and there was great danger of blood poisoning." A second surgery was performed. Returning to the United States in early 1902 to recuperate, Taft had surgery once more. Rectal abscesses have several possible causes, all of them plausible in the early twentieth-century Philippines. Taft might have ingested harmful bacteria, such as E coli; he might have been exposed to it at banquets, and there was no cure for it. He told Victor Heiser that "his intestines harbored a first class zoological garden"—and indeed, he would contract amoebic dysentery in March 1903. Or the illness might have started with severe inflammation, brought on by hemorrhoids or persistent diarrhea. Friction from his heavy clothes and perspiration would have aggravated the abscess in either case.[143] Taft recovered, but he lived with severe discomfort for months.

Dysentery

Nothing signifies a loss of control like rampant diarrhea, and Europeans and Americans in the tropics complained about it constantly. It could be a nuisance, suffered as a feature of life in the colonies, regarded as endemic among Indians and Filipinos. Dysentery was far worse. For many years, there was uncertainty as to its cause. The microscope revealed amoebas in the stools of some sufferers though not all; ultimately bacteria were implicated in other versions. Ingesting food or water that contained these microbes was a sure path to infection, but in the late nineteenth century experts thought there were other causes, all involving contact with pathogenic organisms. "When certain local and climatic conditions exist, and a certain epidemic constitution prevails the disease may . . . become epidemic and highly infective, though *how* I am not prepared to say," wrote Joseph Fayrer, who warned against "exposure of the body, especially the abdomen, during sleep or when perspiring," an endorsement of stomach bands.[144] Many blamed rain or otherwise wet conditions.[145] Chlorinated drinking water came late if it came at all to Indian and Filipino municipalities, and water filters used increasingly in both countries could not screen out amoebas.[146] At its worst, dysentery caused ulcerated colons and abscesses of the liver.[147] Taft contracted dysentery on one of his tours of the archipelago and was treated with benzozone enemas, administered two or three times daily.[148] Doctors had success treating dysentery with ementine, derived from the root of the *Carapichea ipecacuanha* plant (Ipecac), and early in the twentieth century American doctor Edward Vedder and British scientist Leonard Rogers used ementine injections with good results in the Philippines and India respectively.[149] Yet problems persisted in both places. In 1916, a commission found intestinal parasites (not just amoebas) in nearly 95 percent of over a thousand people examined in Pasay.[150] As late as 1938, dysentery caused nearly three hundred thousand deaths in India.[151]

Tuberculosis

Tuberculosis was the leading cause of death in nineteenth-century Britain and the United States; between 1851 and 1910 four million in England and Wales died from it, and at about the same time American-born whites had a tuberculosis mortality rate of 170 per 100,000 of the population.[152] The etiology of tuberculosis was increasingly well understood by the late nineteenth century, thanks to Koch's discovery, in 1882, of the bacillus that produced it. It was well known that the disease swept quickly through poor, crowded neighborhoods, indicating that close contact between people made it spread. Koch isolated its germ in spittle, which led him and others to implicate droplets of moisture—spit and sputum, the discharge from coughs and sneezes and expectorant—as its carrier. Isolation seemed a preventative and, it was hoped, a cure, inspiring the growth of mountain sanatoria in Europe and North America.

Tuberculosis was a ruthless killer in India and the Philippines. Its recognition in India goes back to Vedic texts, which urged those suffering from it to move to a higher altitude. An Indian doctor found that half of the women in Calcutta who died between the ages of fifteen and twenty were victims of tuberculosis, a stunning fact he blamed on the practice of purdah, which crowded women together without access to fresh air.[153] In 1910 the disease killed a higher percentage of Indian prisoners than cholera, smallpox, and malaria combined, and even more than dysentery.[154] Everywhere Britons regarded with horror spat-out betel nut as a likely source of tuberculosis germs.[155] Americans in the Philippines were disgusted and alarmed when local people spat on them.[156] Authorities in the Philippines campaigned vigorously against practices that brought people dangerously close together. They warned mothers against chewing the food or tasting the milk to be given to their children, urged that babies be prevented from playing on floors, discouraged families from sharing a bed, especially if a family member had a cough, directed parents to avoid hugging or kissing their children "exaggeratedly," and entreated teachers not to distribute pencils to pupils every morning and collect them at the end of the day.[157] The windows of houses must be kept open to allow the circulation of air.[158] Tuberculosis patients should be placed in sanatoria.[159] School textbooks condemned spitting: "It is not only disgusting but dangerous. People who have diseases of the lungs, throat, mouth, and nose should be careful to spit only where the sputum will be burned or properly disinfected. Otherwise they are very likely to infect well people. Whether a person is sick or well, he should spit only in a proper receptacle, or in a paper or cloth which can be burned."[160] In Manila in 1908, following the example set by American cities and the US National Tuberculosis Association, authorities banned the depositing of "sputum, saliva, phlegm or mucus upon the floor of any church, schoolhouse, public building or . . . sidewalk," and forbade the sick from working in cigar or cigarette factories or "dancing at a public dance hall," all places where tuberculosis might be contracted and spread.[161]

Plague

The scourge of plague arrived in Bombay via ship from Hong Kong in 1896, and over the next twenty-five years it killed more than ten million Indians.[162] People knew by then that rats carried plague and thus knew to avoid dead ones, but only in 1898 did Paul-Louis Simond establish that fleas served as vectors from rats killed by the plague to healthy rats, to other mammals, or to humans. When fleas bit humans, they regurgitated infected blood onto the skin; when humans scratched the itching bites, they opened their bodies to infection.[163] The plague bacterium attacks the lymph nodes, causing them to swell grotesquely (these are the buboes of bubonic plague), then invades the blood stream. Plague can spread from human to human through direct or indirect contact. The humans it killed were virtually all Indians.

The Government of India moved to contain the disease. Officials in Bombay, writes David Arnold, "simultaneously embarked on a massive, almost comically thorough, campaign of urban cleansing, flushing out drains and sewers with oceans of seawater and carbolic, scouring out scores of shops and grain warehouses . . . , sprinkling disinfectant powder in alleyways and tenements . . . , and, more tragically, destroying several hundred slum dwellings in the hope of extirpating the disease before it could fully establish itself." Plague sufferers were to be taken to hospitals, "by force if necessary."[164] In February 1897 the *haj* to Mecca was canceled, and train passengers were given disinfectant baths when they arrived at stations. Women suspected of having the disease were forced to strip to the waist in order to have their armpits inspected for buboes.[165]

There were some differences in the approach to the plague depending on location. In general, though, the health authorities at first tried to coax victims to go to a hospital, inspected houses believed to harbor the disease, tried to disinfect all such houses, and examined the corpses of victims. The government declared a bounty on rats, offering cash prizes for rat-tails brought into dispensaries.[166] One by one, these measures were modified or abandoned because they proved impracticable, or objectionable to Indians subject to them. People hid family members to prevent them from being sent to hospitals, and they resisted having strangers enter their homes, something the Government's Plague Commission admitted "attacks the domestic privacy of the people," especially as Hindu and Muslim women were not to be seen by outsiders and certain rooms of houses, including shrines and kitchens, might be off limits to nonbelievers.[167] High-caste Hindus would not touch rats.[168] Attempts at disinfection foundered on the inefficiency of the apparatus used to spray houses, the ineffectiveness of standard disinfectants, which could not penetrate rat holes, the effect produced by the disinfectant "New Green Crystals," which left interior walls colored green for days after spraying, and the permeability of Indian houses, which allowed disinfecting vapors to escape through walls and roofs before they could do their work.[169] People were willing to disinfect their houses by burning cow dung cakes, an expedient the government rejected.[170] Inspecting corpses was deeply offensive to the relatives of the dead, and authorities were not sure in any case that one could tell by looking whether a victim had died of plague.[171]

Most of all, the British tried to stay ahead of the plague by vaccinating people at risk of contracting it. Vaccination was profoundly haptic, at once threatening by its penetration of the skin and promising in its ability to transform the recipient from vulnerable to fully protected from the disease. Bacteriologist Waldemar Haffkine was in India when plague struck. He had earlier developed a vaccine against cholera; the authorities now asked for his help with the new threat. Early in 1897 Haffkine injected himself with an experimental vaccine, and thereafter it was hurriedly tested on prisoners. It worked.

The pressure to vaccinate nevertheless encountered sharp resistance. In some instances the injection failed to "take," forcing patients to be revaccinated.[172] This was a hard case to make, particularly since the shot was a painful one and left its recipient feeling "very seedy."[173] Rumors had it that the injection "needle was a yard long; you died immediately after the operation . . . ; men lost their virility and women became sterile; the Deputy Commission himself underwent the operation and expired an hour afterwards in great agony."[174] The plague doctors were "poisoners."[175] As the fall plague season approached the Punjab in 1902, the government attempted an ambitious program of vaccination, hoping to capture some two-thirds of the population in the most affected areas. Officials requested from the Plague Research Lab in Bombay seventy thousand doses of vaccine per day. It soon became clear that there was something wrong with the newly arrived vials: vaccinators complained of their bad smell, and noted that abscesses appeared frequently at the skin's injection sites. On October 30, the lab suspended shipment of the fluid. But it was too late. That day, nineteen people just vaccinated in the Mulkowal District contracted tetanus and died. Vaccination was halted and the families of victims compensated. The disaster shook the faith of the people in the effectiveness of the procedure and undermined the perception of British medicine generally.[176]

American health officials in the Philippines blamed the introduction of plague, as the British did, on ships arriving from Hong Kong. Victor Heiser had observed closely the struggle against plague in India, and in its aftermath he took measures to prevent the spread of disease to the archipelago, building what he boasted were the world's first "ratproof wharves," constructed of concrete and "flashed with steel sheathing underneath" so that "the rat could not find a foothold." The disease slipped in nevertheless, late in 1899. The Americans mobilized a military-style defense against it. Colonel Louis M. Maus, Chief of the Board of Health, carried out an aggressive anti-rat campaign—easier to do in the Philippines than in India, Heiser claimed, because unlike Hindus the Filipinos had no compunction about handling and killing rats.[177] Maus ordered a hundred thousand plates of rat poison to be set out each evening in Manila. Once the rats had fed, they dehydrated and raced for water sources, including the Pasig River, where they drowned. Men brought out carts to harvest the dead, and six crematories then burned the rats.[178] In the meantime, sanitationists went door to door, posting notices of noncompliance with health standards if problems were found, and residents who failed to clean their premises were subject to fine or arrest. Mandatory vaccination orders were issued, and in the end about half the population of the city, most of them from "the lower classes," got shots.[179] The total affected soon diminished, so that after 1905 the only cases of plague still reported were in Bilibid Prison, where men had been accidentally injected with the disease.[180]

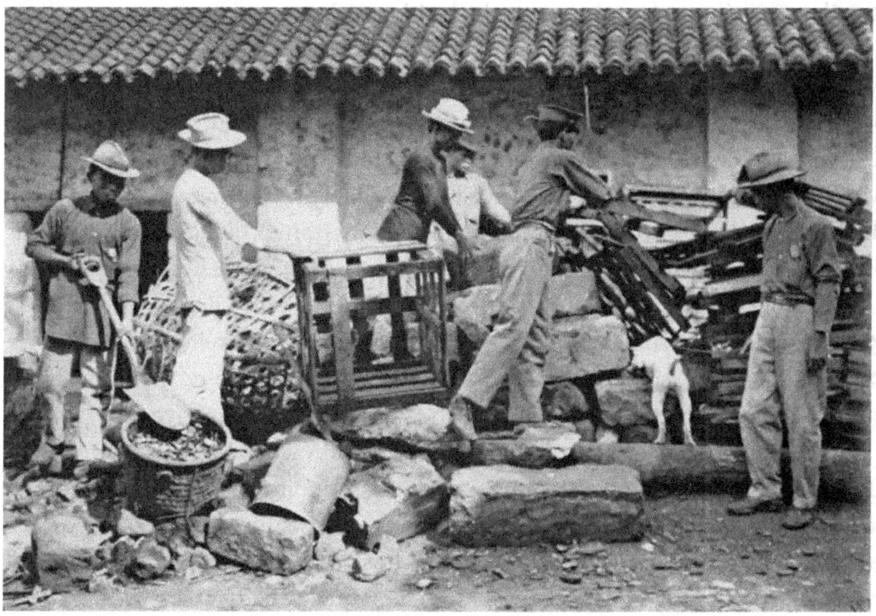

Figure 6.4 Catching rats in Manila. Rats were correctly implicated in the spread of plague, so the authorities pursued them with fervor (and a dog). Courtesy of the American Historical Collection, Rizal Library, Ateneo de Manila University.

Smallpox

Plague came in the fall; in India smallpox was called *basantaroga*, the "spring disease." It was caused by the variola virus. Indians had long tried to protect themselves against the ravages of smallpox through prayer to the goddess Sitala, and by eating, inhaling, or injecting "powdered crusts" from an afflicted person's variolous excrescences, which inoculated the user with some efficacy for at least a year.[181] Smallpox is spread by skin-to-skin contact, through inhalation of viral droplets expelled by coughing or sneezing, and through contact with objects the sufferer has touched, including clothing or blankets. The disease begins like influenza, with fever and body aches and occasionally vomiting. A rash starts in the mouth, then spreads to the whole skin as fluid-filled sores, which become large pustules. The victim exudes a foul smell. After several days the sores crust over, forming scabs. In time these are shed, leaving survivors with pockmarked skin and no longer contagious.[182] British physicians believed that smallpox was fatal in a third of cases, with its survivors often left blind. India was swept by frequent epidemics—in 1868–1869, 1872–1874, 1877–1879, and 1884–1885—resulting in some two and half million deaths.[183] In 1869, British physician Robert Pringle noted that "it has become quite a saying among the agricultural and even wealthier classes never to count children as permanent members of the family . . . until they have been attacked with and recovered from smallpox."[184]

The Indian practice of variolation relied on the transmission of live smallpox viruses, most often through inoculation. The smallpox vaccine, developed by Edward Jenner in the late eighteenth century, contained cowpox, a milder form of the same disease that once contracted provided immunity from the deadlier smallpox.[185] Both methods of disease prevention were intimately haptic. Variolation evolved in India with the sanction of the goddess, and variolous skin crusts might be "sanctified with a sprinkling of Ganges water." Those responsible for transferring matter from afflicted to sound bodies, the *tikadars* (mark-makers), were generally trusted by the people who relied on them. The transmittal of live viruses produced a strong reaction in the recipient, which if survived offered reassurance that the procedure had been effective.

The British were convinced of the superiority of vaccination over variolation. Inoculation was risky, more likely to produce a full-blown and fatal form of the disease and with a higher probability of spreading, since the recipient of live viruses was as contagious as the previous host. Handling the variolous crusts was disgusting and dangerous. But Indians equally had reason to object to vaccination. The vaccine came to India in June 1802 "through a relay of children vaccinated . . . arm to arm from Baghdad to Bombay." Later the lymph was brought in tubes overland or by sea. In both cases, unfamiliarity with the sources and agents of the vaccine, its remoteness from the bodies of Indians, raised suspicions concerning its safety and efficacy. Moreover, removing lymph from the vaccinated child to be prepared for use in further injections was extremely painful. The Sanitary Commissioner for Bengal recorded the scene in 1893: "The child, attended by its weeping mother, is taken round the town or village, and sometimes from one village to another, and after all the lymph has been extracted from the vesicles on its arms, it is a common practice for the vaccinators to squeeze the inflamed base of the vaccine pustules further in order to obtain serum for more vaccinations." The Commissioner argued that calf lymph should replace that drawn directly from humans. But Hindus found such treatment of cows abhorrent.[186]

In 1877, Bombay prohibited inoculation and made vaccination compulsory; the Government of India followed suit three years later. Smallpox deaths declined dramatically, though the laws proved hard to enforce.[187] People associated smallpox vaccination with unsuccessful and sometimes fatal vaccination against plague, resented being told how to look after themselves, and resisted the implementation of a six-puncture system of injection, which left a large scar.[188] Even those *tikadars* who were hired as vaccinators rebelled against working for the state and, they said, usually for less; they preferred to continue as private variolators.[189] British authorities were impatient with what they saw as the Indian refusal to allow their skins to be penetrated for a vitally important health measure. And unless Indians cleaned up their haptic environments, smallpox would continue to kill them. "Until the mass of the people become more civilised in their habits, living in better ventilated houses, more frequently changing their garments . . . no great diminution of the small-pox can occur . . . ; for bad ventilation and dirty habits, both personal and general, have always been allied with epidemic small-pox," wrote the Collector of Belgaum. "Vaccination has done much in eradicating the disease, but to the advance of Civilisation in Europe is due its great diminution, and until well ventilated towns and villages are met with in this country—good dwelling places and more personal cleanliness— . . . will small-pox remain."[190]

The Spaniards had introduced smallpox vaccination to the Philippines in 1805, but Filipinos generally avoided it, and after 1870 the country struggled with almost yearly outbreaks of the disease.[191] Like Indians, Filipinos were inclined to see variolation as more effective than vaccination. The US military vaccinated its troops before they left for the Philippines, then inspected the men as they crossed the Pacific and revaccinated those whose site scar seemed shallow.[192] Smallpox nevertheless erupted among the men soon after they arrived, and serum brought from the United States was insufficient to meet urgent needs. Louis Maus quickly opened two "vaccine farms" with carabao heifers to produce the vaccine, but for a time he was overwhelmed.[193] War displaced populations and spread the disease, with over 14,000 dying in 1902 and more than 20,000 in 1903.[194] Vaccination was gradually made compulsory; Filipino vaccinators, called *practicantes,* accompanied by American soldiers, forcibly vaccinated all those not showing the telltale pockmarks of survivors.[195] While the Americans were for the most part "pleasantly surprised" with the cooperation they received from Filipinos, they continued to fear physical contact with those whom the vaccine had failed to reach.[196]

Malaria

Prevalent in warm, humid, moist climates, malaria was for centuries blamed on miasmas, "poison" produced in soil, borne on the air, and "taken into the body through the skin, the lungs, and the stomach."[197] "Socially," J. B. S. Haldane observed, "malaria is a worse disease than plague or small-pox, because it lasts for years and turns most members of a population into chronic invalids."[198] Its symptoms include chills, sweating, fever, body aches, and nausea, and while many people lived with these for years the disease could also kill. Malaria had a tormented history throughout the world, but by the nineteenth century it was regarded as the particular scourge of the "coloured races" in tropical climates.[199] British scientist Ronald Ross, who was born in India during the first month of the Great Rebellion, found in 1897 that mosquitoes were vectors for the plasmodium parasite that carried malaria. Thereafter, Ross urged the creation of "mosquito brigades" to track down and destroy mosquito larvae. A "superintendent," a "man of good caste," should assemble a team of hunters who would go into yards and homes and fill puddles that housed the insects. "Every man should be given a badge," he suggested. "A diamond-shaped patch of red flannel sewn on the arm or breast is a good one."[200] Malaria could be prevented or cured with quinine, but it was not always available, it tasted terrible, often inducing vomiting, and its many side effects included tinnitus. Researchers experimented with dosage size on Indian prisoners.[201] Here was yet another illness that characterized uncivilized Asian subjects and was transmitted to whites stealthily, treacherously, and by cutaneous penetration.

The British battled malaria in India with their brigades, oiling the watery breeding grounds, and through strong draughts of quinine, even as they fought back nausea. The Americans undertook a similar process in the Philippines. Despite Ross's findings and their widespread publicity, fears lingered among soldiers and civilians that malaria was conveyed by the rain (or the sun) and caught by men who slept in damp clothes. Doctors knew that quinine was the medicine of choice against it and prescribed it widely, but they acknowledged that it rarely reached Filipinos, with the result, guessed Louis Maus, that malaria was "probably responsible for at least one-half of all the

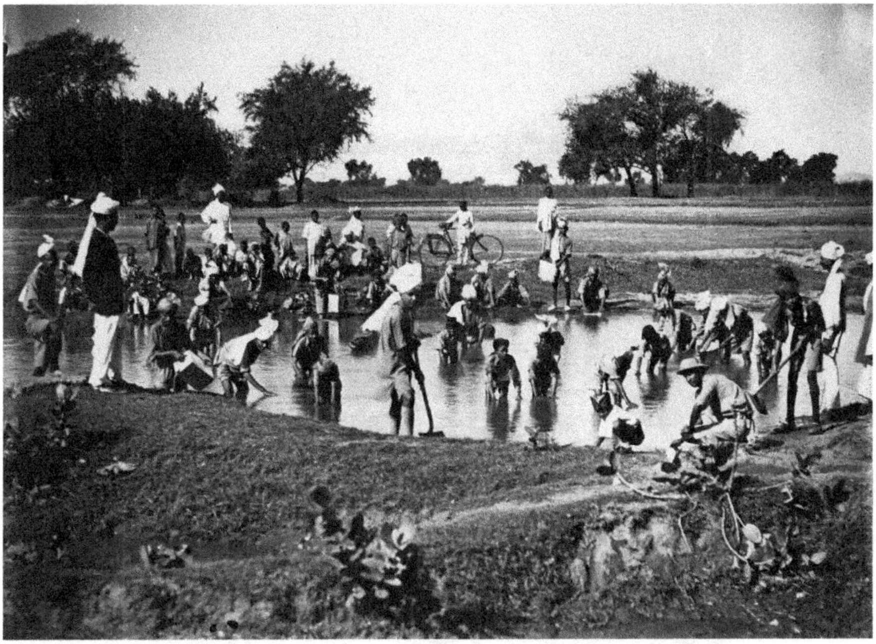

Figure 6.5 Anti-malarial work. These men appear to be dragging the pond for mosquito larvae. Courtesy of British Library, Asian and African Studies.

sickness" on Luzon.[202] The disease could kill: 173 Manilans died from it in 1905–1906.[203] The Americans ultimately understood the connection between mosquitoes and malaria and launched anti-malaria campaigns in the schools, alerting students to the importance of good drainage and mosquito nets and distributing free quinine.[204] As they abandoned the miasmatic interpretation of the illness, they implicated individual Filipinos in its transmission and persisted in avoiding contact with Filipino bodies. Major Charles Woodruff instructed his troops: "You are therefore to consider all apparently healthy native soldiers as possible sources of fatal infection to whites."[205] Appearance might not reflect sickness, making distance the only reliable strategy for staying healthy.

Leprosy

No disease more disturbed the Anglo-Americans than leprosy. It appalled and affronted their every sense: they were horrified by seeing often extreme disfigurement, on hearing the cries of lepers begging or warning off the uninfected, by inhaling the distinctive and pungent smell of the diseased, and by the fear that

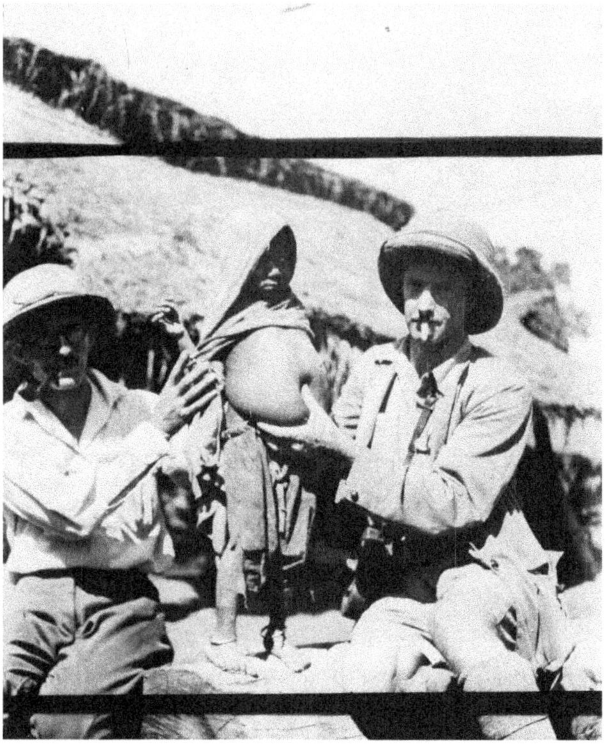

Figure 6.6 A badly bloated malarial child, held and put on display for the camera by British health officials. Courtesy of Library of Congress, Prints and Photographs Division.

their food might have been touched—even prepared—by a leper's suppurating hands. What Britons and Americans feared most of all was being touched by a leper. The skin of the leper's body had been disrupted and torn and therefore trespassed; whatever people in the late nineteenth century did or did not know about how the disease was contracted, there seemed every likelihood that it passed through skin. Leprosy threatened the most monstrous of penetrations.[206]

Leprosy was pollution. Jesus cured lepers when they begged to be clean. Medieval Europeans feared contamination by lepers, who were required to sound a bell as they approached so that the nonleprous could avoid them. Other rules of conduct governed lepers: "I forbid you to ever leave your house without your leper's costume. . . . I forbid you to touch anything you bargain for or buy, until it is yours. . . . I forbid you, if you go on the road and meet some person who speaks to you, to fail to put yourself downwind before you answer. I forbid you to go in a narrow lane, so that should you meet any person, he should not be able to catch the affliction from you. I forbid you, if you go along any thoroughfare, to ever touch a well or the cord unless you have put on your gloves.

I forbid you to ever touch children or to give them anything."[207] American polymath Benjamin Rush speculated that the dark skin of "Negroes" was a variant of leprosy, caused by their "unwholesome diet," tropical homelands, and "savage manners." Well into the nineteenth century, observers believed that diet could cause the disease; among the foods implicated were breadfruit, vegetables, and dried fish. Most medical opinion held that leprosy was heritable or cultural, and assigned it to dark-skinned people living in hot climates. That ought to have changed with the 1874 discovery, by Armaeur Hansen, of the leprosy bacillus, which he found common among Norwegians. Yet leprosy continued to be associated with the tropics. And if leprosy was contagious, it was best, thought medical professionals, to isolate the bodies of lepers, to prevent them from touching the uninfected in any way.[208]

The British had experience with leprosy in their Cape Colony (South Africa). In 1845, they had established a leper asylum on Robben Island for the voluntary confinement of sufferers. But following Hansen's discovery, the colonial government passed the Leprosy Repression Act, which made compulsory the removal of lepers to one of two asylums.[209] Officials in India had much the same impulse. The Surgeon-Major Henry V. Carter, in Bombay, was one of the earliest recipients of samples of leprous tissue from Hansen's lab in Bergen.[210] Such evidence convinced him that "it is most desirable to remove from the sight of, and contact with, healthy men, women, and children, the diseased and repulsive leper, who when a beggar is obtrusive, and who is almost naturally, considering his sad lot, careless of all social restrictions." The danger to the family sheltering the leper was great. Wellesley Bailey, a missionary, was more concerned with what happened to those lepers who were turned out by their families. They were left "to wander about the country in the most pitiable condition imaginable. Their hands and feet drop off bit by bit, joint by joint, until they have nothing but the bare stumps left. As they are unable to work for themselves, they have to eke out their living by begging from door to door, and take whatever is thrown to them—and *thrown* to them it often is, as if they were dogs. . . . The bridge of the nose falls in, and gives them a most forbidding appearance."[211] Surgeon-Major A. J. Laing complained that too often lepers circulated "unchecked . . . with the ordinary population of the country," working in public markets, taking drinking water from city reservoirs, and mingling with crowds at festivals.[212] Reporting from a village in the Deccan, the former Sanitary Commissioner for Bombay found lepers calling out the name of their disease while "push[ing] a small earthen vessel in front of [them] in which passers-by drop a few pice."[213]

No one knew how many lepers lived in India. One estimate put the number at half a million in 1900, but that was probably an undercounting.[214] Traditional Indian understandings of leprosy tended to blame its appearance on karma, eating the wrong foods (especially shellfish), having contact with lepers, laziness, "coitus with fat women," and bad behavior, including disrespect for teachers and "swearing at mendicants." The Hindu *śāstras* permitted the casting out of lepers who showed signs of the disease and denied them inheritance rights, but enjoined the sufferers' families to provide those afflicted with enough food to keep them alive. British policy reflected the decentralized structure of the Raj, which meant that treatment of lepers varied from city to city, state to state. Madrassi Hindus kept leprous family members at home and allowed them to beg or work as they could. In Portuguese Goa, it was customary to massage victims daily with sap from the neem tree, while in the Andaman Islands, off India's southwest coast, a British surgeon directed lepers to bathe, drink a potion of lime water and gurjon oil (also used as a wood sealant against white ants), then rub themselves all over, for up to four hours a day, with gurjon oil ointment. Other wishful remedies were ingested mercury, fumigation with such ingredients as zinc, sesame, and powdered cobra meat, and, increasingly, draughts or injections of chaulmoogra oil, derived from hydnocarpus trees.[215]

Policies concerning the confinement of lepers also varied according to place. Some officials were determined to isolate and confine all lepers. If the leprous were contagious with bacteria, it would be best to remove them completely from the society of the healthy. One collector reported that lepers often sold food and betel in the market or distributed it in temples, and given the leniency shown sufferers by their families and communities such behavior would doubtless be allowed to continue, threatening the health of others. The Madras government struggled to balance such threats with the resistance of lepers and their loved ones to involuntary confinement. A Leper Bill, offered in 1889, called for the hospitalization of "vagrant" lepers without apparent means of support and those who volunteered to be confined, presumably without hope of being cured or lacking sustenance from their families. The government ultimately rejected the bill as too lax, insisting that the "'danger of contagion . . . from those living in respectable houses, who marry and carry on business' was greater than from the 'wandering and outcaste' leprosy sufferers." A more stringent bill, tabled in 1896, called for fining any leper who bathed publicly or drank from a public fountain or who "rides in any public conveyance." This proved too much for Britons and Indians alike. The government settled, two years later, for a Lepers Act that allowed for the "re-arrest and return" to hospitals those who had left without permission. Over two decades later, even this relatively benign policy remained unenforced. Lepers frequently wandered away from hospitals to beg in the bazaars. "The human factor began to be recognized," wrote A. Donald Miller, Secretary of the Mission to Lepers, in 1924, and "it was seen that the normal policeman is not keen to arrest beggar lepers; it was seen that the beggar leper is not keen to be arrested and interned."[216] There were similar problems in Bengal, which called for the detention of "pauper lepers" but gave localities considerable latitude to enforce the law, and in British Burma, where a Lepers Act "has had the good result of cleaning certain places from the sight of leprous bodies," but where the "carelessness which is in the nature of the Burman" too often permitted lepers to prepare food for the market and to nurse nonleprous babies.[217] The British avoided, as best they could, physical contact with lepers. In India, the size of the leprous population and the difficulties of compelling people to remain confined to institutions that could not promise to cure them proved too much to manage anything more.

The situation confronted by the Americans in the Philippines was somewhat different. There were many fewer lepers there than were in India: officially four thousand in 1903, though Victor Heiser thought it more likely that there were between ten and thirty thousand scattered among the islands.[218] Like Indians, many Filipinos preferred to keep leprous family members at home rather than institutionalize them. "We are always, at bottom, opposed to segregation," a politician told Katherine Mayo. "We do not consider the disease very horrible and we want to keep our lepers in our own households at home."[219] The Spaniards had built leper hospitals but largely conceded to such preferences. As in India, those sent to hospitals frequently walked off.[220] In some places lepers formed their own communities, living together in nipa houses, where they were suspected of making cheese and other foodstuffs.[221] Lepers appeared in public, even at markets. Friday was "Leper's Day" in the towns of Bacolod and Cebu, when those afflicted were allowed to beg or "wander around at will."[222]

Not all Filipinos were tolerant of the lepers among them. In José Rizal's *Noli Me Tangere*, a leper is whipped for lifting a small boy out of a canal—after which, the town's mayor yelled, "better to drown than to end up like you!"[223] This was the Americans' view when they arrived in force in the Philippines nearly fifteen years after Hansen's discovery. While they found it repulsive to see or smell a leper, touching one, they believed, could well be fatal. In January 1899, the *New York World* carried the lurid story of a fictional American soldier named William Lapeer (the surname gave it away), recently returned from the Philippines. The story claimed that Lapeer had been captured and drugged by revolutionaries, then injected with leprosy bacteria while he lay unconscious. He was now in agony, waiting to see whether he would contract the disease and "rot to death like the lepers he [had] seen in Manila." Before than happened, he vowed, he would "blow [his] brains out."[224] The previous year, the US Public Health Service had opened an investigation of the prevalence of leprosy in the United States. Popular fears that immigrants carried a disproportionate amount of the disease impelled this decision; Joseph Jones, the president of the Louisiana State Board of Health, worried about Chinese launderers who took water into their mouths, then spat it onto the clothes they were ironing, and recommended that they be confined or returned to China. The commission found only 278 confirmed cases in the country, but recommended the creation of one or two leprosaria.[225] In the Philippines, the haptic anxiety concerning lepers, coupled with the possibility that lepers might be confined to a spot far away from healthy people, led Heiser to establish a leper community on Culion Island, two hundred miles southwest of Manila.

In October 1902, the Philippine Commission approved the Culion site and appropriated $50,000 to get it started. Part of the money was used to compensate and relocate residents of the island to another nearby.[226] Construction began in 1905, and the first contingent of 370 lepers was brought to Culion in May 1906 by a pair of Coast Guard cutters. There was little in the way of personnel and facilities to greet them; those not immediately hospitalized were lodged in shabby nipa huts and languished uncared for. Fifteen months later, Heiser, as director of health, was put fully in charge of the program. The Philippine Commission empowered him "to apprehend, detain, isolate, segregate, or confine all leprous persons in the Philippine Islands" and allowed the police to arrest suspected lepers and turn them over to the health authorities for diagnosis.[227] Heiser embarked on a series of "leper-collecting" expeditions throughout the islands. He contacted authorities in coastal towns and demanded that they gather their lepers in advance of his arrival. The collectors disembarked, examined the lepers (who were called "suspects"), and took on board all those showing symptoms of the disease or testing positive for the leprosy bacillus. They picked up as many as they could find and took them to Culion. Suspects were encouraged to go peacefully. "If a person has leprosy he should not attempt to hide," advised the authors of a popular school textbook on health. "He should go to the nearest health officer and apply for treatment. . . . If he should be placed in a separate place, such as Culion, he will be happier for being sent there. Culion is an enterprising town run by lepers, where lepers are happy and contented. They do not have to hide, but lead happy, normal lives and are not despised or feared by their companions. . . . This is much better than hiding at home and fearing that they may give their disease to those they love."[228]

Once construction at Culion finally accelerated—it was difficult to convince nonleprous workers to spend weeks on the island—Heiser celebrated the colony for its humanity and its facilities. Houses were brand new and solidly built, with roofs ventilated against the heat and the odors of leprous bodies. There was a town hall, a store, a post office where outgoing mail was disinfected, a school, and the Leper Club, including "a piano, a pool table, and many newspapers, some recent, and miscellaneous discarded . . . magazines, unintelligible except for the pictures."[229] Heiser admitted to disappointment with a garden-planting campaign, and while the leper band he formed proved to him the natural musicality of Filipinos he was once greeted with unexpected silence. " 'Why don't you play?' I asked. 'We can't.' 'Why not?' In dumb reply they held up their hands;

they had literally played their fingers off."[230] As for medical treatment, Heiser put his faith in chaulmoogra oil. He first had patients take it by mouth, but it irritated the stomach and induced nausea, and many patients refused to swallow it. Thereafter, and ultimately in cooperation with India's Leonard Rogers, Heiser tried to inject the oil intramuscularly then directly into a vein. This was not entirely satisfactory either, as it produced severe pain at the injection site and fever, such that one practitioner described the treatment as "distinctly on the heroic side."[231] Chaulmoogra oil was of doubtful therapeutic value. It offered some relief from the symptoms of leprosy and occasional remissions, but it was no cure. Not until the development of antibiotics in the 1940s was the disease brought under control.[232]

Heiser claimed with pride that nearly all leprosy patients went willingly to Culion, especially if they had seen a magic lantern slide show illustrating the attractiveness of life there.[233] Evidence suggests otherwise. Again and again, leper "suspects" brought to coastal towns for relocation to Culion ran off, sometimes forcing the collecting party to go after them.[234] On a river trip in Samar, a group including the School Superintendent David Barrows overtook a *banca* (dugout canoe) full of passengers "chanting a melancholy song." They were

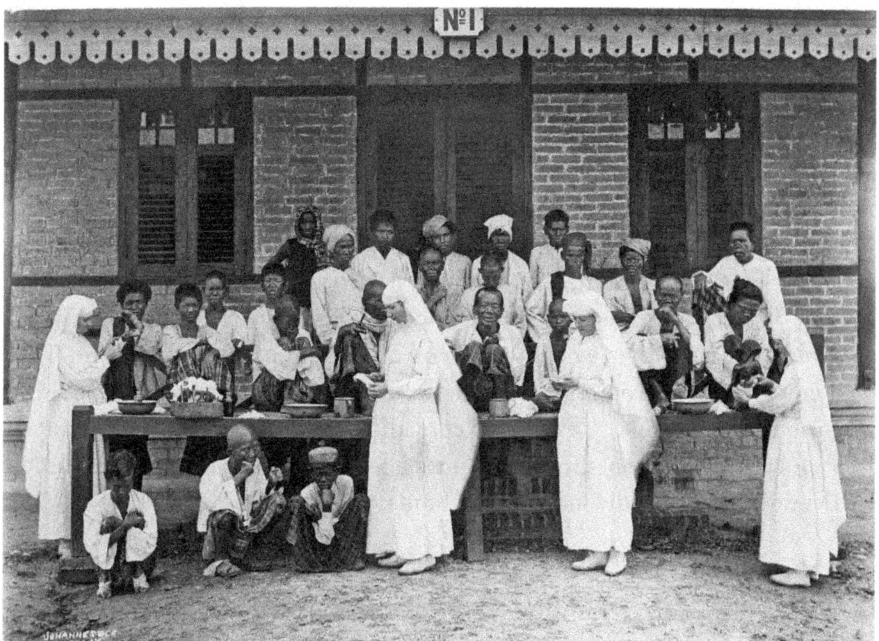

Figure 6.7 Nuns dressing lepers' sores. Though the authorities warned that leprosy spread through casual contact, this happened infrequently. These nuns may or may not have known that. Courtesy of British Library, Asian and African Studies.

lepers on their way to a debarkation point for Culion; "small wonder they were melancholy!" recalled Barrows's secretary.[235] Heiser recorded with exasperation multiple escapes from Culion.[236] Authorities at Culion struggled to manage it. Residents objected to the separation of men and women, and in 1932 a group of men raided a women's dormitory, carried off thirty to forty "girls," and refused to return them for over a week.[237] Officials were unsure whether the lepers should be allowed to marry—and, if so, divorce—and debated whether to force married men to have vasectomies so as to prevent them from having children, who were believed to have a high probability of contracting the disease.[238] When in spite of such efforts babies were born on the island, they were allowed to reach the age of six months and were then transferred to institutions or foster homes in the archipelago, with no real hope that their parents would see them again.[239] What to do with lepers who suddenly tested negative for the disease? Was it ethical to detain them? Release them? Filipino politicians criticized Culion and the treatment of the lepers there. They charged that the "experiment" cost too much in light of its meager results and accused Governor-General Leonard Wood of using the colony as a showcase for his political ambitions.[240] In 1934 the Philippine Legislature, feeling increasingly confident of its autonomy, received the Nolasco Bill, which called for an end to mandatory confinement of lepers and urged instead that they be treated at home.[241]

The lepers of Culion had a song, sung with Spanish lyrics. It began: "I am a leper. I was torn away / From the love of my family. / I live in Culion, exiled / To the Island of pain. / High mountains entomb me / A vast sea imprisons me / It can't be helped; alive or dead / Always, always, I have to be here. / Woe is me! / Always at Culion without cure / And to live / Without parents, native land or home / Without having / Brothers and children of love/ and without seeing / The life of the heart."[242] Yet perhaps the lepers' ultimate power emerged from the frightening condition of their bodies. Guy Henry, the US military governor of the city of Iloilo at the beginning of the twentieth century, found the lepers hard to control "because they would say, 'If you don't want us here, put us out.' They well knew," Henry wrote, "that anyone would dread to physically take hold of them and put them out."[243] Perceived contagiousness by virtue of tactile contact was a surprising weapon, though the presence of thousands of lepers on Culion by the early 1930s vividly indicated its limits.

"Necessary" Intimacies

Avoidance, withdrawal, shunning the body of the Asian Other—these were the most obvious stratagems deployed by the Anglo-Americans to prevent what they regarded as defiling, infectious contact. Whites hid away in their homes and hill stations, washed and disinfected themselves and their surroundings with astonishing determination, covered themselves against exposure to danger from flora and fauna, fought flies and mosquitoes, clubbed snakes to death, and did what they felt they must to purify the bodies of Indians and Filipinos that seemed to threaten rulers and subjects alike with pollution and disease, though often relying on "native" caregivers to do the actual washing, debriding, bandaging, and injecting. Their goal was civilization at haptic remove.

Such a prospect was, in truth, unlikely. The agents of empire could not pretend to be unaffected by the climate that surrounded them. They felt and touched objects and animals and people many times each day. Like the other senses, that of touch cannot be turned off; try as they might, Britons and Americans could not avoid haptic involvement in the new worlds they had entered. Military officers and civilian administrators in India and the Philippines were required to visit all parts of their far-flung districts. They often did this by horse or horse-cart, and by either means they felt the animal and the land under them as they traveled. They stayed in tents for long periods, with the thinnest membrane between them and the environment.[244] The British and Americans were lovers of sport. The former played polo, tennis, and badminton; the latter introduced baseball to the Filipinos.[245] Both spent an inordinate amount of time hunting and fishing, with all the tactile knowledge, exposure to the elements, and haptic discomfort such activities required. They did not wish to be corrupted by the touch or feel of others. Nor would they be cut off completely from them.

There were "natives" to whom they were close, often intimately so. At times they appreciated the touch of their subjects. Sport in India might include Indians: Christopher Masterman got to know "educated Hindus" by playing tennis with them, while E. S. Humphries recalled joining Gurkha soldiers in spirited games of football.[246] The British admired Indian handicrafts, particularly textiles, sought to replicate them in factories at home, and filled their houses with them in India and Britain.[247] As much as Americans deplored the coarse feel of many Filipino fibers used in clothing, they acknowledged that some of the cotton fabric was "delicate" and "exquisite," and the Filipina touch with the sewing needle led the department store Bonwit Teller to commission lingerie "by native needle workers," with "every seam and embroidery done by hand."[248] The strength of the "native" touch was also useful. "The natives have a great talent for massage," wrote Evelyn Beeton, whose Indian bearer rubbed her feet each night before bed.[249] Americans were often carried from boat to shore or across rivers on the backs of small but powerful *muchachos*.[250]

Most Americans in the Philippines could not afford servants, and while leading officials relied on them, Helen Taft at least regarded Filipino servants as "entirely undependable" and preferred to hire Chinese instead.[251] The British frequently experienced haptic intimacy with their servants. Every aspect of

British life in India seemed to require local assistance, from putting on shoes to adjudicating a legal case. Most Britons accepted this and even liked it, as it gave them bragging rights back home: the middle classes could afford help in India that they could not have dreamed of having in England. "You may think and say, 'I have never been used to a maid at home, and can just well manage without one out here,' but do let me advise differently," wrote Mrs. C. Lang in her manual of British life in India. "I said the same myself, but . . . the ayah is a most useful servant and if she is willing and clever will be a tremendous help to you. . . . It is such a comfort when you come in hot and tired to have her to take your shoes and clothes off, and put out what you [need] to wear, to brush, and fold up your things, and generally to look after them."[252] British soldiers used *nappy-wallahs* to shave them in the morning, and the "corn-cuttit *wallah*" trimmed the corns off the men's feet, both of which tasks put servants with sharp objects close to delicate parts of their masters' bodies. Some Britons grew to like the sweepers (*mehtars*) who performed the noisome task of removing the pan from beneath the latrine seat, even while it was occupied.[253] Others, however, recoiled at such enforced closeness to their necessary but unsettling helpers. Evelyn Beeton needed help mounting a horse. Her *syce* [horse groom], she wrote, "clasped me tightly," but as he did "I saw the fleas hop on him. He was filthy." Beeton also complained that servants had difficulty fastening her dress and found it "maddening to feel their black hands fumbling about my neck and back."[254] Another British woman ignored her servant's warning that she was about the step on a snake, so he "did a thing absolutely without precedent in India—he touched me—he put his hand on my shoulder and pulled me back." She knew he might have saved her life, but the episode left her uncomfortable, and soon after she dismissed him.[255] What most discomfited Britons was their frequent need to employ Indian women, often of the lower castes, as wet nurses to suckle their infants. At best wet nurses needed constant supervision; at worst they threatened British children with pollution, for one could not know what they might have ingested and put into their breast milk or vouch for their cleanliness.[256]

There was one other common intimacy: sexual contact between colonizers and subjects. British and American authorities were sometimes embarrassed and inevitably worried about sex in their empires, for liaisons between (usually) white men and dark-skinned women ran afoul of metropolitan mores, angered local societies, and threatened to debilitate soldiers and others with sexually transmitted diseases, which they persuaded themselves were endemic in Indian and Filipino women. Yet both civilian officials and military officers tended to assume that men would be men, and that the apparent alternatives to sex with Asian women—masturbation ("lead[ing] to disorders of both body and mind") and homosexuality (subversive of morale, and scandalous)—were even less acceptable.[257] Britons and Americans insisted that living in the tropics increased the sex drive, which explained the alleged lustiness of Asian women and eliminated any cause for shame among the westerners who patronized, molested, or assaulted them.[258] Sex was thus a necessary evil, or simply necessary.

"The monotony of life, and the apathy of mind, so conspicuous among Europeans in hot climates . . . too often lead to vicious and immoral connexions with Native females, which speedily sap the foundation of principles imbibed in early youth," lamented James Johnson in his guide to life in India.[259] This was in 1813, years before the Great Rebellion, when British bodies were not yet closed entirely to contact with Indians. On the whole, the lower classes of Britons in India were considered likely to pursue sex with "native" women, while the upper classes were expected to disdain such contacts as beneath their station and a blot on their masculinity.[260] Between 1820 and 1870, as many as a third of the British soldiers in India were diagnosed with syphilis.[261] Other British men entered into monogamous relationships with Indian women, who were "to look after them and their houses," as the tea planter J. L. H. Williams recalled. These "Old Women," or "Keeps," as they were known, produced "Eurasian" children who were often shunned by Britons and Indians alike, and left in limbo when abandoned, as they often were, by their fathers.[262] When Vere Ogilvie's grandmother arrived from England at her husband's station in Punjab, she found the "compound full of native women with whom he had solaced his solitude, and several suspiciously pale-faced children running about." Her presence put a stop to it.[263]

The relative tolerance for such mixing mostly ended after the rebellion. The British and Indian governments now actively encouraged British women to come to India, either with husbands or men to whom they had become engaged, or as single women (the "Fishing Fleet") with the opportunity to meet and marry the increasing numbers of single British men come to India to run the empire.[264] The authorities also regulated prostitution. What might have been tolerated earlier was now viewed by the government as dangerous to the soldiers and civilians whose job it was to keep order in a demonstrably disorderly place. The prostitute was an easy, disreputable target.[265] The 1868 Indian Contagious Diseases Act, modeled on British legislation, required the registration, medical inspection, and, if necessary, the isolation and treatment of prostitutes in "lock hospitals" and put certain areas off limits to them.[266] The Anglican Church blocked efforts to create authorized "comfort stations" for men.[267] None of this ended either prostitution or the practice of living with Indian women out of wedlock. Orphanages dedicated to sheltering the children of these unions remained full.[268] Still, the government had registered its disapproval of what it saw as promiscuity, even while blaming it fully on Indian women and confining its consequences to them.

The pattern was similar in the Philippines. The Spaniards had established a system by which prostitutes were to be examined by a physician (at Saint

Lazaro leper hospital) and detained there if found to be infected with venereal disease, but enforcement of this policy was lax.[269] The US Army that arrived in the archipelago starting in 1898 teemed with STDs, perhaps involving half of all soldiers.[270] The Americans' response to this was nevertheless to place full responsibility for infections on Filipina prostitutes.[271] The military took charge, in several towns organizing the trade in prostitution by setting up red light districts in which the women, often brought in from other Asian countries to avoid offending local people, were frequently inspected for disease. In at least one instance their male customers were examined too and issued certificates if found free of STDs.[272] The Spanish system of confining infected prostitutes in lock hospitals was expanded by the Americans; the women were charged up to a dollar for their examination and placed in wards according to nationality.[273] Officers worried as much about their soldiers having sex with "respectable" Filipinas. "I deem it the duty of each officer," wrote Maj. General Adna Chaffee in 1901, "to personally caution the soldiers of his command that the honor of the men is at stake and reputation of their regiment also and that it is far from a soldierly quality to debauch the wife or daughter of any native in these islands."[274] Such edicts were seldom enough. There were numerous complaints of rape lodged against American soldiers by women in the town of Candelaria in 1902.[275] Sex scandals swirled around General John Pershing, who served in the islands from 1899 to 1903, and Judge Henry Clay Ide, a member of the First Philippines Commission.[276] The Wood-Forbes Mission in 1922 heard that some 18,000 "mixed-race" children had been born in the Philippines since the Americans had arrived. Nearly all had been abandoned by their fathers.[277]

Haptic Subjects

Some of the haptic practices of Indians and Filipinos seemed at first glance small things, and to the Anglo-Americans who observed them they were often little more than sources of annoyance or amusement. So, for instance, did Indian and Filipino men walk arm in arm and women with hands clasped, even if they were apparently not lovers.[278] Indian therapies often relied more fully on the sense of touch than did their European counterparts: massage, often with herbs and oils, was an important part of curing the sick.[279] Britons marveled at the sight of Indians who drank from tumblers by pouring directly into their mouths, without touching their lips to the edge.[280] Dramatic haptic inversions of caste occurred during the spring holiday of Holi, when the Ramoshis of the Central Provinces, according to a British observer, "pour mud out of a pot on any respectable man they chance to meet, and challenge him to a wrestling match; the next day cow-dung is flung on all well-dressed people."[281] In the Philippines, families shared beds.[282] Filipinos were inclined to believe that disease was less the result of morbific contact or even miasmic emanation than of seasonal change or visits from spirits, which were best confronted by closing doors or windows after dark. But when illness did come, several of the likeliest cures, including fumigation to produce sweating, and massage, involved touch.[283]

British and American health officials in India and the Philippines were rarely patient with their subjects' insistence on remaining close to the diseased or even dead bodies of their relatives. Indians and Filipinos often lived as extended families.[284] They resisted removing their pregnant or their sick to hospitals, remote and hostile places that were said to conduct sinister operations, and to which they would have to relocate in order to feed and nurse their kin until they recovered or died.[285] "Most of them have the notion," wrote an Indian reporter, "that to go to a hospital is to die, that British doctors mercilessly hack and hew the body instead of treating as the native doctor does, with drugs and balsams."[286] They preferred to attend the afflicted at home. Indians and Filipinos welcomed visitors to domestic sick rooms, risking, westerners objected, the spread of smallpox, tuberculosis, and plague. In Indians' and Filipinos' views, the sick would die without care and company, and if the victim was to die, then family members and friends must be in attendance.[287] N. Mukerjee, Chairman of the Calcutta Corporation, told British authorities that "people would prefer to die of plague rather than consent or submit to the removal of their mothers, wives, daughters or sisters to hospital."[288] Indians tried to protect themselves against spirits or devils, especially when there was illness at home, by closing windows and stopping up all forms of ventilation.[289] The same was true in the Philippines. The American doctor Paul Clements described a sickroom in the town of Taytay. "The patient lies on a mat on the floor, usually with a cotton blanket over him. He is entirely dependent upon the family and neighbors for attention, and gets plenty of it such as it is, but much of it is misdirected. The prevalent idea that currents of air are not good for the sick causes them to shut up the house as tight as possible. . . . The room and indeed the entire house, is filled with sympathizing neighbors at all hours of the day and night if the patient is suffering from an acute and dangerous disease."[290] The dead also needed attending, by prayer alone or by proper removal and attention to rites of cremation (required by Hindus but abjured by other Indians and Filipinos) or burial. Hindus would not abide the practice of autopsy; in one case, a group abducted a body from the autopsy room at a Calcutta hospital and took it to a burning *ghat* along the river for immediate cremation.[291] Americans abhorred the Filipino practice of sitting up all night with a corpse, no matter what the cause of death.[292]

In India, thus, there was faith in touch, but only of a certain kind. Local healers applied leeches to patients with eye disease.[293] In March 1878, the King family's cow took ill; "she refused to eat, and a great swelling came in her throat." The servants summoned three village holy men. One of them stroked the throat of the animal with a neem twig while he chanted. The second pierced the cow's ear with a sharp needle. The third made a ball of sugar, got a dog to lick it thoroughly, then fed it to the cow. The animal recovered.[294] Indian health practitioners felt for not one but six of their patients' pulses.[295] The arrival of the stethoscope in India proved a boon to male doctors and female patients, as it allowed women to stay concealed behind a curtain and to place the diaphragm of the instrument on their chests, without being otherwise touched, while the doctor listened unseeing through the earpieces.[296]

Other kinds of touch were considerably more problematic. While Britons worried about contact with an Indian, many Indians were equally concerned about the likelihood of pollution should they be touched by the wrong person. They were most apprehensive having to do with inspection, poisoning, penetration, or vivisection. After all, wrote the *guru* Swami Vivekananda in 1901, westerners were "lustful; drenched in liquor, having no idea of chastity or purity, and of cleanly ways and habits; . . . whose Atman [soul] is the body, whose whole life is only in the senses and creature comforts."[297] Contact with such a person would surely be corrupting. Villagers practiced *chalauwa*, by which they meant to transfer human disease to a bit of food or an animal, then offer the newly infected object or creature to the appropriate deity in propitiatory sacrifice.[298] The introduction of bathtubs and seat toilets to India baffled the inhabitants: who would think to get clean by sitting in increasingly dirty still water, and why would someone wish to occupy a seat frequently used by others to perform unclean acts? (The British complained about finding sand on toilet seats where Indian users had squatted on them.)[299]

The haptic violation that most worried Indians was vaccination against disease. Inoculation against smallpox long antedated the British presence in India. Still, a host of objections met British efforts to vaccinate the population. Nineteenth-century vaccinations were rather like surgery done without anesthetic, "comprising several deep incisions into which pulpy vaccine lymph was then inserted. Targeted mainly at babies and young infants, these vaccinations produced pustules and inflammation," along with persistent pain and occasional sepsis. "Weak" lymph, especially common in the countryside, demanded even deeper gouging of the skin, yet frequently failed to "take," which required revaccination. Smallpox vaccine, increasingly drawn from cows, was resisted mostly by Hindus but by other Indians too, who objected to the pain inflicted on animals and wondered at the cleanliness of the process by which the lymph was derived.[300] Health authorities tried various ways to calm fears, hiring Indian vaccinators, including women who would inject other women, and reminding people that injection was nothing new and was recommended in traditional ayurvedic practice.[301] These efforts were seldom sufficient, undercut as they were by widespread reports of the vaccine's ineffectiveness and its dangers. Attempts to demonstrate that the vaccination process were sterile failed to convince audiences; Gandhi excoriated vaccination as "filthy . . . little short of eating beef" in its wrongheadedness.[302] Even the preliminaries of taking the patient's temperature and swabbing clean the injection site were met with suspicion, unwanted and polluting instances of alien touch.[303]

Filipinos were, on the whole, somewhat more willing than Indians to accept the healing touch of westerners. They understood the importance that American men attached to hand contact—or so it seemed to Taft, when the lawyer Mario Crisóstomo visited him in the hospital following surgery in late 1901. "My wish, Honored Sir," Crisóstomo wrote before coming, "is to have an opportunity of grasping your beneficent hand before your departure. . . . I doubt not that I shall be able to shake hands with you before long"—and Crisóstomo added that he hoped to kiss Taft's hand before leaving the room.[304] The hapticity of their Catholicism—the giving of communion, the touch of the priest's blessing—may have accustomed Filipinos to more vigorous tactile involvements. Or it may have been that Spanish attempts to vaccinate Filipinos, however haphazard, better prepared residents for American health campaigns dedicated to eradicating disease. Filipinos were less happily disposed toward medical inspection of women, and their refusal, similar to that of many Indians, to relinquish control over contact with sick and dying bodies in their homes suggests resistance to the new haptic regime. Certainly those living outside of cities and towns were suspicious of vaccination. When Igorots heard that vaccinators were coming to a town near them in May 1902, many of them "t[ook] to the woods" to avoid injection; those who stayed and got shots scratched themselves bloody with the itching.[305] Bicolanos believed that sorcery and spirits caused illness and that injections would make things worse.[306] Victor Heiser found prejudice against smallpox vaccination widespread. "It is alleged," he wrote, "to produce baneful effects during menstruation, pregnancy, lactation, early infancy, or some other equally absurd reasons are given in protest. These superstitious ideas are frequently respected even by the best of Filipino vaccinators."[307]

There is one important difference between Indian and Filipino senses of touch, and it has to do with the existence of caste in India. Caste is defined in good part by respect or contempt for the senses. In its most rigid applications, those of the lower castes or subcastes must not look directly into the face of a high-caste Brahmin. Caste carries a proscription against food sharing, or commensality. And caste lines were not to be crossed through touch.[308] Marriage across caste was proscribed. Members of the lowest caste were called "untouchables." Only the lowest castes were allowed to touch polluted objects.

Caste made it difficult, Britons argued, to keep people healthy, for when Indians resisted certain kinds of touch they prevented the examinations necessary to discover disease and to administer life-saving vaccinations. In 1903, the Home Department heard the complaint of the Imperial Anglo-Indian Association about the differential treatment given arriving ship passengers during a plague epidemic. Inspectors treated gently those "who were of white complexion and claimed to be Europeans," giving them but "the usual slight examination supposed to suffice for persons of respectability adopting clean habits of life," while those of the same class but "of a brunette complexion," were forced to wait with "lascars [seamen] and other dirtily clothed persons and to be subjected to the disinfection of [their] very garments," a double haptic insult.[309] Perhaps in response, the government worked out an elaborate set of rules for inspecting train passengers: "First and second class passengers and *purdah* ladies traveling third class will ordinarily be examined in their carriages. Other female third-class passengers will, if time permits, be taken for examination to a special room or in other cases will be examined in their carriages. Male third class passengers will be required to alight for examination on the platform." If plague was suspected, secondary examiners would be present, and would include "women and caste-neutral 'menials' . . . to do the touching."[310] Who gave plague or smallpox vaccinations to whom required constant sorting out. Using upper-caste vaccinators would have solved the problem, but most refused to take this sort of work, which would have meant intimate touching of an unclean patient.[311] All of this was inconvenient. But what rankled most of all was the knowledge that Hindus, and probably all Indians, privately regarded Britons as unclean, beneath caste, and therefore untouchable. The British deplored Indian sanitary habits, but it was they who were polluted: many Hindus would not eat with them or shake hands, and if forced to do so they washed themselves vigorously as soon as possible thereafter.[312]

C. E. Tyndale-Biscoe came out to Kashmir in the last decade of the nineteenth century. He was a missionary and a teacher, and he was determined to use schools, twelve of which he founded, to teach his students (all boys) life lessons in hygiene and social equality. Though the upper-caste students shunned contact with him it was, he said, they who were unclean, of which "the nose gave distinct evidence." When one pupil refused to sit next to another of a lower subcaste, Tyndale-Biscoe and his British teachers shoved the recalcitrant boy into the lap of the other then vigorously rubbed their heads together. When he came into the assembly hall each day, Tyndale-Biscoe noticed that the boys, seated on the floor, parted to let him pass without contact. One day, he brought his dog, Taffy, with him to school, and after walking untouched to the front of the room ("as the lane filled in behind" him), he whistled for the dog, who "immediately came bounding over the assembled school to join his master. The cries, the moans, the horror and disgust were indescribable. Taffy was no respecter of persons, and day after day were they well and truly 'dogged' till they could at last bear the touch of their Principal without a shiver."[313]

Filipinos did not generally reciprocate American disgust at physical contact with themselves. They did not always know how to respond to haptic invitations; William Freer encountered two "Negrito" men and thrust out his hand in greeting, and while the men took Freer's hand they registered "no more response than a wooden hand might give."[314] The Americans regarded Filipino ideas about touch, and medical practice, as governed by superstition. Emily Conger, who was trained as an osteopath, gained a reputation for her laying-on of hands. People came from miles around in search of her healing touch: "I had divine power," she wrote.[315] Worried about the impression Filipinos would give a visiting American Congressional delegation in 1905, an editorial in the newspaper *El Renancimiento* urged people to be mannerly, thus to convince the visitors that "beneath the rough dress and skin browned by the sun, may be found a good people, upright, capable and anxious to be correctly appreciated and understood by the great American people."[316]

Most of all, Filipinos and Americans quickly reached an understanding that certain kinds of touching between them were acceptable. Torture, beatings, and rape, all too common, were not among them. But Edith Moses received enthusiastic embraces on leaving Filipino friends in Apalit.[317] And Americans and Filipinos often danced with each other at the *bailes* put on by local people or their visitors every time a group of US officials stopped in a town. Governor Forbes gave a ball for girls living in dormitories in Manila. Each was to invite two boys, and Forbes himself led off by dancing the *rigodon* with a Filipina named Francisca Tirona.[318] More than twenty years later, Governor Theodore Roosevelt Jr., was urged by an aide to dance with the niece of the provincial governor. "I was afraid if he failed to dance at all perhaps they might think he did not like the baili [*sic*]," the aide recorded. Afterward, "I heard much favorable comment on his having danced with a Filipina. 'Muy sympatico,' they said."[319] Three American women teachers in Malolos were invited to balls and parties, where "they were popular, and danced with young Filipinos, and I am sure no one could wish for a more attractive partner or more graceful dancer than young Señor Arnedo, of Sulipan, who was the life of the party." Edith Moses founded a social club in Manila, whose requirements for American membership included a promise to dance with Filipinos.[320]

British and American efforts to bring haptic discipline to their imperial possessions would continue up until the time of independence. Improvements were made. The land remained rough, but there were more roads and railroads and vehicles had better suspensions than the carts of the late nineteenth century. The heat and moisture did not change, yet there was electricity in more places, which meant that fans were increasingly reliable, and the westerners flocked to hill stations to escape the worst of the weather. The bodies of subjects were provided with more soap, their surfaces with more disinfectant. In the capitals, men learned to shake hands. Many of the diseases the westerners had encountered, and many they had brought to their empires, were declining in frequency, as people learned or were compelled to avoid physical contact with the sick and accepted ministrations of touch, including vaccination. The British still used violence against the stubborn bodies of Indian nationalists. Indians and Filipinos continued to resist the crudest haptic violations committed by the imperialists. But there was more talking now, less grappling. And the Americans danced away the last years of their rule of the Philippines.

7

Nourishing

Imperial Foodways

Unpretentious or uncouth? It is clear that tastes in food cannot be considered in complete independence of the other dimensions of the relationship to the world, to others and to one's own body, through which the practical philosophy of each class is enacted.

—Pierre Bourdieu, *Distinction: A Social Critique of the Judgement of Taste* (1984)

Colonial politics often spoke in an indisputable visceral tongue. Its experiments, engagements, and traumas were experienced in the mouth, belly, olfactory organs, and nerve endings, so that the stomach served as a kind of somatic political unconscious in which the phantasmagoria of colonialism came to be embodied.

—Parama Roy, *Alimentary Tracts* (2010)

Even less than other senses does taste stand alone. The appearance of food or the witness of its preparation contributes to its appeal or its ability to repel. How a substance sounds in the mouth may be the difference between enjoyment or rejection of it: some are put off by the squeak of cheese curds between the teeth or the loud crunching of pretzels by someone nearby. Smell, as Immanuel Kant put it, is "taste at a distance"; there is no sense of taste without the complicity of odor.[1] Foods are embraced or spurned because of their texture—while some regard the mouth feel of a ripe avocado or a plate of okra as succulent and enticing, others recoil at what seems to them disgustingly slippery or slimy. Taste is thus the most intersensorial of the five senses, acutely subject to the opportunities for delight and disgust that all five together inspire.

Along with smell, taste is an intimate sense, one drawn deep into the body by its presence in the mouth and through the nose. It profoundly affects perceptions of Others: we are what we eat, as the saying goes, and so are they, and if what and how they eat is regarded by us as amusing, bizarre, or disgusting, then the consumers perforce become these things. Eating, writes anthropologist Sidney Mintz, "is not merely a biological act, but a vibrantly cultural activity as well," and as such it is frequently "encumbered with moral overtones" and entangled with identity.[2] The taste of food and drink elicits powerful emotions. Certain tastes inspire memories and, as the madeleine dipped in tea did for Proust, may produce overwhelming pleasure. Others bring unpleasant surprise. "How do you 'step back' from the sensation of a just-dried mussel on your tongue?" asks Lisa Heldke. "From the odor of durian?" Tastes, she concludes, "both remind us who we are and point out to us who we are not."[3] Human infants learn taste (and language) before learning other things.[4]

The first tendency of those newly arrived in an outpost of empire was to resist ingesting local food and drink, and to rely instead on provisions sent from home or another familiar place. Britons and Americans were often revolted by the food and drink of India and the Philippines and by the way local people prepared, served, and ate or drank them. Bourdieu emphasizes the class basis for taste, but it is surely true that food made and consumed by those of another race or ethnicity is even more likely to elicit disapproval and even disgust.[5] There was much at stake in tasting, for unlike what is seen or heard, what is eaten can kill. Unboiled water carried deadly diseases. Indian curries, laced with hot chilies, made from pigs or cows or goats fed on garbage, and prepared by cooks who, said the British, were strangers to soap and water and stirred pots with their fingers and toes, could not only be unappetizing but possibly dangerous. In the Philippines vegetables were fertilized with human feces, flies attended in droves the open air markets where people bought their food, and the unsuspecting American traveler in the highlands might find on his plate boiled grasshoppers or a haunch of dog.

Metaphors of empire were haptic, but also gustatory. The British and Americans "devoured" or "swallowed" their imperial possessions; "the taste of empire is in the mouth of the people," enthused the *Washington Post* as the United States annexed the Philippines.[6] Opponents of empire objected that tropical nations inhabited by those they alleged to be racially inferior were indigestible. Subjects spurned the alleged nourishment provided by their conquerors—Mohandas Gandhi fasted frequently in protest of British policies—or feared that the imperialists would consume them: Damien Pascual recalled that Filipino children in occupied towns were urged to "stay indoors or the Americans will eat you."[7]

And yet it is impossible to insulate oneself permanently from local foods. They hold temptations that the tongue cannot altogether resist. Stubborn as it is, taste can change, of necessity and through learned preference. The bottled peas of home were simply not as good as fresh vegetables cooked with Indian spices, as the British finally admitted. Fruits canned months earlier in the United States instantly lost their savor when compared to fresh papayas, mangoes, and pineapples that grew abundantly in the Philippines. The Anglo-Americans struggled, in their view heroically, to revise the sensory epistemes of their subjects, to alter how and what they saw, heard, smelled, and touched or felt. Such revision seemed to them essential if they were to civilize Asians. It was in the realm of taste where a kind of sensory compromise was first reached. In spite of themselves, Britons and Americans acknowledged that Indian and Filipino foods were usually more enticing than theirs. The strange might be made familiar or might be exciting in its strangeness. The Anglo-Americans would not abandon their own foods, which they believed connected them securely to home and civilization. Instead, their imperial menus offered a combination of tastes, with roasted meats served with rice and *dhal* in Calcutta, with Australian beef accompanied by bananas and shark's fin soup in Cebu. Or they might eat local foods for lunch and "western" ones at dinner. By the second decade of the twentieth century, and in spite of themselves, Britons and Indians and Americans and Filipinos were eating hybrid cuisines that foretold a sensory accommodation achieved less by coercion and manipulation than by the common ground Selves and Others seem so often seem to find in food and drink.[8]

What They Ate

Tastes in Britain and the United States in the late nineteenth century were shaped by tradition, French food fashion, and changing technology and market forces that enabled increased agricultural production, the preservation and canning of food, refrigeration in railway and marine shipping, and the incorporation into diets of products from empires and beyond, most prominently sugar.[9] The British tended to resist new foods, fearing that changes in their diet by way of imperial foodstuffs would damage national identity.[10] Middle-class Britons ate eggs, toast, and jam for breakfast, and for lunch and dinner roast beef, lamb chops, sausage, poultry, fish, and meat pies, butter and cheese, quantities of potatoes, soups, and puddings made with milk. Milk was also added to chocolate and tea or drunk straight, especially by children. The British drank a good deal of beer, whiskey, and fortified wine.[11] They ate limited numbers of vegetables and fruits—cabbages, cucumbers, peas, celery, apples, cherries, pears, and berries—in good part because they considered such things luxuries, "feeble and female foods which were unlikely to help in turning out real men."[12] "To be reckoned a civilised person," concludes historian Lizzie Collingham, "one had to eat beef and consume alcohol."[13] American food preferences were on the whole similar to British ones. By the late nineteenth century, beef, sugar, and bread had supplanted, at least for the urban middle class, salt pork, molasses, and corn meal mush.[14] Americans ate regional dishes including brown beans and brown bread, shellfish, and chili peppers, at least as many dairy products as their British counterparts, seasonal favorites including stuffed turkey and pumpkin pie, and, for recent immigrants, foods reflecting their national backgrounds.[15] Americans drank more coffee than tea and, like the British, a great deal of alcohol.

When Britons first arrived in India, many of them agents of the East India Company, they formed a tiny minority of the population. Most were men, often without benefit of full access to their own food.[16] Experts advised them to adapt their bodies and their sense of taste to the tropical climate and the food favored by the "natives." James Johnson, whose 1813 book on life in India was widely consulted by Britons going there, suggested that rice and curry was "a salutary dish for the sick." "That vegetable food is better adapted to a tropical climate than animal, I think, we may admit; and particularly among unseasoned Europeans," he concluded. The European in India should eat a simple breakfast, stick to boiled rice made with local spices, and eat only limited amounts of unfamiliar fruits, including mangoes ("which not seldom bring out a plentiful supply of pustules, or even boils, on the unseasoned European") and pineapples, though Johnson admitted that both were "delicious."[17] To some extent, British men took this advice. While the merchants of the company refused to give up eating enormous quantities of meat when they could get it—a surgeon estimated that more animals were killed each month to feed the British in India than were slaughtered in a year to feed the country's Muslims—many Britons nevertheless moderated their diets and adjusted to their circumstances. The early British grandees acted like Indian princes (*nawabs*), opening their bodies and their senses to the environment and its food.[18] Percival Griffiths left it to his bearer and cook to prepare his meals, "a nice hot chicken curry for lunch and mulligatawny soup and roast chicken for dinner."[19] Peter Mundy ate "dopiage"—that is, "dopiaza," or "two onions," likely made with chicken—with rice, "kegeree" (a dish with Indian spices, rice, fish, and eggs) and pickled mangoes, while Robert Clive, the victor at Plassey in 1757, and his fellow officers chewed *paan* and had their own betel-sets and spittoons.[20] In his novel *Vanity Fair*, William Makepeace Thackeray has Jos Sedley, late of India but now back in England, torment Becky Sharp with a spicy curry he has taught his mother to make.[21]

Such practices had their limits. "Going native" in their deportment or their consumption of food and drink exposed British officials to presumptions of familiarity by their Indian subalterns and, they worried, to comestibles that were not in the end good for them. There were reports of Europeans dying after drinking tainted arrack, a potent liquor made from coconut, and an excess of pineapple was implicated in the death of Rose Aylmer in Calcutta in 1800.[22] Britons ascribed what they saw as the effeminacy of Bengali men to their "enfeebling" diet, and in particular to the absence of meat from Hindu tables.[23] Even before the germ theory took hold, all food and drink in India was suspect: water and milk had to be boiled to be safe, fresh fruits and vegetables were washed in potassium permanganate (called "pinky"), and meat and fish must be eaten the day it was butchered or caught.[24]

After the Great Rebellion, Britons felt that by "going native" they had let down their guard, allowing themselves to adopt dangerous culinary habits and otherwise to trust those around them. They claimed to have been repaid with treachery. Their cooks and servants could poison their food, under cover of unfamiliar substances and spices new to their palates. Arriving at a new understanding of their role in India as bringing civilization, they could not adopt local foodways; their need to maintain status meant that "curry and rice were demoted" from their menus.[25] "The molten curries and florid oriental compositions of the olden time," wrote a Briton from Madras in 1885, "have been gradually banished from our dinner tables."[26]

Thus earlier suspicions about the safety, wholesomeness, and tastiness of Indian fare grew enormously after 1857. The food itself, the British now claimed, lacked quality. The recipes used by Indian cooks led to barbarous dishes unfit for consumption by civilized people. The means used to prepare food and drink were unsanitary, the result of ignorance concerning hygiene or the willful filthiness of those charged with their preparation. And Indian table manners were revolting to see or hear, for "native" diners served and ate with their fingers or full hands and slurped from their (dirty) plates and cups in sonically disgusting ways. It was best after all to stick to one's own foods, brought from home, and to British recipes one could trust. If preparation by Indian cooks was necessary—that is, if the foods were not tinned, which required only opening and serving—the choice was either to supervise the process closely or ignore it altogether, trusting to luck or faith to avoid getting sick.

The British indictment of Indian food and foodways was broadscale. In the immediate aftermath of the Great Rebellion, a correspondent for the *Times of London,* recently arrived in India, expressed dismay at local eating habits: "Everything that grows and is fit for food of man or beast is cut, carried off, sucked or chewed, or boiled or roast, or eaten raw."[27] Britons complained that the Indian plantain tasted like "an indifferent mellow pear," the mango "like turpentine," and the guava "an almost equal mixture of raspberry jam and garlic," edible separately but never in combination.[28] A dish as innocent as porridge could be polluted by the presence of worms in the semolina used to make it.[29] Indian chickens were tough and stringy and "one got sick to death" of eating them, beef had the qualities of "lean, tasteless flabbiness" and was of "wretched quality," and veal was "far from attractive."[30] Sausages, made in part from soy flour, were (according to Anne Bremner) "revolting"; camel, eaten raw by some in Rajasthan, nauseated the British with its look and smell.[31] At a rajah's palace near Raipur, Edgar and Carol Hyde were served "leaves and ants rolled and wrapped in leaf gold which tasted horrid."[32] Breakfasts in India were "horrible meals" because

Indian cooks did not understand how to prepare fish and meat, which were "of poor quality" in any event.[33] Bread, made from arrack, had a sour taste and was so mushy "you could squeeze it like a sponge."[34] Of the Tamil-speaking workers on his tea plantation in the early twentieth century, J. L. H. Williams wrote: "Some of their dietary habits were peculiar." They ate snakes and rats and venison even if it was "rotten and stinking," and tiger meat, considered inedible even by "primitive . . . jungle tribes," but which they claimed gave them "heart and strength."[35]

Dining as guests in the homes and palaces of Indian princes or other dignitaries tested British politesse and social diplomacy. A visitor to the court of Sadaat Ali Khan was distressed to find milk served in chamber pots.[36] At a nawab's table, George Atkinson reflected that his host's cooks were "not adepts at Christian cookery," which meant that "trifling irregularities greet the senses. The salad indicates the presence of cod-liver oil, and we have faint suspicions that 'Day and Martin' "—a shoe polish—"has been introduced as a sauce." Like others he was served, these were "brazen dishes" with a "pungent odour which, penetrating our olfactories, reaches to the very roots of our hair."[37] At a garden party in Lahore, Evelyn Beeton confronted "native" food, including "various sweet stuffs and stale looking cakes, most dangerous and repulsive looking."[38] Lady Chapman had dinner at the Mir's palace in Hyderabad (Sind) in 1913. "We may have used our fingers," she recalled, "and I remember my mother's warning looks as some of the dishes went round, and her scarcely concealed horror when we took some bright yellow twisted sweetmeats which we had already seen in the bazaar but had never been allowed to sample."[39]

As these examples suggest, it was not just Indian food itself, nor the perceived ignorance (or sadism) of cooks who prepared it, that troubled British eaters. Indian kitchens and cooks seemed to them unacquainted with hygiene or uninterested in observing its rules. By the early twentieth century many Britons understood the connection between bacteria, conveyed by undercooked food and unclean beverage, and serious disease. Sanitary kitchen practices and good table manners would lessen the possibility of getting sick, and the latter was in any case a sign of civilized behavior that the British middle class had adopted even before the perils of eating with one's fingers, sharing food, and spitting at the table were appreciated. Britons ate off plates, drank from cups, and used utensils to serve themselves from common platters and their own forks to eat what they had taken. Their vessels were best made of china, which resisted contamination.[40] They discouraged noisy eating. The British hoped to impose this sense of culinary propriety on Indians.

For a time, they despaired of doing so. Indians, Britons said, did not seem to understand how important it was to maintain clean hands, surfaces, and utensils in the kitchen. Flora Annie Steel and Grace Gardiner, who published the much-consulted manual *The Complete Indian Housekeeper and Cook* in 1888, observed multiple abuses of culinary hygiene. British *memsahibs* "never go into their kitchens," they wrote, "for the simple reason that their appetite for breakfast might be marred by seeing the *khitmutgâr* [a table or kitchen servant] using his toes as an efficient toast rack (*fact*); or their desire for dinner weakened by seeing the soup strained through a greasy *pugri* [turban]." Indian kitchens, they said, were notorious for their poor drainage, leaving "offal" and sewage on the floor. Yet "even supposing the kitchen is kept in a cleanly state, it by no means follows that the food will be cooked cleanly, and the mistress must always be on her guard against the dirty habits which are ingrained in the native cook. The strictest morning parade will not prevent him stirring the eggs into a rice pudding with his finger." Steel and Gardiner then addressed the servants. Avoid placing milk or water near a foul-smelling drain; to do so would risk "poison[ing] your master or your master's child, as surely as if you had put arsenic in their food. Cleanliness," they admonished, "is no mere fanciful fad on the *sahib-logue's* part. It may be a matter of life and death. Never forget this." Servants should keep a bar of soap and a clean towel at hand and avoid cooking in woolen clothes, which retained odors and dirt.[41] Another culinary and housekeeping adviser, "Chota Mem" ("Little Memsahib," Mrs. C. Lang,), urged British women to inspect the kitchen on occasion "when the cook is not expecting you. I am afraid you will get some shocks, but it may make him have cleaner ways."[42] George Atkinson agreed: it must be done. "Look into an Oriental kitchen," he wrote. "If your eyes are not instantly blinded with the smoke, and if your sight can penetrate into the darkness, enter that hovel, and witness the preparation of your dinner."[43]

Britons feared that Indians served guests food with their dirty fingers; Emily Eden quietly deposited a pair of broiled quails, "a great lump of sweetmeat," and a handful of pomegranate seeds beneath her seat after these foods were handed to her by her host in Amritsar.[44] Strong smelling food likely betrayed its unsanitary handling. Rosamund Lawrence was embarrassed to discover that fish purchased and given to guests by her servants was obviously spoiled, while Margery Hall, who secretly liked Indian food, was nevertheless put off by a meal at a rest house that "had a very strong taste of cowshed."[45] As they were tempted to avoid visiting their own kitchens, so were Britons put off the butcher's shop in the bazaar, "headquarters of the village flies."[46]

Britons worried especially about the effects of tainted food and drink on their children or the infirm. Milk, the staple of the British child's diet, was untrustworthy in India, drawn from dirty or sick cows, handled with sanitary indifference, then served in bottles or vessels that were themselves unclean. Many families kept special "nursery cows" to produce milk for children. Parents insisted that the cow be brought around to the verandah to be milked, that a house servant inspect the hands of the *cow wallah* before he did the milking, and that the milk then be boiled thoroughly. British children brought their own bottles of milk, wrapped in tissue paper, to parties, because few parents trusted that other households were as fastidious as theirs.[47] Florence Marryat worried that Indian food was less nutritious for children than British, and that an Indian diet put stress "upon their delicate nervous systems."[48] Parents were warned to keep their children away from spicy Indian curries.[49] When Iris Macfarlane was sent to Indian schools, she was not allowed to eat "curry lunches" with her classmates, "but sat on the hillside eating hotel sandwiches" packed by her mother.[50] The purported inadequacy of an Indian diet was a leading reason why most parents sent their children to Britain when they were still very young. "Few sights are more pleasing," wrote an English observer, "than to see these puny, pallid, skinny, fretful little ones *converted, by British food and British meteorology,* into fat and happy English children."[51] Britons who were ill were advised to stay away from Indian food, which would only upset their digestion, cause fever, nausea, and inevitable diarrhea, and might even produce cholera or dysentery. Bland British imports, among them "Granose flakes" and "Sanitorium Fruit Crackers" served with Bovril (beef paste) or boiled milk, were the usual prescription for intestinal illness.[52]

The British in India could not abandon Indian food; in the end they liked it too much to give it up entirely. As they tried to withdraw their bodies from Indian society, they embraced British food as never before. There was more safety than savor in it, and for a while at least they allowed curries to remain on their menus at breakfast and lunch. But dinner was a time to be British, with the protections and status privileges that implied, and if Indians were invited to dinner, as was sometimes necessary, they would learn to partake of British food in British style. A dinner given by the Viceroy, Lord Reading, for the installation of the nawab of Bahawalpur in the northwest in the early 1920s was a formal English meal including soup, tinned paté, tinned salmon, roasted poultry, caramel custard, and coffee. Afterward, the Indians confessed to each other that they were "greatly disappointed" with the experience. The food seemed to them tasteless, and they were forced to use utensils with which they were unfamiliar.[53] Yet the British would maintain decorum even in the remotest places and show the Indians by example how culinary civility looked and smelled and tasted. And they sought constantly to remind themselves by their food who they were. "And sure enough did they drive away from the Club in a few minutes," wrote E. M. Forster in *A Passage to India,* "and they did dress, and to dinner came Miss Derek and the McBrydes, and the menu was: Julienne soup full of bullety bottled peas with the cutlets, trifle, sardines on toast: the menu of Anglo-India. A dish might be added or subtracted as one rose or fell in the official scale, the peas might rattle less or more, the sardines or vermouth be imported by a different firm, but the tradition remained: the food of exiles, cooked by servants who did not understand it."[54]

The British ate from bottles and tins, like Forster's characters peas and sardines, but also other vegetables and fish, French *paté*, and haggis "for the homesick Scots."[55] Tinned food had a metallic taste and lacked nutrition, but it promised safety and was handy when traveling.[56] They served jam from home, cheeses from France, and beef from Australia; on Christmas Day they resorted to tinned turkey.[57] For bread they did what they could, often shunning Indian *chapattis*—"food for dogs," declared one Anglo-Indian.[58] Craving ice for drinks and food storage, the men of the Raj arranged for their "coolies" to place on the ground during cold nights large shallow saucers filled with water. At three in the morning, the coolies ("poor shivering wretches") would chip the ice out of the saucers, pack it, and store it for later use, including for ice cream.[59] Britons drank what historian K. T. Achaya charitably calls "a fair amount," in his estimate a bottle of Madeira with dinner and three bottles of claret afterward for men, and a bottle of wine each day for women, along with the gin they all had at home or their clubs.[60] Menus for dinner parties given by the British indicated the turn toward European food after 1858. An ordinary gathering with friends might include soup, fried fish, mutton cutlets with bottled tomato sauce, roast chicken, caramel custard, and the inevitable sardines on toast.[61] Hilda Bourne described a more elaborate luncheon for fifty to sixty people: cucumber sandwiches, tomato sandwiches, a dish of *paté de fois gras*, a pair of two-pound cakes, five dozen *petit fours*, one pound of chocolates, another of "mixed sweets," five dozen macaroons, three dozen "Queen cakes," and three dozen "Rock cakes"—all requiring a hundred pounds of ice for preservation and display.[62] After these affairs the men retired to smoke cheroots, which replaced the hookah in European circles by the late nineteenth century.[63]

Recipes for curry disappeared almost entirely from British household advice books.[64] As their food became more British, so did Anglo-Indians resolve more firmly to practice the table etiquette being followed back home. For their parties they wrote menus in French. They ate off the good china and set their tables with silverware, fancy glassware, linen tablecloths, and white napkins folded into the shape of peacocks and placed in wine glasses. Indian food was generally served all at once, but since Europeans brought food to the table in courses, that is what the British in India did. And, in spite of the heat, the British dressed for dinner, even if there were no guests. Women put on dresses with petticoats. Men wore "boiled white shirts, white waistcoats, black or white ties, and tail coats or dinner jackets" in black and made of wool.[65] Such habits were a vital part of preserving and exalting British identity in a strange and hazardous place, regardless of the effort it entailed and the haptic discomfort it produced.

The Americans who came to the new empire in the Philippines after 1900 were less often inclined to similar displays. They were not themselves royalty or viceroyalty, nor were they among princes whom they felt the need to impress.

But they were, like the British, anxious about their position and the food and drink they consumed. And they were as determined to civilize the Filipinos' sense of taste as they were to correct and refine their other four senses. Their own tastes and foodways had changed only recently and not in every class; no doubt many of the soldiers who came to fight in the Philippines ate at home more salt pork than beef. When in the early nineteenth century British visitors joined Americans at table, they were appalled by their behavior. Dining at an inn in Nashville in 1831, a British army officer remarked on the manners of his tablemates: "Each man helped himself with his own knife and fork, and reached across his neighbor to secure a fancied *morceau*. Bones were picked with both hands; knives were drawn through the teeth with the edge to the lips; the scalding mocha and souchong were poured into saucers to expedite the cooling. . . . Beefsteaks, apple tart, and fish, were seen on the same plate the one moment, and had disappeared the next!"[66] By the latter part of the century, according to historian John F. Kasson, American table manners had improved considerably; they were now no less than "the supreme test of refinement, character, and to use the catchall term so dear to the hearts of nineteenth-century advisers, 'good-breeding.'"[67] Americans now ate with forks (rather than knives), dining room servants covered their thumbs with a napkin while they served, and diners were told "not to scratch their heads" or "pick their teeth" at the table, and to "keep their hands below the table when unoccupied."[68] The Americans would attempt to export their newfound manners to allegedly uncivilized Filipinos. Reform of Filipinos was a Progressive enterprise, and thus part of the effort to curb noise, refine the skin, and improve food hygiene, eating habits, and table manners. "Brutes feed," asserted one authority on etiquette. "The best barbarian only eats. Only the cultured man can dine." Cities began to pasteurize milk: by 1914, New York had fifty-six "milk-stations" that did this.[69] In 1906 President Theodore Roosevelt signed the Pure Food and Drug Act, and the following year the Federal Meat Inspection Act, both designed in part to prevent the adulteration of food products.

Fear and contempt were the first American impressions of Filipino food and water. Soldiers were supplied with rations, which were rarely satisfying and often ran out. These included hardtack, beans, canned salmon, canned fruit (peaches, pears, and prunes), canned beef, canned butter ("like Vaseline in consistancy [*sic*]"), "milk toast made with condensed milk, which is nasty," and beverages that could be boiled for safety, including coffee and hot chocolate.[70] Occasionally they did better, finding a well-stocked mess with a competent cook and reporting with enthusiasm on meals that included oatmeal, pancakes, poultry, and perhaps a small steak or pork chop.[71] Living off the land, which usually meant looting, yielded eggs, chickens, fruit, and *camotes*, Philippine sweet potatoes that brought many more complaints than praise. Officers tried as far as possible to prevent their men from eating local food. "If we eat like natives," one declared, "we will become as stupid, frail, and worthless as they are."[72]

Civilians who arrived in the archipelago during and after pacification agreed, at first, that Filipino food was largely unpalatable. Food in the Philippines was strongly influenced by other Southeast Asian cuisines, and also included dishes borrowed from China, Mexico (the popular *adobo* originated there), and Spain. Though it varied widely by region, rice was at the center of the Philippine diet, and Americans wearied of its constant presence.[73] If they ventured into the Philippine hinterlands beyond Manila, as many teachers did, for example, they encountered dishes and ways of eating them that shocked or amused them. Herbert Priestly found the food in Bicol "not of a kind or quality to support white people."[74] The Igorots of the Luzon cordillera ate strong-tasting foods heavy with garlic and oil. Dean Worcester discovered in an Igorot commissary line nothing but "some wads of sticky, unsalted, boiled rice which our Igorot carriers had inside their hats, in contact with their frowzy hair! We ate as much of this as the Igorots could spare, killing its rather high flavour with cayenne peppers picked beside the trail."[75] Chicken was a staple and a source of protein, as it was for most Filipinos. Americans soon grew tired of it and were especially appalled when Igorots used every part of the bird, including the feet and head, "to yield whatever nourishment they might contain."[76] There were insects on offer, including grasshoppers, fried and sold by the bushel in the market, and beetles, discovered by teacher William Freer with their "wings and legs removed" and "floating about in the liquor in which they had been stewed."[77] Unable to drink water in the countryside for fear of getting dysentery, Americans resorted to green coconut water, beer, or, in a pinch, *tapoy*, the Igorots' "disgusting rice wine."[78] It was difficult to avoid eating the wrong thing in Igorot country for fear of offending one's hosts, and many Americans tried at least to sample the food and drink they were offered. Charles MacDonald recalled a "queer dinner of shark-fin soup . . . along with grasshoppers, bad eggs, snails, rice-bread, young goats and coconut juice." A Filipino band played throughout the meal "in an endeavor to make the diner forget the menu (perhaps)."[79] Bishop Charles Brent was for the most part accommodating, but after consuming, among other things, "eggs fried in rancid olive oil and some rank sausage," he returned to Manila with amoebic dysentery. There were times Brent simply declined invitations for fear of having to "eat and drink some of their good things."[80] Most revolting to the Americans was the consumption of dog by some Igorots. Americans demurred from eating dog if it were offered, and officials tried to dissuade the Igorots from eating it, seeing it as symbolic of the upland peoples' barbarity.[81]

A crisis arose in 1901 when the Manila office in charge of military commissaries announced that American teachers would no longer be issued permits allowing them to make purchases at the stores. Governor-General William Howard Taft

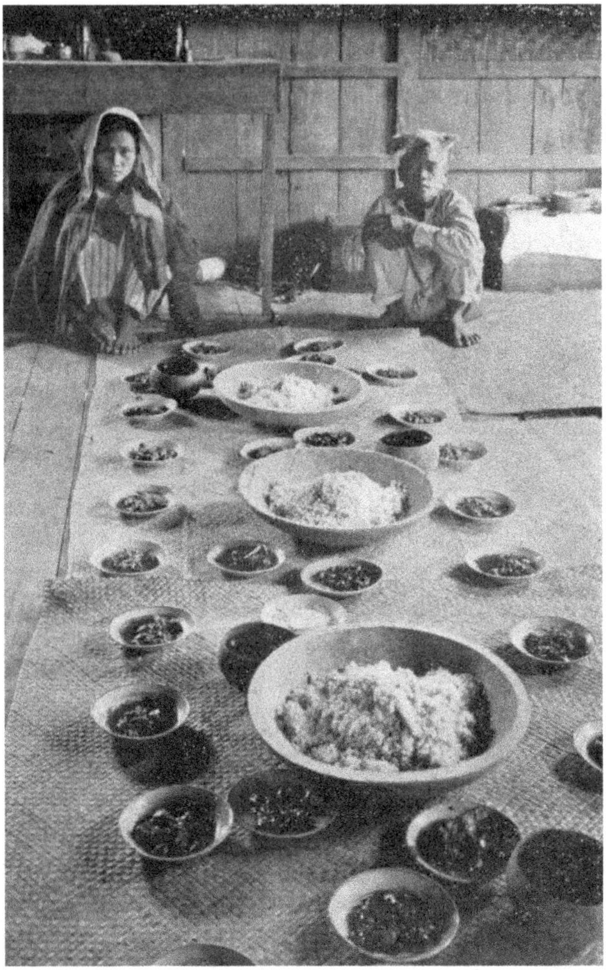

Figure 7.1 The caption of this photograph is "A Strange Couple." In it, the Filipinos have laid on a feast—rice and its accompaniments—according to Dean Worcester, in memory of a dead child. From Dean C. Worcester, *The Philippines Past and Present*, Volume II (New York: The Macmillan Co., 1914), p. 946.

received a number of letters from aggrieved officials and teachers and from Fred W. Atkinson, the Superintendent of Public Instruction in the islands. Atkinson pointed out that the teachers had been recruited and sent to remote towns on the assumption that they would be able to buy American food at the commissaries, and that there had been no hint that the policy would be discontinued. "Teachers cannot live on native food," Atkinson wrote. "If teachers are sent out in towns where they cannot procure proper food, the result will be disastrous to many of them by breaking down in health; and the usefulness of all will be much lessened." From Union province, a Mr. Tompkins wrote that "on account of the scarcity of stores here it is impossible for the three teachers and myself to procure anything to eat this side of Manila except rice and fish." In Tarlac, Sydney Hopson noted that there were no restaurants, and R. J. Fanning claimed that his "physical condition [was] threatened" by his need to eat "native food, which is not agreeable or conducive to health."[82] Benjamin Neal was saved by a local military officer who invited him to dine in his mess—"a Godsend to me as the native food was ruining my health."[83] Ultimately, civil commissaries were established to allow Americans to buy staples in all but the most remote places.[84]

In Manila, there was a chance to get better and safer food. Americans in the city were closer to supply lines from the United States, Australia, and Japan, from which more familiar foods came, and like Britons in India they strongly preferred these. "White flour, red meat, and blue blood make the tricolor flag of conquest," wrote journalist Woods Hutchinson in 1906, and Americans in the Philippines heartily endorsed his view.[85] As of 1902, the US military consumed each month 900,000 pounds of beef and mutton, 60,000 pounds of butter, and 15,000 pounds of cheese, all from Australia.[86] The quality of canned goods evidently improved, or was higher when sold on the open market rather than issued as rations to soldiers.[87] Distilled water was widely available in the capital.[88] And it was possible to get a good meal in Manila, if one belonged to the right mess, had a good cook, was well connected or well off, or attended the right parties. The Tafts received apples from Japan and oranges from California, and American whiskey and French wine via Hong Kong.[89] In September 1902 they gave a dinner featuring an all-French menu, including "Potage," "Filet de boeuf a la Perigord," "Chapon aux champignons farcis," and "Glace Vanilla."[90]

But few could afford such luxuries. Most Americans in Manila and other large towns complained about their provisions, if somewhat less frequently and a bit more philosophically than their counterparts in the countryside. Businessman Charles Morris found the city's restaurants "primitive in character" and with monotonous menus, providing "little more than rice and fruits for sale." "I have yet to see a soldier who would tackle any of the cooked dishes," wrote John Clifford Brown, "and a soldier will try almost anything."[91] Some vegetables were reminiscent enough of those at home, but all seemed more trouble than they were worth, requiring careful washing in rare untainted water, and often prolonged cooking, which depleted their flavor and nutrition. Among fruits mangoes and bananas won some praise; their thick skins protected them from the worst bacteria present in the environment or on the hands of Filipinos who picked or sold them.[92] *Camotes* were "watery and stringy," watermelons and paw-paws lacked taste.[93] The most common local meat came from the water buffalo, or *carabao*, but Americans found it difficult to digest.[94] "Manila is a hard old town," Robert Carter wrote his father. "The eating is [bad]; nearly everything has a suspicious smell." Carter refused to drink milk because he had heard all the cows were diseased, and dairy products were in any case hard to keep fresh in the heat, while "rice gags a man" and failed to stop his chronic diarrhea. "The eating out here," he concluded, "is the worst feature of life."[95] "It is said that if you are careful [in] what you eat and drink, and live a regular life, you can be as well here as anywhere," noted Daniel R. Williams, who staffed the Philippine Commission, in June 1900. "The only trouble about this is that you cannot always be sure just what you are eating and drinking."[96]

Emily Conger despised Filipino food. Children ate "little rice cakes, thin, hard, and indigestible as bits of slate." The islands' garlic and tomatoes were "inferior" to those at home. On board a Spanish steamer from Manila to Iloilo, she was offered a Filipino meal: "There was a well-prepared chicken with plenty of rice but made so hot with pepper that I threw it into the sea; next, some sort of salad floating in oil and smelling of garlic; it went overboard. Eggs cooked in oil followed the salad; last the 'dulce,' a composition of rice and custard perfumed with anise seed oil, made the menu of the fishes complete." She preferred the apparent safety of American food: "I now gladly opened my box of crackers and cheese, oranges, figs and dates." On July 4, 1900, Conger made for US soldiers the foods of holidays at home: "eighty-three pumpkin pies, fifty-two chickens, three hams, forty cakes, ginger-bread," and more.[97]

Like Anglo-Indians, Americans in the Philippines recoiled at the way food was overseen, prepared, and eaten by the local people. Markets where food was sold were particular sources of hygienic anxiety. Victor Heiser, the Philippines health director, tried to clean up the public food market in Manila, prohibiting the sale of "low-growing vegetables" which he feared had been fertilized with night soil, providing forks at the butcher stalls, and placing a barrel of mercury bichloride solution at the entrance and requiring that all vendors and shoppers wash their hands in it.[98] Years later, in Cagayan on a leper-collecting trip, he discovered a newly reconstructed market "not kept as well as it might be. Flies were literally found swarming everywhere; no food screens in use. . . . The tables from which meat and fish were sold were filthy, some having galvanized iron tops, very rusty. Apparently no proper disposition of waste made."[99] Frank Laubach took in the Dansalan market on Mindanao. Vendors sat on the ground and placed their wares, including foodstuffs, alongside them. "There are troughs containing brown sugar and coarse salt, which look as though they must be swarming with germs." Sugar and salt were sold from sacks made of bark or leaves.[100]

Nor could Filipinos be trusted to cook and serve and eat food cleanly. The cholera epidemic that struck Manila in 1902 seemed to Americans sobering evidence that Filipinos were not boiling water or thoroughly cooking foods washed in it.[101] Neither Filipinos nor the Chinese who sometimes handled food could keep their fingers out of others' drinking water or dairy products; in 1934, most

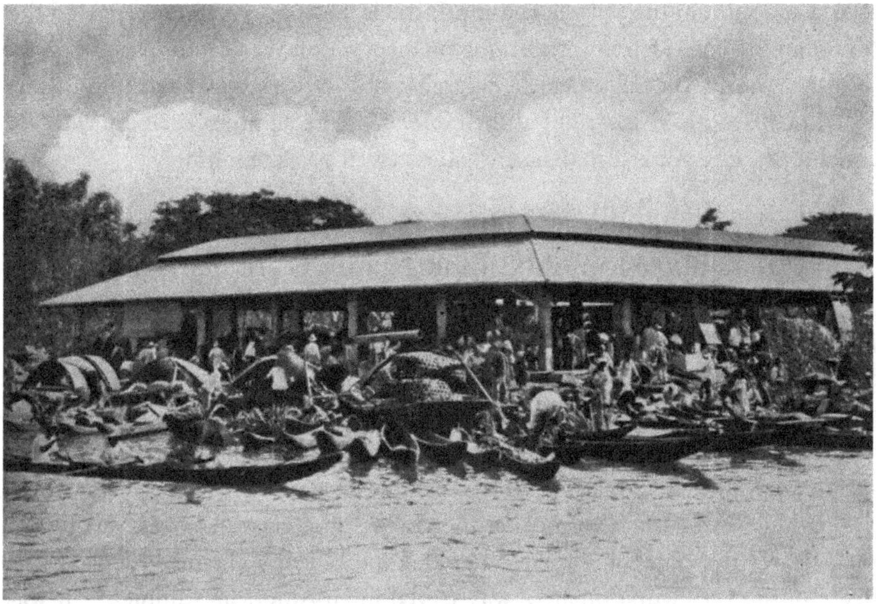

Figure 7.2 A market in the Philippines. Americans were fascinated and appalled by the condition of the food for sale in the open-air stalls. Courtesy of Library of Congress, Prints and Photographs Division.

of the staff of the Malolos Provincial Hospital got food poisoning from eating poorly prepared pineapple ice cream.[102] When they ate, said the Americans, Filipinos put their hands into the common rice pot; when they drank it was from coconut shells dipped repeatedly into a single vessel.[103] William Freer's cook, Clemente, was willing to take cooking instruction (less garlic, softer rice), but "could not wean himself from the habit of using the kitchen floor for the purposes of a table while preparing the food or washing the dishes."[104] Canned sardines should have been safe, but Ruth Hunt watched them being processed on the beach: "It looked most unappetizing. The final packing is done in old Standard Oil cans. All this is coupled with the appearance and unsanitary condition of the packers [and] made me decide never to touch local sardines!"[105] At a Filipino home, Edith Moses looked forward to a promised dulce for dessert, only to discover that it was a can of corn dusted with powdered sugar and passed down the table hand to hand.[106] Ralph Buckland suffered through a difficult dinner at a Manila hotel, including "soup that looked a mystery" and "some rather poor bananas," but was most put off when the waiters used a dirty cloth to wipe plates and utensils between courses. Weeks later, he had dinner on board a ship staffed by Filipinos. There was good fish but the beef was tough, and for dessert the cook produced a can of guava jelly, with a teaspoon placed in it. "The jelly can began on the Filipino end of the line," Buckland wrote. "The first one took a spoonful of the jelly, licked it off, stuck the spoon back, and passed the tin on up the line, each in turn licking off a spoonful. We did not eat any guava jelly that meal." The Filipinos then gargled noisily with water, making "a sort of hydraulic tooth-brush, right at the table. We were all pretty well put out," he concluded. "Our American delicacy had received a severe jolting."[107]

Teaching Moments: Table Manners and Famines

Just before the Great Rebellion, a British officer took his seat at the table of Nana Sahib of Cawnpore. His napkin was "a bedroom towel." The dishes were an assortment of plates, bowls, and cups seemingly stolen from the army mess or discarded by an English household. The knife had a bone handle, the fork and spoon were silver, from Calcutta. The vegetable serving dishes were mismatched, the pudding came on a soup plate, the cheese on a glass dish that was meant for dessert. The claret, brought too cold, appeared in a champagne glass; the beer, "of the very worst quality," was served in an American tumbler.[108] It was amusing, disheartening, and it indicated to the British in attendance how little even the wealthiest Indians understood of etiquette, one of the small but significant signs of civilization. Along with other inappropriate behaviors the British noted among Indians at table—bringing out all the courses at once, serving and eating with one's fingers, spitting, chewing noisily and with open mouth, loudly clearing one's throat—the inability to set a table properly, with matching china and silver, proved that Indians had no respect for a civilized sense of taste.

To the extent they felt was possible, Britons tried to teach Indians how to be more mannerly at the table. Following 1858, the F and C Osler Company, makers of glass and dishware, saw an opportunity to enter the Indian market. The company, founded in Birmingham in 1807, had established an office in Calcutta in 1844. "I am very anxious to introduce or try to introduce native dinner sets in crockery," one company executive wrote to another in 1879. "I have been making enquiries about it and the result is favourable. The 'orthodox' Hindoos are not very likely to adopt innovation at first, but 'young Bengal' is not quite so strict as their fathers were. Most of them still retain the native way of eating—with their fingers, but the old custom of smashing pots and pans made of clay after they have been used once is not now considered so necessary as it used to be."[109] British residents hired to tutor Indian princes taught their pupils "table manners, drawing-room etiquette and an appreciation for European food and liquor," and these lessons gradually took hold.[110] On the other hand, it was considered a mistake to spoil servants with unfamiliar food. This was especially true for wet nurses who, if given such luxuries as tea with milk, were likely to get indigestion and induce "green motions in the babe" they were suckling.[111]

The most important and sobering lesson the British thought to teach their Indian subjects was to live frugally and conserve food. In the absence of these measures, they warned, there would be hunger. India, or areas of it, was periodically devastated by famine; Jon Wilson estimates that between twelve and thirty million people died of hunger in the last quarter of the nineteenth century, many of them during the famines of 1876–1878, 1896–1897, and 1900–1901.[112] British policies exacerbated problems caused by the failure of the monsoon, or during years in which the weather was dominated by the El Niño-Southern Oscillation (ENSO) weather pattern. British India overall did not lack food. But the authorities failed to distribute it across regions, allowed grains to follow demand and higher prices out of India and into world markets, built railroads to serve wealthier, urban areas, and denied funding for catchments and dams that might have allowed for water storage against dry years.[113] British officials were not prepared to accept their complicity in mass starvation. Economizing with food was a moral imperative for the poor in a country of limited means—or so Britons told themselves. If Indians went hungry it was because they were fatalistic or lazy, traits that no amount of government compassion or intervention could overcome. A writer for the *Edinburgh Review* concluded in 1877 that Hindu resignation was largely to blame for the mass starvation, and their stubborn adherence to the caste system and misplaced loyalty to their villages meant that people refused to leave their jobs and homes to search for sustenance elsewhere.[114] A year later, Mrs. King was philosophical about the Indians' plight: "Terrible . . . as is a famine, it doubtless makes more room for those who are left, and it seems to be Nature's way of adjusting the balance between food and population."[115] During the Bengal famine of 1944, European restaurants in Calcutta served lobster, caviar, and champagne, and while there was food rationing Europeans got larger shares than Indians.[116] Here, then, was a failed teaching moment, one that relied on exhortation and scorn rather than an honest conveyance or exchange of information.

In the Philippines, famines were shallower and less dramatic than in India, but people were nevertheless faced frequently with undernourishment. During the Insurrection the US military targeted food supplies for destruction or removal, with the likely consequence that the insurgents fought with greater desperation.[117] After pacification, the Americans tried to educate Filipinos to raise and eat more meat (though not dog) and vegetables, drink more milk, and avoid eating polished rice, which had been stripped by polishing of vitamin B and thus could not prevent the onset of beriberi.[118] Reversing the British formulation, Dean Worcester was convinced that what most observers regarded as Filipino "laziness" was in fact "the direct result of physical weakness due to improper and insufficient food."[119] "In the Philippines," one author charged, "the big bulk of the native population eat[s] food which is not calculated to promote health in the

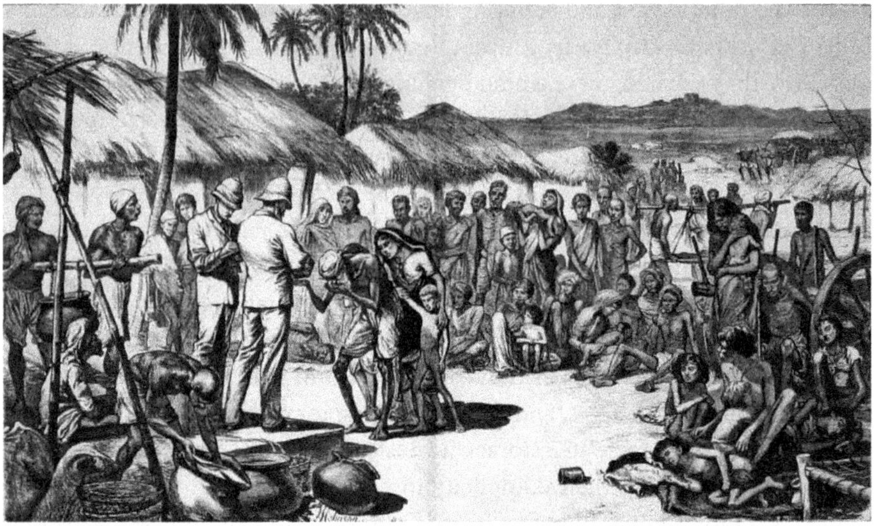

Figure 7.3 British authorities distribute food to hungry Indians in Madras during the famine of 1877. Abjection appears to have been a requirement for assistance. From *Illustrated London News*, May 26, 1877. Wikimedia Commons.

body and we see the consequence in feeble, skinny children, and weak men and women."[120] Officials urged the upland people to cultivate crops, while the government Bureau of Education commissioned advice books for schoolchildren, which provided instruction in proper habits of cultivation and consumption. Students in the first grade learned the benefits of canned condensed milk over carabao milk, those in grade two were taught etiquette, third graders were instructed in the importance of calcium, and fourth graders memorized the nutritional content of whole grains, fruits, and vegetables. At the University of the Philippines women students took two courses in home economics, including nutrition and cooking, while men studied the farming of food crops such as sugar and coconuts.[121] "Unwholesome food is food which does not make good red blood and which is likely to make one sick who eats it," wrote Alice Fuller. "Green fruits, wilted vegetables, fish which has been dead a long time without being cured in some way, lard from a sick hog, meat of animals that have been drowned or have died of sickness, half-cooked rice, very hard corn, and many other things commonly used as food, are not wholesome."[122] Leonard Wood lectured health care workers on the need for "a better balanced food supply," including more green vegetables.[123] Recipes showed cooks how to turn fruit into "whip," marmalade, and jelly.[124] The government endorsed the establishment of "food booths" at festivals, wherein cooks could demonstrate hygienic techniques and display various ways to prepare vegetables.[125] An American livestock broker wrote to Governor Taft urging him to acquire some "Cincinnati cows" for the islands: "I think that the milk of the cows will get the blood of the inhabitants in such condition that they will act like civilized and accomplished people." Taft thanked the man and agreed with his conclusion, though the cows, unused to conditions in Southeast Asia, would have been poorly suited to life there.[126]

Nearly as important to the authors of advice manuals were the table manners of Filipinos. Despite the seemingly favorable influence of Spanish foodways, Americans accused Filipinos of having sloppy and unhygienic habits during the preparation and consumption of meals. Dining with the "natives" was less enjoyable when they cut vegetables on the kitchen floor, ate with their fingers from a common dish or put knives in their mouths, talked about their bodily functions, slurped their soup, or chomped their meat. American school teachers tried to instill better table manners in their students, hoping the lessons would go home, and officials established "Knife and Fork Societies" to convince Filipinos to stop eating with their fingers.[127] The authors of the textbook *Elementary Home Economics* advised that table manners were not trivial but "the long-continued practice of thoughtful people." Napkins should be placed in the lap, not tucked

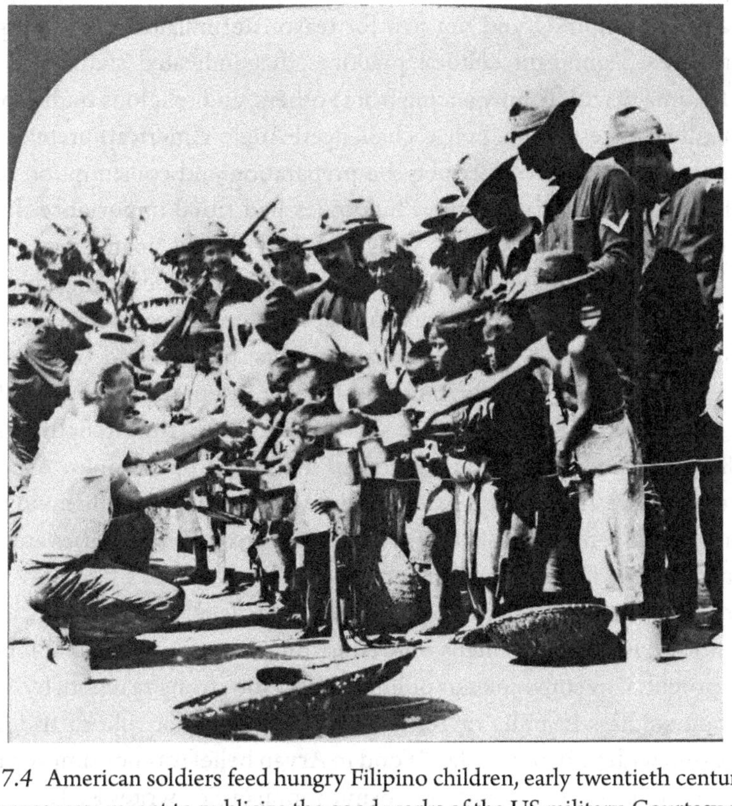

Figure 7.4 American soldiers feed hungry Filipino children, early twentieth century. Such images were meant to publicize the good works of the US military. Courtesy of Library of Congress, Prints and Photographs Division.

into the collar like bibs. "Dip soup away from the body and sip it without noise from the side of the spoon. Do not cool soup or any other food by blowing on it." Lips must be "closed when chewing," and those at table should take small bites and avoid speaking with their mouths full. Diners must use forks "to convey solid or semi-solid food to the mouth." Toothpicks should not be used at the table.[128] Another text advised readers that "it is best to eat from a table" rather than the floor, since "food on a table is not so likely to be contaminated as food on the floor." Diners should have their own place settings, and it was "particularly important" that the serving platter have on it a dedicated serving utensil. "Do not eat you food rapidly and ravenously. It looks ill-bred and is bad for your health. Take your time and chew your food thoroughly." And the authors thought it necessary to admonish readers not to share with others food that "has been in the mouth of somebody else or which has been bitten by another person."[129]

Indian and Filipinos Foodways

Britons and Americans did not always suspect it, but food was vitally important to Indians and Filipinos, and not just for reasons of nutrition. In both places, foodways were significant cultural practices that indicated status, the possibility of intimacy with (or distancing from) others, and religious traditions that, while hardly timeless, nonetheless challenged Anglo-American pretensions to civilizational monopoly concerning the preparation and consumption of food and drink. Food in India and the Philippines had ritual importance. In India it connected human beings to the gods and the cosmos: "man is what he eats and . . . purity of thought depends on purity of food," according to anthropologist Jack Goody.[130] Filipinos, as Americans came to recognize, used food and drink to distinguish themselves from others, both in and outside of the archipelago, and as social lubricants designed to demonstrate hospitality to strangers, and thus their openness to social intercourse. The strength of Indian and Filipino foodways more than matched that of European ones; Asian consumption practices insisted on recognition by the agents of empire and helped to inspire hybrid senses of taste that breached the anxious boundaries erected by westerners against feared contamination.

Fears of contamination by ingestion invoked deeply held beliefs in both Hinduism and Islam that humans were constituted from food and that food thus had the potential to consecrate or pollute. Recall the strong reaction, by Muslim and Hindu soldiers in India in 1857, to rumors that their rifle cartridges had been greased with pork or beef fat. "Food in Aryan belief was not simply a means of bodily sustenance; it was part of a cosmic moral cycle," writes K. T. Achaya.[131] The gods enjoyed food: Krishna ate butter constantly, while in its representations the elephant-headed Ganesh held a bowl of sweets.[132] *Darshan*, whereby humans and gods look upon each other, is at the core of Hindu worship.[133] Yet as Sylvain Pinard has pointed out, the practice of mutual gazing is preceded by the lustration of the image with ritually pure foods, including honey and clarified butter, which is likely then to be consumed by priests and worshippers.[134] Sanskrit texts prescribe an elaborate set of practices around food, including what should be eaten, and when, and by whom.[135] Diet determines health: while British ayurvedic medicine dismissed the importance of dietetics, well into the twentieth century neither Hindu nor Muslim doctors would prescribe medicine without proffering advice about what food or drink should or should not be taken with it.[136] Smallpox could be caused by "disharmonious combinations of food, such as meat and fish, rotting foodstuffs; pungent, sour, salty and alkaline foods."[137] Tastes are specific and of great significance. English provides four words for taste: sweet, sour, salty, or bitter. To these Sanskrit and Hindi add two more—pungent (*katuka*) and astringent (*kashaya*).[138] Aesthetic experience in India, observes art historian B. N. Goswamy, is defined as "'the tasting of flavor' (*rasavadana*)," the root of which, *rasa*, refers in part to "taste, flavor, relish . . . a state of heightened delight."[139]

Taste, or the consumption or nonconsumption of certain foods, also demarcated the boundaries of caste. To eat the wrong sort of food, prepared by the hand of a cook from a caste lower than one's own, or in the company of caste inferiors, was considered highly polluting. Cooks must occupy a caste rank higher than that of those for whom they are cooking. The kitchen must be purified, and the cook must bathe and put on clean clothes, preferably without exposed seams, before starting in. The cook must not taste the food while preparing it lest it retain her saliva. It was best to serve on ephemeral plates, made from banyan or banana leaves. In traditional Hindu homes men precede women to the table, and while leftover food (*jutha*) is counted as "the remains of *some one*" and thus considered vile, it may be eaten by young children or the lower castes, who display a practical "lack of fear against saliva pollution." For the Hindu, according to anthropologist R. S. Khare, "it has been a case of ordering and controlling one's sensorium towards food, not always because of its unavailability but for raising and handling it as a totally moral construct." Foods help Hindus manage "greetings, farewells, distinctions of status and rank precedence, and reciprocity."[140] These proscriptions did not just apply to caste-conscious Hindus. In May 1902, the Sikh Amar Singh went to tea with Zorawar Singhjee, a fellow Sikh, and Mohammed Khan, a Muslim. He was appalled when the two men shared a plate and Zorowar offered him food from it. "Now I will never eat with Zorowar Singhjee," he confided to his diary, "because he eats with Mohammedans and out of the same plate too. . . . He must be crazy to think we would accept his mouthfuls from out [of] the plate in which a Mohammedan is eating. How foolish and ridiculous."[141] Nor were the British immune from caste sensitivities surrounding food. Nora Scott came to the aid of an Indian girl who had been beaten. The girl accepted from Scott's servant raw food which she then cooked herself, but she refused Scott's offer of tea because "she was too high caste for that."[142] High-caste Hindus "will not consent to eat with us," wrote Monier Williams, "or to drink water touched by us or our servants." Such habits, he complained, impeded "social intercourse."[143] Helen and George Browne, the protagonists in Sara Jeanette Duncan's 1893 novel *The Simple Adventures of a Memsahib,* asked for milk in a small village. Milk was available but the Brownes could not be allowed to drink from the villagers' cups, so "the outcast sahib bought a new little earthen pot for a pice [coin], breaking it solemnly on a stone when they had finished" drinking, thereby sparing people on both sides the embarrassment of putting their lips to the same vessel.[144]

Indians were curious about British food and foodways. Some of the wealthy adopted European food and its manner of presentation. Just as curries made their way back onto British menus by the early twentieth century, so too did Indian princes incorporate into their culinary practices written menus, serving in courses, the use of individual knives and forks, and eating off plates designed for London dining rooms.[145] Following custom that food was to be offered to superiors for purposes of honor or propitiation, Indians brought comestible gifts to British officials. The collector Robert Moss King had a rule that only fruits or vegetables were acceptable tribute. When a man brought him a pair of turkeys and King remonstrated, the donor insisted that these were "*vegetable* turkeys" and thus within the rules.[146]

On the whole, though, British foodways did not much penetrate India. Apart from such breakfast items as porridge, tea, and perhaps toast with marmalade, the British contribution to Indian food was largely confined to biscuits and lackluster white bread.[147] A maharajah refused to allow the Bombay to Calcutta train to pass through his capital "because travelers might be eating beef in the restaurant car."[148] "As a rule the Englishman's dinner is plain and monotonous," wrote Behramji Malabari, who visited England in the 1890s. "The cook knows nothing of proportion in seasoning his food; knows little of variety, and has a rough slovenly touch."[149] Certain British foods inspired puzzlement or mockery. When Irene Bose grew tomatoes and lettuce in her garden, the neighbors were appalled. Eating tomatoes was "unlucky" because they were the color of blood, while the "raw leaves" of lettuce were suitable only for goats.[150] British table manners were hardly the last word in civilization for cultivated Indians. In his 1911 manual *Hints on Indian Etiquette, Specially Designed for the Use of Europeans,* S. Iftikhar Hussain offered gentle lessons to British hosts and guests. In India, one washed hands before *and* after meals. When dinner was announced, the host did not lead the way to the table but followed after his guests, and while he was expected to sit at the head of the table the others could find their own seats—here was a subtle dig at the fraught British practice of seating everyone according to understandings of rank. Dishes arrived from the kitchen all at once, Indians did not talk much during meals, and young men were not to smoke or drink in front of their elders. Most important was to avoid serving pork when Muslims were present and beef if there were Hindus.[151]

Indeed, the question of meat consumption preoccupied Indians, especially nationalists, who sought at once to mobilize power against the imperialists and yet distinguish themselves morally from them. Since the British recognized neither the Muslim prohibition against pork nor the Hindus' against beef, Indians were confronted daily with the slaughter of pigs and cattle for British tables. By the late nineteenth century, some in the nascent Hindu nationalist movement called for eating beef at least as a means of self-strengthening. Meat consumption had long been associated with masculinity in North India, and meat was often eaten by men before battle.[152] Many remembered with humiliation that the British had, in the aftermath of the Great Rebellion, forced condemned Muslims to eat pork and Hindus beef before executing them.[153] In Bengal especially, there were calls to imitate the British; if they were to be resisted, it was imperative that their Indian opponents match them in the physical strength possible only through the consumption of meat. "Which is the greater sin?" asked Swami Vivekananda. "To kill a few goats, or to fail to protect the honor of my wife and daughter?" The answer was clear: "Let those who belong to the elite, and do not have to win their bread by physical labour, shun meat."[154] Calcutta scientist Chunilal Bose argued that the Bengali diet lacked protein. This made for an effeminate people with a "disinclination for physical exercise and any kind of active work," weakened "powers of endurance," and an overall "lowering of vitality"—confirmation of what the British had said for years. Men needed to eat more chicken, beef, and pork if they were to convince the British of their fitness for self-rule.[155]

The other side of this argument was made most persistently by M. K. Gandhi. As a young man Gandhi had eaten meat, even endorsing the view that its consumption was necessary for a "culinary masculinity" required to resist the British. Before leaving India to study law in London in 1888, he promised his mother that he would become a vegetarian. He struggled at first to avoid meat, but once he discovered vegetarian restaurants in the city and Henry Salt's book *A Plea for Vegetarianism*, he embraced the practice with enthusiasm. Following his return to India, Gandhi placed vegetarianism at the center of his nationalism. Far from seeking to match the British in masculine toughness, he insisted, Indians should celebrate their civilization, in which the spiritual mattered more than the material, and wherein refinement meant, in part, avoiding the cruel practice of slaughtering animals for food. Restraint in matters concerning food and in other types of bodily conduct would reflect India's superior virtues and shame the British into withdrawing from the subcontinent. To achieve this, nationalists must never respond to British provocations with violence. The libido must be mastered, and so must the palate. The ultimate power rested with the man who could exercise full self-restraint; "so overpowering are the senses," Gandhi wrote, "that they can be kept under control only when they are completely hedged on all sides, from above and beneath." In gustatory terms this meant a willingness not only to deny oneself meat but to fast, giving up food entirely in protest against the British and thus placing one's life in the hands of those who fostered the oppression of his people. In his lifetime Gandhi undertook seventeen hunger strikes that threatened to be unto death, all of them aimed at effecting changes in British policies.[156]

In the Philippines, the Americans came to understand the strong association between food and hospitality in Filipino homes. A standard greeting in Tagalog is *Kumain kan na?*—Have you eaten?[157] Long before the Americans arrived, it was common for Filipinos to offer dinner and a *baile* to friends and political supporters.[158] The Americans, usually officials, were important visitors, and their hosts pulled out the stops to impress them with the quality and quantity of food and drink and the graciousness of their service. Food closely reflects status in the Philippines, so the approach of distinguished visitors and facing the prospect of getting a meal wrong could be highly stressful.[159] Anticipating a visit to her province by Governor Francis Harrison in the fall of 1913, teacher Paz Marquez recounted for her fiancé a discussion by the women's committee formed to host the event. "Someone proposed a typically Filipino lunch. But no! the idea is ridiculous. We wish to convince the Americans that we are civilized enough to be independent, and we shall be refused if we eat off banana leaves." "Yet," she wondered, "is it very uncivilized to eat from banana leaves?"[160]

Such questions were left to the relatively well off to ponder. That food was so closely bound up with status meant that it defined group boundaries within the archipelago, and that it became connected intimately to the development of national consciousness. The Americans needed to see that Filipinos ate the right sorts of food in polite ways, and it would not (or might not) do to serve them chicken on banana leaves. It surely would not do to have them associate Tagalog foodways with those of the mountain people or Filipinos from the remotest provinces. Not all residents of the archipelago ate the same foods. Nurse Rosa Balunsat, who worked at a sanatorium for tuberculosis patients, recorded in frustration that "it is very hard to please the patients regarding the food. There are foods that the Ilocanos ate but the Visayans would not eat, and vice versa. . . . What is 'mansarap' [delicious] for some may be 'muy detestable' for others."[161] Among Tagalogs, meals consisted of boiled rice and that which went with it, the *ulam*. This included most of all fish and shellfish or sauces derived from fish, but also vegetables, eggs, poultry, and pork. People ate a lot of bananas, which were abundant, and the middle classes developed in the 1920s a taste for American apples. Filipinos generally avoided cold milk—many are lactose intolerant—but did cook and serve cooked milk-based desserts, including *leche flan*. A meal often ended with coffee and cigars or cigarettes, which over time largely supplanted betel use among the respectable class.[162]

This was civilized food. Even more than Americans, Tagalogs distinguished it from food consumed by outlanders and particularly Igorots, whom Americans encountered frequently on their travels to Baguio. There were Filipinos, for example, who imagined that a meal need not include rice; by Tagalog standards such offerings amounted at best to snacks.[163] Alcohol in the mountains rarely bore scrutiny—Victor Heiser drank an Ifugao fermented rice liquor called *bubud* and pronounced it a "vile tasting mixture."[164] Most of all, Americans were titillated and revolted by Igorot consumption of dog. They tried to get the Igorots to substitute other foods for it, including canned salmon.[165] Tagalogs were mortified by it. When Carlos P. Romulo, later a distinguished diplomat, was asked why the people of the Cordillera ate dog, he replied: "The Igorots are not Filipinos."[166] The Americans must understand that the state true Filipinos sought was one that did not countenance such barbarities. The independent Philippines would be constituted by those who ate proper food properly, the sort of people the Americans had come to know, and whose food and foodways they had come in some instances to enjoy.

Adaptation

Revulsion, disgust, rejection—all of these at some point characterized British and American responses to the food and drink they encountered in their colonies. Indian and Filipino foodways seemed to the Anglo-Americans to entail the worst habits and most barbarous tastes of uncivilized people. The food was intrinsically bad. It was poorly sourced, unsafely prepared, treacherously served, and eaten with such disregard for decency as to dismay any civilized person forced to witness or engage in its consumption. In this way tasting and eating seemed, much like the other four senses, logical targets for reform by more bodily enlightened westerners. And to some extent, Britons and Americans attempted to change Asian foodways. When Asians were invited to join imperial officials or military officers at meals, they were shown by example what sorts of food and drink they ought to consume and especially how to consume them. Indian cooks faced constant correction of their culinary practices, assuming their employers could brave entry into their own kitchens. American food companies advertised vigorously in the Philippines, promising such safe and attractive offerings as Heinz ketchup and Lea & Perrins Worcestershire sauce.[167] Filipino schoolchildren were instructed in the ways of civilized eating. If they did not wish, to echo the words of one American, to "become as stupid, frail, and worthless" as the "natives," Britons and Americans had to avoid eating and drinking as the locals did.

But they were in Asia to devour empires, and this they could not do without consuming some of their food and drink. Despite themselves, Britons and Americans were drawn to Indian and Filipino food. Out of the need to rely on it at times when supplies of their own comestibles ran out, and increasingly because they acknowledged its pleasures, the agents of empire created with their subjects hybrid cuisines, clumsy yet frequently enticing, sometimes by including samples of each type of food on menus, sometimes (and more often in India) creating dishes that incorporated ingredients and seasonings from both traditions. The boundaries that agents of empire constructed around their bodies in order to distinguish their refined Selves from uncivilized Others were rendered most permeable in the realm of food and taste.

Britons and Americans did not find the foods of their colonies altogether surprising. They had long had access to spices from Asia via trade routes adopted by the Portuguese, Spaniards, and British throughout South and Southeast Asia.[168] New World foods with which they were familiar, including chilies, guavas, tomatoes, and potatoes, had for centuries circulated to India and the Philippines and entered those countries' cuisines.[169] East India Company ships bore such names as *Clove* and *Peppercorn*, and their owners hoped to increase into Britain the importation of these spices along with cumin, caraway, cinnamon, and nutmeg, all of which were used heavily in British cooking and as preservatives.[170] The English custom known as *voidee* involved offering departing dinner guests a handful of spices, much as Indians provided *paan*.[171] American cooks had long used the Asian spices ginger, nutmeg, and mace.[172]

By the late nineteenth century, British and American foodways had been strongly influenced by the presence of immigrants and, in Britain's case, by those returned from imperial service. Interest in Indian cooking, or really any cooking outside of the British tradition, coincided with a nationwide soul-searching campaign aimed at the poor quality and taste of English food. Commentators blamed social unrest in Britain on the awfulness of British meals and the discontent they inspired in the working-class and poor. British cooks ruined good meat with "boring preparations and poor cooking techniques," complained one writer. Foreign cooks tried to make meat tender, while the aim of the British seemed to be "to make it hard." "Don't tell me the hardness is in the meat itself," the writer declared. "Nothing of the kind; it's altogether an achievement of the English cuisine." As an essayist in the *Examiner* put it: "A bad dinner in humble life has for its common consequence a quarrel with the wife, and recourse to the dram-bottle or the publichouse"; thus did poorly prepared food contribute to the decline of morality among workers.[173] Meanwhile, Indian food was making inroads in British society. The first Indian restaurant in London opened in 1809, and Richard Terry published a popular Indian recipe book there in 1861.[174] By the 1920s there were several places to get Indian food in the capital, and the handful of Indian expatriates and many more Britons who had served in India patronized them frequently. "Eating a curry was an opportunity to relive old times," writes Lawrence James. "British customers liked to be called 'sahib' and referred to the waiters as 'bearer.' "[175]

Gustatory practices in the metropole corresponded to the erosion of barriers the British in India had tried determinedly to erect between their bodies and curry after the Great Rebellion. Try as they might to maintain strict British decorum in their kitchens and dining rooms, more and more the British allowed Indian dishes to creep back onto their menus. It was convenient to eat Indian food while traveling or in camp, places to which large amounts of tinned food and roasting ovens could not always follow. While some Indian hosts served western food (generally French) for their British guests, others offered Indian food, and often, their British guests admitted, they preferred it.[176] Hilda Bourne and other Britons about to leave their post near Rajahmundry were given a farewell dinner by a Mr. Venkataralnam. "And what a meal!" Bourne exclaimed. It featured vegetables, "balls of highly spiced meats in thick gravy," then "the most delicious pilau I have ever tasted." Full as she was, Bourne had seconds, leaving barely enough room for the fruit and a piece of cake baked to resemble a palace.[177] Curries persisted at breakfast and lunch. And they edged back in at some dinners too, occasionally appearing alongside European dishes, including in the messes of ships carrying Britons to and from India or when Indian guests were present at the table.[178] By the 1920s large train stations had on their platforms three dining rooms: European, Hindu, and Muslim. "Anybody with any sense avoided the European restaurant," recounts David Burton, "except perhaps to buy a lukewarm soda or beer, for the food was as horrendous as it was over-priced." From the Muslim restaurant wafted "the delicious aromas of kebabs and pilaus," a temptation to Europeans "provided they could turn a blind eye to the kitchen conditions out back."[179]

In the nineteenth-century United States, home cooks celebrated the simplicity of meat and potatoes while outwardly denigrating the foods of immigrants—even while serving macaroni and chop suey to their families.[180] More than Great Britain, the United States was increasingly a nation of immigrants, and American foodways reflected it. Italians imported wine, figs, and olive oil; the French brought to California walnuts and cuttings from prune trees; Norwegians introduced fruits and vegetables that they missed from home. Chinese farmers in Hawaii stocked streams with Asian fish species and in California created an

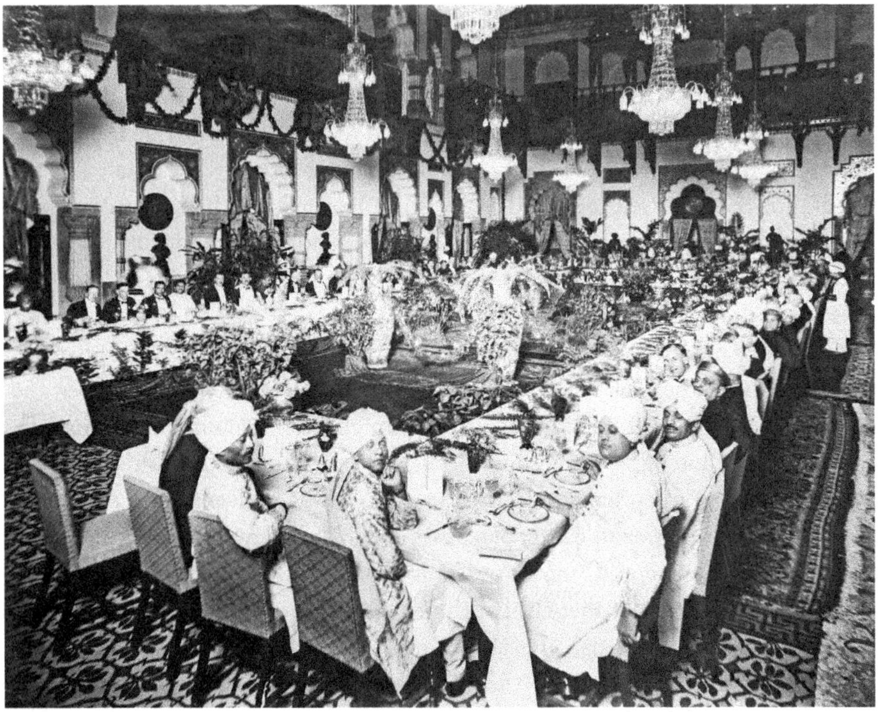

Figure 7.5 A banquet in Ooty (Ootacamund), a British hill station in south India. The British ultimately succumbed to the pleasures of Indian food, and the two peoples socialized over lavish meals such as this one. © Phil Yeoman/BNPS.

enormous demand for imported rice; the Japanese added napa cabbage and daikon radishes and bought from Japan quantities of pickled plums and gluten cakes.[181]

There is of course good evidence that Americans often recoiled from what they saw on their plates, or on Filipino plates, in the Philippines during the early decades of the twentieth century. Such a reaction might be explained by the food's setting: ethnic food in the United States would have seemed safer than such food prepared and served in a foreign land, where there seemed little way to control any part of the cooking process and the context of difference surrounding meals was generally disquieting. Ethnic food in the United States was minority food, which could be sampled for its exoticism but if need be quickly abandoned. In the Philippines, Emily Conger threw her dinner into the sea, Ralph Buckland drew back from a shared jelly spoon, and Albert Sonnichsen thought that the local watermelons tasted like "bread soaked in water."[182] But again and again, Americans in the archipelago showed at least grudging appreciation for local food and drink, and sometimes much more. In Bohol, four hundred miles south of Manila, two Americans were given breakfast by a local *presidente*. "The meal was elaborate, well cooked and good," wrote George Percival Scriven. There was abundant meat and fish and a "good Spanish wine" along with tuba, the potent coconut liquor.[183] In Iligan (five hundred miles from Manila), one local aristocrat had three cooks—Chinese, Spanish, and Filipino—and though his host apologized ritually for the meanness of the meal, Willis Bliss Wilcox was delighted to discover well-prepared boar meat, venison, beef, bread, potatoes, chocolate, and coffee, accompanied by canned goods.[184] "Dinner was served at eight, and it was indeed a feast to remember," wrote Daniel Williams from Apalit in 1900. "A great mahogany table glittered with the finest china and linen, its entire length being set off by massive bouquets, pyramids of fruit, wonderfully ornamented cakes, and stands of most elaborately carved toothpicks. The number and variety of courses were amazing, creating a sense of wonder as to where and how they were all produced. There were wines of all kinds and color, the effect of which doubtless added to the conviviality of the occasion."[185]

What accounts for this apparent contradiction between often-expressed contempt for Filipino food and foodways and the frequent admiration for them? First, eating Filipino in the Philippines provided Americans with their only opportunity to get fresh food. They might complain, as Mary Fee did, about "flavorless" bananas, and deplore the dangers of eating uncooked vegetables, but they also recognized that the tropics that so frightened them also produced an abundance of fruits, vegetables, and fish that offered nutrition, satisfaction, and sometimes superb taste.[186] "Excellent food everywhere," recorded Leonard Wood in his diary during a trip upcountry in 1921. "Mangoes, and such bananas as one only sees when in the country where they grow. We had for dinner a most remarkable fish." Even the steaks served in Fuga won Wood's approval.[187] Early in the American occupation Helen Taft had to grow her own tomatoes, cauliflower, and beans, but the soil and sun at Malacañan Palace yielded enormous quantities of all three.[188] The opening of the Benguet Road to the temperate hill station of Baguio in 1905 brought to Manila fresh peas, beans, summer squash, and strawberries.[189] Back in the capital after touring the provinces, Edith Moses lamented her return to American fare. "Civilization and the civilized are a bit slow after the experiences of the past weeks," she wrote. "I find that I miss sweet peppers, *chili con carne*, and various other native dishes I learned to like on the southern trip. Our American menu lacks 'color.' "[190]

Second, much of the Americans' admiration for Filipino food was inspired by a belief that it wasn't actually Filipino at all, but an inheritance from Spain. Americans in 1900 were perhaps not convinced that the Spaniards were as civilized as themselves, tinged by a Catholicism that made them seem sinister, perfidious, and rapacious.[191] Yet depraved as they might be, the Spaniards were always represented as human, and if swarthy, nevertheless recognizably Caucasian. After all, they were Europeans. They did not dwell naturally in the tropics. They wore "western" clothes, spoke a Romance language and listened to opera, and seemed (and smelled) clean. Their food was recognizable too, often very good, and they prepared and ate it as civilized people did.

What Americans praised most often about food in the Philippines was its apparent similarity to Spanish food and its presentation. Philippine ingredients were unavoidable, but if they were turned into meals by cooks familiar with Spanish recipes the results were usually well worth eating.[192] To the basic rice and fish diet of Filipinos the Spaniards, by their own account, had added dishes of great variety and taste: "Catholic-style stews," sausages and cutlets, breads, techniques of marinating and pickling, drinking chocolate, and milk puddings and custards.[193] They seasoned the rice and added to it chicken and chorizo to make *arroz Valenciana*; they ate cheeses, olives, and paté imported from Europe; they brought to the islands their strong wines.[194] At a *baile* in Bayombong William Freer ate "course after course . . . —fish, venison in several different modes and courses, chicken, goat's flesh, patties and other dishes which have no English names." Dessert was "a rich pudding made of native chocolate, sugar, *carabao's* milk, eggs, and rice flour," and "all of the food was well prepared, very palatable and nicely served." That Christmas in Solano, Freer had another feast, this with some fifteen courses including "soup, roast chicken, roast pork, croquettes, fried chicken, sausages, pork cutlets, venison, roast beef, deer liver" and so on—and both meals had been "prepared in the Spanish style."[195] William Cameron Forbes enjoyed eating ice cream, or *sorbete*, "Spanish fashion," using a rolled wafer as an edible spoon.[196] Multicourse banquets, heavy on meat and wine, were the rule when American officials arrived in town, and they were inspired by Spanish cuisine.[197]

Finally, even if Americans were sometimes puzzled by what was put on their plates or in their glasses, they came to regard Filipino efforts to please them as genuinely felt acts of hospitality. "When Americans hosted parties," historian Paul Kramer writes, "they were inviting Filipinos to collaborate in the new state; when Filipinos hosted, they were recognizing the commission's power." In Filipino homes and streets and in town halls where banquets were served, American visitors "were forced to recognize and adapt to Filipino customs."[198] They learned, with Edith Moses, to pick an olive off the tines of a fork aimed at her by a neighbor at the table, to accept at least a small amount of everything served, and to appreciate even the carabao meat, warm champagne, and "queer sweets, rather sticky and clogging to the American taste," because they were served with so much sincerity and good will.[199] Without enough waiters to serve the American visitors, organizers of a banquet in Cebu in April 1901 employed a Philippine judge to help out. After each course, he removed the place settings from the table, wiped them off with a single towel, and then returned them to his guests. Moses kept her knife and fork after she witnessed this, but she registered less disgust than warm amusement at the honest effort to please.[200]

In these ways taste, while always contested, nevertheless became the gateway sense for imperial encounter and a frequent site of accommodation between rulers and subjects. Britons and Americans did not stop worrying about what they ingested in India and the Philippines, and they retained some of their contempt for Asians' foods and foodways. Yet they acknowledged the tastiness of Indian and Philippine food, and if they could not altogether ignore the dubious methods of its preparation and presentation, they learned to accept these as the price of their genuine gustatory enjoyment. The variety of foods offered during meals seemed itself a virtue, or at least a sign of status: the poor may have only bread or rice, but a selection of dishes drawn from several food groups indicates the prosperity and breadth of taste of middle-class diners. "A meal incorporates a number of contrasts, hot and cold, bland and spiced, liquid and semi-liquid, and various textures," observed Mary Douglas.[201] Such was the British experience with curry, the savor of which they resisted until they simply could not. And historian Donna Gabaccia concludes that Americans have never been conservative in their tastes for food. "In a bountiful society where fears of cultural difference nevertheless persist," she writes, "food remains the least controversial, the most typical and reliable, and cheapest of all ways to find pleasure in life"—such that Americans' "multi-ethnic eating . . . proclaims our satisfied sense of affiliation with one another."[202] A common interest in good food allowed rulers and subjects in India and the Philippines to relax just a bit in each other's presence, and opened the possibility that reconciliation might also take place in the realms of the other four senses.

Conclusion

The Senses at Empire's End

> In nineteenth and twentieth-century India, migrants from the antipodes to the centre, from the Rann of Kutch, Cape Comorin and Chittagong to Calcutta, Bombay and New Delhi, turned into imperial Britons by mastery of their tongue and technology, filling their houses with European and American books, furniture, art, glass, china, drink, wearing western-style clothes, reading English-language newspapers and listening to English medium broadcasts. The successors to the proconsuls were . . . proconsuls.
>
> —Roderick Cavaliero, *Strangers in the Land* (2002)

> We are not of the Orient, except by geography. We are part of the western world by reasons of culture, religion, ideology, and economics. Although the color of our skin is brown, the temper of our minds and hearts is almost identical with yours.
>
> —Philippine President Manuel Roxas, speech in the United States (1946)

How does a nation leave its imperial possessions? There are complicated logistics involved. The apparatus of government must be turned over to those only recently subject to its control. Papers are discarded, burned, or carried off; art and maps are removed from walls and nameplates taken as keepsakes from the tops of desks; keys are given up. Law courts change hands as judges from the metropole relinquish their dockets to local justices. In the homes of colonial officials servants are bid goodbye. Soldiers and officers take their leave, though some linger by invitation of the new regimes, or by choice. Departures are about packing. Furniture is sold off; clothes, housewares, books, and keepsakes are crated for the journey home. There are individual ceremonies of departure—a last circuit of a collector's district in central India, a final banquet and *baile* with Filipino colleagues, an evening ride on a favorite horse or one more visit to Manila's Luneta park. Planned handovers of power and celebrations of independence provide a formal coda to empire. Then the ships and planes depart, and new nations are left to determine their course. Thousands of the colonizers' dead, buried in cemeteries in Lucknow and Manila and more remote places too, stay behind.

While no one should mistake for genuine empathy the Anglo-Americans' nostalgia for privileges lost, there is no question that the five senses, fully engaged in the pastimes and projects of imperial control, created lasting affective bonds between rulers and subjects in India and the Philippines and made leave-taking difficult. Empires are emotional communities, and emotions are triggered by the senses. Britons missed the sights of India—"such colour!"—and the lights of the bazaar at night.[1] They recalled with fondness the sound of bells tinkling on ox carts at twilight, the smells of dust after rain, of incense and curry, and of wood smoke, "the most gorgeous smell in the world."[2] There were moving moments with servants, who seemed (at least) to lament their masters' departure, often grasping their hands or kissing their feet. Returned Britons "create[d] little Anglo-Indias" in their homes, according to E. M. Collingham. "They attempted to reproduce the distinctive curry and rice, and chutneys and pickles of Anglo-India," and they brought with them furniture, textiles, photographs, incense, and bells that reminded them of their service to the Raj, by way of every sense.[3] There was less fondness in the recollections of Americans who had served in the Philippines; they rarely embedded themselves as deeply in Philippine society as the British did in Indian. Yet Americans bonded with Filipinos especially during the shared experience of the Second World War with Japan. As the Insurrection had done years earlier, the Pacific War heightened senses and intensified feelings among soldiers, though this time they brought Americans and Filipinos together. American and Filipino soldiers suffered alongside each other during the Japanese siege of Bataan and the subsequent "death march," during which their captors assaulted and murdered men of both nationalities. Filipinos and Americans together formed resistance groups in northern Luzon, sharing food and drink and walking barefoot when their shoes gave out.[4] A wartime comedy skit performed by a Filipino troupe in Manila contained this exchange: "*Sino ba ang hinihintay mo? [Who are you waiting for?] Si Uncle [i.e., Uncle Sam]*"; it infuriated the Japanese.[5] Filipinos had hurt feelings about what seemed to them the abandonment of the archipelago by General Douglas MacArthur, but the general promised to return and he did, directing the bloody liberation of Manila in early 1945, after which a Filipino band serenaded the exhausted troops with Sousa marches and "God Bless America." MacArthur was fond of many Filipino leaders—an affection that, for all its undeniable paternalism, was evidently reciprocated.[6]

Yet leave the Britons and Americans did. Independence was conferred on the Philippines on July 4, 1946, and on India on August 15, 1947. These dates were important, especially symbolically, as we will see. But they were not watershed moments. The decisions for independence were in fact made piecemeal, over time, and if they did not always move India and the Philippines inexorably toward liberation they nevertheless trended in that direction. It is true that India's independence seemed to come abruptly in 1947. Lord Mountbatten, who was named the last Viceroy in February 1947, was instructed to guide India through the transition to freedom by June 30, 1948, and it was he who decided, on arriving in India, to accelerate the timetable considerably. That he did so was in part a result of his understanding that much had already been done to distance India from Britain's ambit. From the first, there had been a shallowness to the Raj. Even after 1858, the British did not control the Native States: the Rajput Agency, Kashmir in the north, Hyderabad, and Mysore, among others. Goa was Portuguese, Pondicherry French. As of 1910, the British formally held sway over just over half of the subcontinent's land mass. Even within the area of their dominion, the British sensed the limits of their power, confined as it was to towns and cities.[7] In 1882 Viceroy Lord Ripon had authorized the devolution to local and district governments of new powers of decision, free of central control, with councils to be elected by rent-payers, and concerning such matters as education and sanitation—the rationale being that it was desirable for the British government "to train the people over whom it rules more and more as time goes on to take an intelligent share in the administration of their own affairs."[8] The First World War increased pressure on the British to make further reforms. Indians made great sacrifices for the empire. Indian divisions were sent to Mesopotamia and the trenches of Europe; nearly four thousand were killed in one night's fighting at Ypres in April 1915. India supplied substantial funding for the war effort, thousands of rifles, and the jute for the sandbags of the western front. Britons who might previously have been recruited to service in India became officers elsewhere, which put more Indians into vital administrative positions.

The changes brought by World War I intensified Indian demands for greater autonomy, which in turn prompted a harsh reaction. In April 1919, General Reginald Dyer ordered his troops to open fire on an unarmed crowd gathered for a protest in the city of Amritsar, killing more than a thousand. Parliament passed the Government of India Act eight months later. Written chiefly by Edwin Montagu and the Viceroy Lord Chelmsford, the Act reformed the Indian constitution, modestly extending the franchise and further strengthening local councils, all of them now with Indian chairs, creating a two-house legislature in Delhi meant to debate proposals made by the central government, and in the provinces introducing the principle of "dyarchy," which reserved power over some issues for the elected bodies. The educated men of India, Montagu and Chelmsford said, were "intellectually our children" who had "imbibed ideas which we ourselves have set before them." These reforms did not amount to independence. Enormous struggle lay ahead. Yet they did no less, writes historian

Jon Wilson, than help "create pockets of official power which directly challenged the will of the imperial hierarchy."[9] Throughout the 1920s and 1930s the nationalist Congress Party increased its pressure on the British to leave India. Mahatma Gandhi led marches and boycotts of British goods and undertook fasts; British-trained political leaders, among them Jawaharlal Nehru, demanded further concessions; Gandhi, Nehru, and hundreds of other organizers were jailed. In 1929 the Viceroy Lord Irwin promised India dominion status, and five years later the India Bill made the provinces self-governing and established an Indian federation, which the princes were invited to join. Irwin recognized, as historian Roderick Cavaliero has observed, that India was now "set irreversibly on the road to self-rule, not immediately, as the more extreme nationalists were demanding, but over a suitably protracted period, while Indian politicians learned their trade."[10] World War II brought matters to a head. India was threatened with Japanese invasion, and the British tried frantically to mobilize the Indian military to resist. Men, capital, and goods were conscripted for war on an unprecedented scale. By the end 180,000 Indian soldiers, all volunteers, had been killed, wounded, or taken prisoner.[11] The Nationalists were unwilling to be exploited in these ways on behalf of an empire they despised. "For God's sake leave India alone!" cried Gandhi.[12] This the prime minister, Winston Churchill, was disinclined to do. He loathed Gandhi—"this one-time Inner Temple lawyer, now seditious faqir, striding half-naked up the steps of viceroy's palace, to negotiate and parley on equal terms with the representative of the King-Emperor"—and resented the nationalists for taking advantage of Britain at the moment of its greatest vulnerability.[13] He rebuffed attempts, including by the Americans, to persuade him to make concessions. Authorities in India struggled to keep order, certain that the nationalists meant to sabotage the war effort, but unsure they could prevent this.[14]

In the end, of course, independence came, to India and Muslim Pakistan, whose founder, Mohammed Ali Jinnah, would not countenance minority status in a Hindu-majority state. It was worse than messy; in their haste to depart, the British left borders in flux and extremists to set the religious parties at each other's throats, and at least a million people were killed during riots that followed partition. But the instruments of independence had been in the crafting for decades, and the British were by 1947 in some measure resigned to their fate. Soon after independence was declared, John and Nora Scott were sitting on a bench in the Bombay sun when they were approached by an Indian friend, Rao Sahib Mundlik. "Well, Rao Sahib," said John. "England's day is over." Nora: "I shall keep my English umbrella, I cannot give that up." John (waving his umbrella at Mundlik): "Yes, we'll cling to my umbrella, the last sign of English power—the last rag. . . . Exit the Rao Sahib, laughing."[15] The First Cameron Highlanders were less playful as they left for home, chanting: "Land of shit and filth and wogs /

Gonorrhea, syphilis, clap and pox. / Memsahibs' paradise soldiers' hell. / India fare thee fucking well."[16]

In a similar way did the United States move toward conferring independence on the Philippines. Most American officials, who were at first convinced that Filipino backwardness would prevent the archipelago indefinitely from achieving independent status, came around to thinking that their rule had a shelf life. Even the US military in the midst of war conceived local governments chosen and run by Filipinos, and Governor William Howard Taft formalized their presence, with the argument that American democracy itself was founded in such federalism. Taft also proposed the creation of a national assembly. Congress approved, and one was elected in August 1907 and convened that October. Its first act was to recognize American supremacy. But the Assembly would become an incubator for politicians and parties, and Filipinos also gained the right to place two of their own in the US House of Representatives, with one each chosen by the Governor and the Assembly. The election of Woodrow Wilson and a Democratic Congress in 1912 improved prospects for Filipino self-rule. With a determined assist from Manuel Quezon, one of the two Filipino representatives in Washington, the president appointed as Governor-General Francis Burton Harrison, a New York Congressman who quickly committed himself to a policy of "Filipinization" of the islands. The policy was given legislative ballast with the passage of the Jones Act (1916), for which Quezon served as amanuensis. The act replaced the Philippine Commission with a senate and the assembly with a house of representatives, to be elected by Filipinos, albeit only male property holders. The governor retained a veto over legislation. Trade between the United States and the Philippines would remain unfettered by tariffs. It was not independence, but it was a long step toward it, and in truth as much as many Filipino *ilustrados* wished for the time being to undertake.[17]

American conservatives were harshly critical of Wilson's policy and especially Harrison's execution of it. William Cameron Forbes, Harrison's predecessor, accused Harrison of corruption and moral turpitude. Yet Forbes, who remained strongly attached to the islands, allowed in 1921 that progress had been made toward empowering Filipinos, and he saw no reason to reverse course—a view endorsed even by General Leonard Wood, Harrison's tough-minded successor. The Wood-Forbes Report of 1921 noted that while much remained to be done, particularly in the areas of public health, agriculture, and the probity of civil servants, Filipinos had made strides over the previous five years.[18] In 1934 Congress passed, and President Franklin D. Roosevelt signed, the Tydings-McDuffie Act, or Philippine Independence Act. It announced the independence of the Philippines within ten years, establishing in the interim the Philippines Commonwealth. The United States for the time being retained its military presence on the islands and strictly limited Filipino immigration. The Philippines was to have a constitution, and an election in September 1935 for a president, vice president, and members of the National Assembly. The Americans hoped the process would unite the country by including the upcountry people and the Moros, who remained apprehensive about *ilustrado* domination. Quezon was elected president; he was inaugurated on November 15, to the tune of "Hail to the Chief," but he was disappointed to receive but a nineteen-gun salute—a sonic demonstration of his continued inferiority to American heads of state.[19] Full independence would come eleven years later, following the trauma of war, Japanese occupation, and violent liberation. It would seem in some respects an anticlimax.

There were many reasons for the timing of these decisions for independence. In the British case, the ravages of World War II made it clear that a small island could no longer hold in thrall a people increasingly determined to control their own destiny. Indian nationalists demanded that the British "Quit India," given their manifest inability either to protect or govern the country, as continuous riots and mutinies seemed patently to demonstrate. The British were heavily in debt to India and militarily overstretched. They would settle for India and Pakistan accepting roles within the British Commonwealth. The Americans had

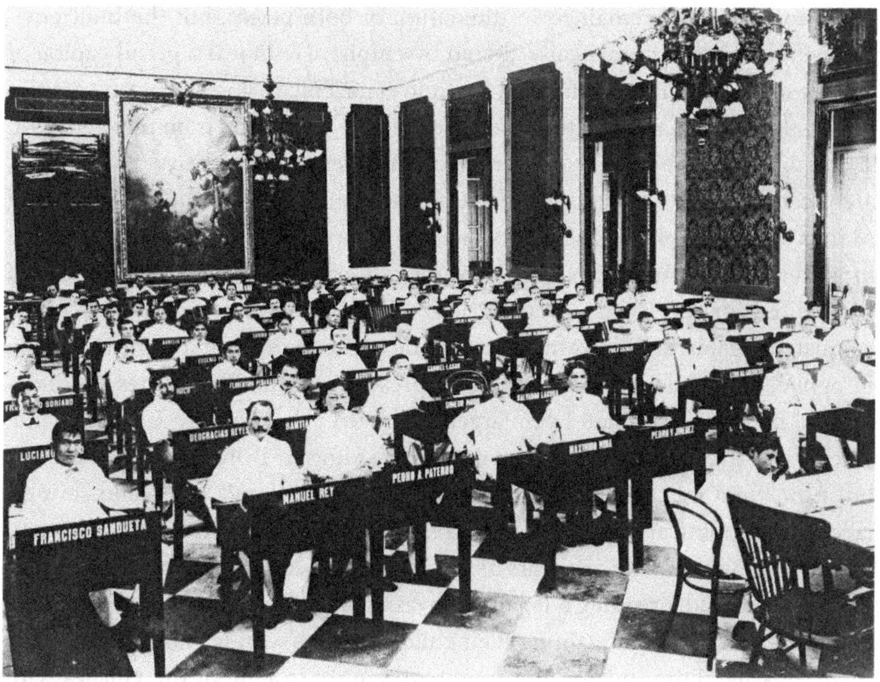

Figure C.1 The Philippines legislature, 1930s, clearly prepared for a larger role in governing. Courtesy of Library of Congress, Prints and Photographs Division.

promised independence to the Philippines in 1934. Never comfortable with the label of imperial power, the United States sought ways maintain influence in the Philippines without formal governance, and it was this model that the Americans embraced after their flag descended in Manila in 1946. The United States retained, by treaty, military bases on Philippine soil, and continued to exercise economic dominance over the islands.

But as Indians and Filipinos organized their governments and confronted the promise and perils of self-rule, their recent masters took satisfaction in the improvements they claimed they had brought to sensory and bodily practices in both countries. Efforts to refine the senses of elite subjects had been, the British and Americans judged, at least partially successful, and their own accommodation of the sensory habits of these subjects—the achievement in some instances of hybrid sensibilities enabled by their admiration for some aspects of Indian and Philippine sensoria and especially the adoption of Indian and Filipino foodways—allowed them to persuade themselves that they had done what they set out to do: civilize their backward charges. Indians and Filipinos of the best sorts might now be entrusted to govern in part because they showed sufficient respect for the body and the senses.

The appearance of the land and people had changed in India and the Philippines since the late nineteenth century. Stark landscapes and colors both bleak and saturated remained in the nature of both places, but the built environment had been dramatically altered by empire. Delhi was a grand capital of British-made buildings influenced by Indo-Saracenic forms. Great universities dotted the cities. Railroads traversed the country, providing train travelers with sights that few had seen before, and from a different perspective.[20] In Manila, architect Daniel Burnham opened promenades and vistas to the water, ringing Manila Bay with plazas and parks, and lit its streets at night. "Manila is the most thoroughly American typical American city I have ever visited outside the United States," wrote a visiting journalist.[21] In both countries, successful campaigns against smallpox meant a decline in the number of disfigured people in public, and while leprosy remained a presence, in the Philippines those deformed by the disease had been largely removed from sight, to Culion Island. Deceit and trickery no doubt remained, according to Britons and Americans, but now there was no war as there had been in 1857 and 1899, and serious, face-to-face political negotiation had replaced visual evasiveness and gestural mendacity. Anglo-American fears of turning dark in the tropical sun had mostly vanished. Instead, dreading a Japanese invasion of India in 1942, British parents entertained fantasies of "staining their children's faces with walnut juice to make them look like little Indians and sending them off to hide in the villages with their *ayahs*"—shades here of British soldiers trying a similar subterfuge during the Great Rebellion.[22] In the Philippines magazines ran ads for Lux Toilet

Soap, offering color portraits of white American film stars in exchange for four wrappers, in this way connecting proper hygiene to whiteness.[23] Right up to the moment of their departure from India, the British continued to try to make the land and its people legible. They strained especially to mark boundaries between India and Pakistan, or between religious communities within both states, and between India and the remaining principalities that Delhi had resolved to absorb. "The settlement was going ahead," recalled an observer during the summer of 1947. "Every morning the procession would set out," led by the official Philip Tollintin and attended by a coterie of Indians, making "their way from village to village. Everything had to be written down, measured, and recorded. A mistake, or a wrong decision, could lead to bitter feuding or even murder."[24] As independence became inevitable in the Philippines, leading Americans dismissed as exaggerations the supposed racial, and thus physiognomic, differences between Filipinos, as if to reassure themselves and their subjects that imminent rule by a group principally constituted of Catholic Tagalogs would not inspire conflict. "Actually," wrote anthropologist H. Otley Beyer, "if one travels from northern Luzon to the southern islands, he sees a relatively homogeneous people throughout the lowland or Christian provinces." There were differences between the majority and those living in the mountains and in Mindanao, but the encouraging trend overall was "a smoothing out of racial and cultural differences and the building up of that type of blended and developed culture which we think of today as 'Filipino.'"[25] Governor Frank Murphy was even more reassuring as the Commonwealth dawned. "The increasing homogeneity in the population is not a mere altruistic hope," he told the final session of occupation legislature. "There is strong scientific basis for holding that seemingly discordant and nonfusable elements not only can be but are *being* fused. . . . The pagan, Moro, and other non-Christian peoples possess essentially the same racial traits and innate psychology as the majority of the inhabitants of the Christian provinces."[26] Leaders of the mountain people in the 1930s "retained their 'ethnic identities,'" but also entered national politics and more and more considered themselves Filipino—or so the Americans claimed.[27]

There were sonic changes too. As with those involving vision, these were incomplete: Mary Chenevix Trench and her family were driven off their sleeping verandah on a hot night at Bikaner Palace in late 1946 by "the noise and coughing and spitting," while an American observer found that Filipinos remained in 1930 too susceptible to "having their ears tickled by political fireworks," and concluded that as ever, "flaming oratory, however bombastic, hypocritical, and mendacious warms them into chemically manufactured passion."[28] Yet encouraging sounds now sometimes replaced or overrode noise. Brass bands and orchestras in both countries had improved since the days of their discordant tones and willfully disjointed rhythms.[29] The sounds of construction, of civilization, echoed from sewer projects in India's cities and the Benguet Road that drew Manila closer to the American hill station at Baguio; "up and down the huge canyon," wrote William Cameron Forbes, "can be heard the sound of the pick, the rattle of rocks bounding down the mountain, then a loud splash in the river, the booming of dynamite and powder as the great blasts go, and the strange cries of men."[30] Radio began in India in the 1920s, and the India Broadcasting Company, which was overseen by the BBC, launched in July 1927. The service had thousands of subscribers by the late 1930s, listening mostly to broadcasts of Indian classical music.[31] There were radios in many homes in the Philippines too—politicians made use of them for campaign speeches during the run-up to Commonwealth status—and long distance telephoning was "quite the usual thing" in Manila by the mid-1930s.[32] Concerts in the islands blended western classical music with occasional Philippine songs; a performance at the Central Student Church in Manila in fall 1934 featured the violinist Ernesto Vallejo playing his own composition "Viennese Love."[33] The English language had taken hold among elites in both countries. In India, Rabindranath Tagore translated many of his Bengali poems into English, while both Gandhi and Nehru wrote and spoke extensively in English. Despite its being the medium of instruction in Indian schools, English remained at the time of independence largely the preserve of a small educated class, and Nehru thought it would soon be replaced by Hindi as the national tongue. "But . . . the English language stood its ground," according to historian Sarvepalli Gopal, as residents of southern India especially opposed the spread of Hindi, which they did not speak.[34] The American determination to teach English to all Filipino schoolchildren led to a broader diffusion of the language in the islands.[35] "The English language is now spoken in every barrio in the Archipelago by people of all ranks of life," proclaimed Governor Murphy, and if that exaggerated the extent to which English had spread, it nevertheless reflected a basic truth about the direction of the Filipino soundscape by 1946.[36] "English had become a status symbol," according to historian Renato Constantino. The most successful politicians in the archipelago were those who used the language in the most florid forms of oratory—who spoke the newly imported tongue with the oratorical flair and drama long expected by Filipinos of their leaders.[37]

It is likely that the odors of India and the Philippines changed over time, and even more likely that British and American perceptions of the odors changed. "You've got to go to a place, see it and smell it, before you can say what's got to be done about it," wrote Clement Attlee in 1927, confirming what generations of India hands had long known.[38] The advent of sewer systems in the big cities funneled underground the scent of excrement, though visitors to Bombay and Calcutta, to Manila and Capiz, still complained about public defecation ("nuisances") and the stench of the streets and waterways. Villages remained redolent with the smells of animals, rot, and human wastes; the authorities continued their campaigns to install latrines in the countryside and to persuade residents to use them.[39] Estimates done in the early 1930s showed that sixty percent of Filipinos living in the provinces still lacked access to toilets or latrines.[40] Yet Anglo-Indians who returned to Britain after 1947 tended to remember the best of Indian smells, with a rose-tinged nostalgia suggesting that their sensibilities, and not the odors, had changed. Sir Frank Pearson recalled "the spicy smell of the village bazaar, the wonderful still of the evening with the old men sitting round the Pipul tree."[41] "I think it is true that anyone who lived for any time in India under the British Raj absorbed the country into their blood," reminisced Lady Chapman. "Even after half a century, the smell of woodsmoke evokes a picture of driving through an Indian village at dusk with the smoke curling from wood and cow-dung fires, and smell of curry."[42] There is none of this among Americans who served in the Philippines. But when Governor Murphy recorded his first impressions of Manila in the mid-1930s, he commented on the heavy commercial use of the city's *esteros*. Unlike Americans before him, he did not mention their smell.[43]

Imperial hapticities were the subject of negotiation as time went on, with sufficient satisfaction offered the Anglo-Americans that they had altered Indian and Filipino practices regarding touched and touching bodies. Just as landscapes were resistant to visible change, so was the felt environment stubbornly durable: westerners could alter their style of dress, stay out of the sun, or use fans, powered by humans (India's *punkahs*) or electricity, but they remained in the tropics, where it was hot and moist. In other ways, though, touch, active and passive, could be corrected. Railroads and roads smoothed the surface of the land and improved the speed and comfort of travel. William Cameron Forbes exulted: "One does not now find long stretches of cogon grass and brush with numberless gullies and washouts in places where good roads were located a few years ago. One is not stopped at out of the way barrios until a neglected surface road dries out sufficiently to permit the passage of the vehicle he is employing."[44] Mortality from diseases of contact declined in both colonies through the first half of the twentieth century, as municipal governments and health boards, increasingly run by local people, persuaded their constituents to use toilets, accept vaccination, allow for the isolation of contagious patients, and exterminate rats, mosquitoes, and flies.[45] Elites in India and the Philippines increasingly turned western medicine to purposes of their own.[46]

The Indian hill stations and their Philippine counterpart at Baguio were always both exceptions to and models for haptic contact between rulers and subjects. Simla, Ootacamund, and the others were intended to separate Britons from Indians, rising above the hot moist tropics to provide a respite from the enervation and pollution said to threaten European bodies in India's lowlands. Over time, however, the British in the hills found themselves yielding to their insistent dependency on Indian servants, laborers, and, increasingly, officials with whom they came grudgingly to share power in the years after 1919. In Baguio, the Americans had, by contrast, included Filipinos almost from the start, inviting members of the *ilustrado* elite to buy property and join the country club. Hosting Filipinos, offering them social patronage, would, the Americans hoped, provide opportunities for the cultivation and moderation of reckless political views. "We are accustoming [Filipinos] to certain phrases of democratic simplicity of a sort that hitherto have been quite unknown among Oriental peoples I believe," Forbes wrote to Rudyard Kipling. "For instance our highest officials, including the Governor-General, wear the same clothes as other civilians, walk the streets and enter into games and sports with natives and others on a basis of equality."[47] Hill stations became sites of encounter in which agents of empire hoped their sensory practices would rub off on the "natives."

As Forbes suggested, haptic cultures found commonalities in the texture of commodities and the ways people learned to dress. In 1875, Arthur Lasenby Liberty opened the Liberty Department Store on Regent Street in London. He stocked a variety of Indian textiles intended to merge the Orientalized exotic with the European, exciting his customers without frightening them; thus, Indian carpets reflected Asian craft but "European tastes," and silk patterns from Mysore were given names—Rangoon Poppy, Poonah Thistle, and Allahabad Marigold—meant to suggest, writes Saloni Mathur, "hybrid blends" of Indian place names and familiar English flowers. Silk pajamas were "exquisitely soft" and "very light," and carpets of a texture that a bare foot could encounter "without a feeling of instinctive recoil." But the feel of an Indian object or person could not always be so easily domesticated. In November 1885, Liberty sponsored a group of villagers from India to recreate a "living village of Indian artisans" in London's Battersea Park. The event was badly mishandled. The artists nearly froze in the cold of an early English winter, and the snake charmer's cobras died from exposure. Visitors could not keep their hands off the two women dancers. Liberty admitted his mistake. His store continued to be successful, selling to Londoners the textiles it placed at the haptic junction between India and Britain.[48]

By the end of the nineteenth century the production of fine, hand-woven textiles in India had declined, replaced mostly by machine-made cloth manufactured in Britain. Wealthy Britons were looking for items that were unusual products of village craft; more and more middle-class Indians preferred mass produced clothing from Europe, or clothes sewn in India from coarse imported thread. Fashionable Bengali men seemed to think, according to S. C. Bose, that their "adaptation of the European style of dress could bring them the benefit of 'modern civilization' by 'wearing tight pantaloons, tight shirts and black coats of alpaca or broadcloth.'" These clothes were harsh against the skin and a restraint on the body; such were the haptic costs of imperial respectability.[49] It was against this sort of thinking, the beguilement of the "civilized," that Gandhi initiated his campaign for the weaving of homespun cloth (*khadi*) in 1918. He meant to support weavers whose lives were threatened by the intake of British cloth, and to emphasize his own intimacy with the touch of the spinning wheel and the feel of a homespun *dhoti* against his skin. Gandhi appropriated the sense of touch that came from the making and wearing of textiles.[50]

Filipino tastes in clothing, and those of Americans in the Philippines, divided by gender. American men continued to shun dark wool suits except on the most formal occasions, preferring the relative lightness and coolness of white linen against their skin. Filipino political leaders for the most part adopted this custom, though were more inclined than the Americans to wear dark-colored suits or jackets, surely in an effort to prove themselves even more respectable than their tutors. More interesting was the surge of interest in Filipino fabrics and clothes for women. Notwithstanding their doubts concerning the feel of coarse cloth against the skin, American authorities had long admired Filipinas' dresses and defended them when employers insisted that women wear clothes "in American or European style."[51] When Henry Stimson was governor-general of the Philippines (1927–1929), his wife, Mabel, wore Filipina clothing to dances, delighting Manilans.[52] By the early 1930s, women's fashion aimed at "the fragile effect so admired this season," featuring such traditional Philippine fabrics as organdy, organza, and "our old friend, *pique* . . . now making its appearance in evening dresses. Ideal for Manila!"[53] And, as ever, physical contact cemented relationships between Filipinos and Americans, who by the mid-1930s seemed to be in the process of departing. On the day Quezon was inaugurated president of the Commonwealth, a photographer snapped a picture of him shaking hands with Frank Murphy, the governor about to become US High Commissioner. A columnist for the *Philippines Herald* later noted Murphy's "restrained smile," indicating "good cheer," "inspiration," and "concern." "He knows the dangers ahead awaiting the frail bark of the Philippine Commonwealth, but there is strength in that grip that he is about to give his friend and associate, Manuel L. Quezon, and the strength in that grip will by contagion infuse confidence into the heart of the man who is about to shoulder the manifold worries of a rising Filipino state."[54] Such, the columnist hoped, was the power of vigorous touch.

In their efforts to put the senses right in India and the Philippines, Britons and Americans found themselves for the most part contented with their failures to do so regarding taste. At minimum, Britons got used to Indian food.[55] At home, in clubs, in barracks, and at camps, the British succumbed to the irrefutable logic of the tongue: tinned and preserved comestibles from home could not compete with fresh foods in India, prepared with local spices by chefs who knew far better how to cook vegetable *kormas* or mutton *rogan josh* than a roasted joint of beef with a side of brussels sprouts. "It was best to keep to the dishes which the cook could manage without guidance," thought Mrs. H. A. Barnes. "Curry with dahl [*sic*] (lentils) and chapattis; nothing nicer or safer. Fresh fruit in season was plentiful."[56] Even before 1947, Britons returned from India craving the savory foods they had eaten there. The notable London Indian restaurant, Veeraswamy's, opened in 1926, which the repatriated agents of empire patronized in search of the spices and obsequious service they had come to expect in India. Amidst "Indian carpets, chandeliers, punkahs . . . and other decorative accoutrements intended to connote the luxurious 'East,'" diners relished the chance "to eat again a real curry and remember the days when they were important functionaries on salary instead of 'retired' on pension," as historian Elizabeth Buettner has written.[57]

In the Philippines, the Americans had some modest successes in their efforts to reform the sense of taste. Imports of American apples, dairy products, and canned foods, most notably Spam, changed Philippines tastes.[58] Historian René Alexander Orquiza Jr. notes that a menu from the Manila Hotel from 1936 included very few Filipino dishes; most "were so classically French that you easily could have been in a hotel in New York or London." Such food was for elite Manilans "a marker of class and refinement." This perception was reinforced

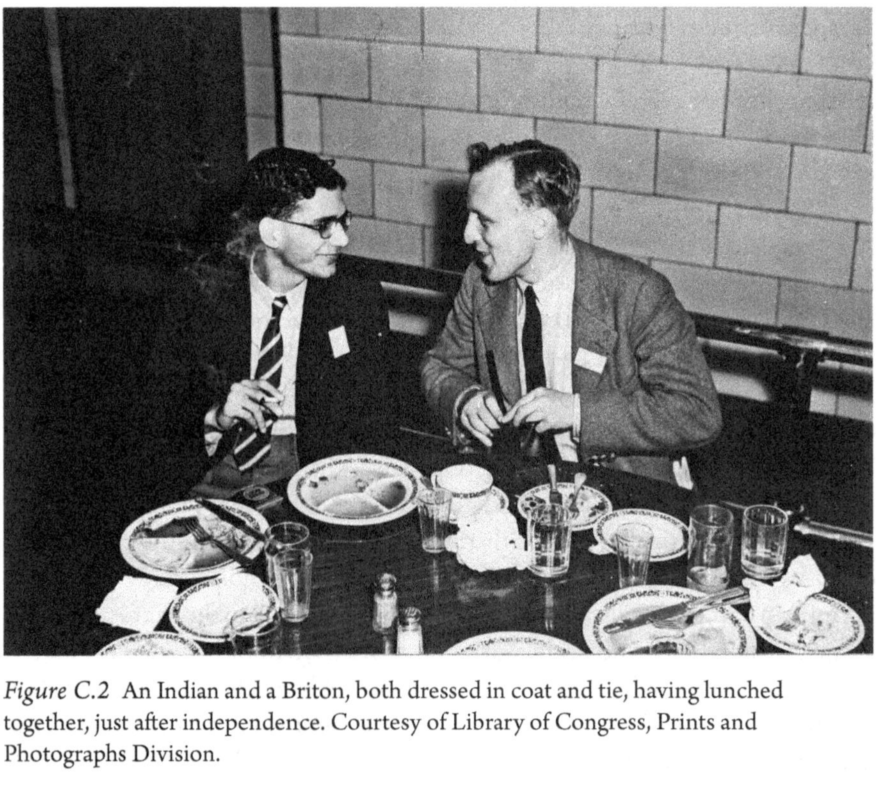

Figure C.2 An Indian and a Briton, both dressed in coat and tie, having lunched together, just after independence. Courtesy of Library of Congress, Prints and Photographs Division.

by magazine advertisements that extolled the superiority of American food products suitable for domestic use. American drinking chocolate was safer than its competitors, Horlick's malted milk imparted "the glow of health to pale cheeks," and the best way to prepare *lechon*, the Philippine spit-roasted pig, was with Heinz ketchup and Lea & Perrins Worcestershire sauce.[59] Leading Filipino politicians were dissuaded from chewing betel.[60] American social workers urged even urban Filipinos to plant vegetable gardens.[61] Nicholas Roosevelt took stock in the mid-1920s: "One of the most interesting developments in the Philippines," he observed, "is the effect of improved diet on the health and physique of the Filipino peoples." Eating wheat as well as rice, more meat, and better quality vegetables had made for enormous improvements in Filipino bodies.[62] Yet menus used at meals for Frank Murphy aboard the steamship *S. S. Mayon* as it bore the governor and his guests through the waters of archipelago in June 1934, and several others for the weeks surrounding Thanksgiving that year, included Philippine dishes as well as American ones, and if these were not so numerous as those inspired by European cooking, they were nevertheless an indication that Americans were no longer altogether averse to unfamiliar foods. Alongside lamb chops, navy bean soup, and English steamed pudding, Murphy found chow chow, Sinigang de Pascaco (a tart fish soup), anchovy paste, Carne Estofada con salsa Rubia (meat stew with tomato sauce), buttered chayote, mango, papaya, and coconut pie.[63] Americans and Filipinos had, by necessity and by choice, developed hybrid tastes in the Philippines.

On the whole, Britons and Americans were satisfied with Indian and Filipino sensory transformations. The leaders of India's Congress Party and Filipino *ilustrados* now seemed to see the world as westerners did, dismissing as nonsense conjurers' tricks of vision, avoiding gugu eyes, looking at the world logically, if not always in precisely the same ways that Britons and Americans did. They sounded better and heard things properly because they spoke English. Champions of sanitation, enemies of foul odors, they urged their people to keep themselves clean and continued with vigor campaigns on behalf of underground sewers and against public defecation. They ate with knives and forks, not fingers, and some were as happy eating western food as curries or *adobos*. Against their skin they placed western-style clothes, and they endorsed efforts to isolate the diseased and the dead, avoiding contact with the polluted others of their lower castes and classes almost as strenuously as the British and Americans had once sought to avoid touching them. Subalterns learned "western" manners, hoping not to offend the senses. Iris Macfarlane, the wife of an English tea planter in Assam, decided she would learn Assamese. She hired a teacher, who brought as his textbook "a book of etiquette, which, when I could read it, I discovered to be full of instructions about which hand to use for shaking and how to blow one's nose into a piece of cloth and put it into one's pocket; a revolting idea to Indians, but white men did it."[64] And Filipinos, observes Stanley Karnow, "readily accepted American styles and institutions. They learned to behave, dress and eat like Americans, sing American songs and speak Americanized English."[65] Indians and Filipinos were not of course to be considered Britons or Americans. But the habits of elite groups in both India and the Philippines had seemingly become more civilized.

Were they civilized enough to stand alone, to manage their own affairs? Were their senses tamed and ordered? Were their bodies under sufficient self-control? Could they keep their people safe and fed and avoid offending or antagonizing other nations with primitive understandings of the world? There were those in the metropoles who thought not and who were thus unreconciled to Indian and Filipino independence. Some Britons had what scholar Francis Hutchins has called "illusions of permanence" regarding India, the belief that they should and must stay on forever. The Cambridge professor Sir John Strachey told his undergraduates that India as a polity was a fiction: "There is no such country, and this is the first and most essential fact about India that can be learned."[66] British soldiers and officials in India in the 1940s still routinely referred to Indians as "niggers," "wogs," and "black-bellied bastards," noted the filth in the streets and the apparent indifference to it, and believed, for racial reasons, that no progress toward civilization had been made or was possible.[67] Winston Churchill's attitude toward Indians is well known. In 1931, he decried the possibility of relinquishing the Raj as "a hideous act of self-mutilation," and he called Indians "the beastliest people in the world next to the Germans," even while he abetted the starvation of thousands in Bengal in 1943–1944.[68]

Yet in the end even Churchill grudgingly conceded that the time for India's independence had come, as long as India and all states emerging from it remained British dominions.[69] World War II had finally and irrevocably broken the boundaries that the British had since 1858 tried to erect between their bodies and those of Indians, having feared bodily offense or even contamination by uncivilized sight, sound, smell, touch, or taste. Mountbatten was the first viceroy to allow Indians freely into his residence, and he and his wife visited Indians in their homes.[70] Whatever its shortcomings, the Indian elite had persuaded the British government that its representatives knew how to behave in a civilized way. They had learned to respect the senses.

Much the same thinking characterized the Americans in the Philippines. Here, too, skeptics remained. Nicholas Roosevelt acknowledged that while "a few thousand Filipinos know and understand something of American civilization . . . the rank and file have no idea of what America is or stands for," disqualifying the islands for independence. It was necessary "to accept the obvious conclusion that independence is out of the question for two or three generations at least; and to shoulder our burden courageously, carrying through the thankless task to completion."[71] Such sentiments were shared by many Republicans at home, by the businessman L. P. Hammond, and by the health and sanitation expert Victor Heiser, who in 1928 insisted that "dealing with officials" in the Philippines was "like dealing with the immature mind of boys"—yet incredibly, "the world professe[d] to believe that the Filipinos as a whole are ready to run the complicated machinery of a 20th century government."[72] Paul McNutt, who would become the last US governor-general and the first US ambassador in the Philippines, argued in a 1938 radio address that progress made in the archipelago would be wasted if the Americans left too soon: "If we scuttle, if we run away, our monument will be destroyed. The things we counted on, our aspirations to point the way to a new benign colonialism . . . will perish."[73]

But again, as with British India, most American officials had decided by the end of the war that the time for occupation had passed. Both countries had had enough of it, and the Filipinos had for the most part demonstrated their loyalty and determination to be free during the horrors of Japanese rule. The Americans had long admired aspects of Philippine culture and had glimpsed in it the seeds of civilization. The Wood-Forbes Report of 1922 had praised the Filipinos' "many attractive qualities." They were "happy and care-free," generous to a fault, and "naturally an orderly and law-abiding people." Filipinas were "strong" and "hardworking" domestic caretakers. There remained work to be done: Filipinos had a "disregard for sanitary measures" and were "still rather oriental in their attitude toward disease and questions of public health and sanitation."[74] But there had been improvements along these lines, and independence was imminent. The High Commissioner Frances Sayre told an audience in Manila in late 1939: "Philippine independence surely will not mean the end of American co-operation. Civilization goes forward when different races and different cultures join hands and make their contributions to each other."[75] The Americans were not leaving, completely; their military would remain in the islands. Yet they trusted their Filipino counterparts to be their partners in the quest for civilization now defined not as the imposition of one culture on another, but, as Sayre had explained, as an interracial and intercultural community.

Much of the impetus for sensory reform came from local elites. It is not surprising that the men who occupied positions of immediate subordination to their imperial rulers would have an interest in replacing those who had governed their country. It is also unsurprising that local groups would find it expedient and even attractive to mimic the behavior of those in power.[76] Appearing "western" in style and deportment, speaking English with the prescribed inflection and accent, avoiding excessive sniffing, smelling of soap, shaking hands that were presumed free of germs, and eating European or American (or hybrid) food as it was eaten in the metropoles—all of these were ways to convince a man's masters of his fitness for self-government. One might learn by going to Britain or the

United States how best to behave. This had long been true for Indians. All of them, writes historian Michael Fisher, "made choices about how to present themselves through their comportment as well as their words. They selected sartorial styles to identify themselves visually and practised dietary customs which shaped their social intercourse with Britons and other Indians." Gandhi and Nehru took law degrees in England and learned to argue their cases (and air their grievances) alongside the brightest colonialists of their generation. Indians abroad socialized with Britons, read their newspapers and books, and lived in their rooming houses. "Thus," Fisher concludes, "being present in Britain meant the power to know Britons and address them directly."[77] No one was more mortified than an Indian to see one of his countrymen begging in London's streets.[78]

In the Philippines, Governor Taft decided to send each year a few bright young Filipinos to the United States for study. Alex Sutherland accompanied the group that sailed from Manila in October 1903 and reported back to Taft. The students were an intellectually curious group who wrote "a great many letters," and Sutherland soon witnessed "visible improvement both in the matter of their general personal neatness and appearance, and also in the matter of behavior at the table."[79] Manuel Quezon, Sergio Osmeña, and other Filipino politicians who came to the United States during the colonial period were on what their hosts considered their best behavior, dressing in suits, speaking English, and eating American food. Most Filipinos immigrating to the United States—some 150,000 (including Alaska and Hawaii) by 1946—were poor and battled to overcome prejudice against them for their habits. They had "a low standard mode of housing and feeding," complained a judge in California. Perhaps for that reason, Filipino-Americans were acutely conscious of the impression they were making. An angry group of them in Stockton's Little Manila stopped a cook at a Filipino diner from grilling dried fish, the odor from which had suffused the neighborhood.[80] A Filipina named Gloria had related worries in New York. "One time," she confessed to an interviewer, "my office supervisor made a surprise visit to my house. I had just cooked *binagoongan* [a pork dish made with fermented shrimp paste]. The whole house reeked of shrimp paste. It was so embarrassing."[81]

More often, the leaders within each country—the *bhadralok* (gentlemen) in India, the *ilustrados* or *caciques* (political bosses) in the Philippines—demonstrated a willingness to undertake practices and comport themselves with the manners their rulers expected of civilized men. Imperial efforts to improve Indian society carried within them the seeds of the empire's destruction. Leading Indians bested the British at their own game. They learned impeccable English, studied the law and ethics, and conducted themselves with more social grace than most Britons could hope to do. The cultural mimicry deployed by the *bhadralok* brought about what historian Harald Fischer-Tiné calls "a complete assimilation of the indigenous population," or some number of it, "to the culture of their colonial masters in dress, behaviour, language and ways of thinking," and subversively "blurred the line separating the colonizers from the colonized," in small ways and large.[82] So, for example, did upper-class Indians begin to infiltrate the hill stations, places of privilege for the British who nevertheless found it increasingly difficult to keep the "natives" out. The Indians became partners in rule with the British. The racism that had earlier sustained the stations' virtual segregation did not disappear, but by the early twentieth century its effects were had been mitigated by the elite's acceptance "of some of the same values and practices" adhered to by the British.[83] Challenged by the British to compose their own version of government if they thought it was easy, members of a committee led by Tej Bahadur Sapru and Jawaharlal Nehru's father Motilal quickly wrote a constitution that called for a bill of rights and the centralization of power.[84] The *bhadralok* embraced technology, science, and the pursuit of public health and sanitation.[85] It proved all too easy for Indians in positions of power to treat their subordinates as the British had often treated them. A mutiny by sailors in the Royal Indian Navy in February 1946 targeted a British officer named F. W. King, but the mutineers also complained bitterly that fellow Indians who were their immediate superiors had called them "bastards" and generally abused them.[86]

Mohandas Gandhi lived his life as if in deliberate rejection of the British quest to civilize Indians. Despite his British education, Gandhi refused to embody the essential characteristics of Britishness. He wore only a *dhoti,* with a homespun shawl on cold days. He often spoke in the vernacular, confounding British ears. The authorities were loath to touch him, exposed as he was, and there seem to be no photographs of the Mahatma shaking hands with British officials, only those depicting his offer of *namaste* with his palms placed together. The activist Gandhi drank no alcohol, consumed only a few foods and never meat, and always ate with his hands. Jawaharlal Nehru was different. His father Motilal equated civilization with westernization, and sent his son to England for his education. He advised Jawaharlal on the best ways to wear western clothes and how to make British friends, and on the masculine necessity of learning to shoot and even getting into "a real fight" from time to time. British classmates called Jawaharlal "Joe."[87] As an adult he became what he called "a queer merger of East and West, out of place everywhere, at home nowhere," but most contemporaries seemed to think that Nehru handled himself as well during audiences with Lord Mountbatten as in speeches given to masses of Indians in Delhi. He generally wore Indian clothes but managed, wrote the American journalist John Gunther, "to appear courtly and impressive even when shrouded with yards of cheesecloth apron"—that is, while wearing a *kurta* with a homespun jacket that would come to bear his name. Nehru was tall for an Indian, light-skinned, a polished writer and speaker of English. He recited British poetry and subscribed to a variety of British, American, and French newspapers and journals. He swam and skied.

Religious display made him uncomfortable. Unlike Gandhi, Nehru smoked cigarettes, drank wine, and occasionally ate meat.[88] When officials came to arrest him early one morning in August 1942, he insisted on eating his breakfast—cornflakes, eggs, bacon, toast, and coffee—before he would agree to be taken off to prison.[89] And Nehru's chief Muslim rival, Mohammed Ali Jinnah, affected an even more obvious western style, dressing himself in Saville Row suits and smoking through a cigarette holder.[90]

Filipino leaders, the *ilustrados* who would rule their people once the Americans had handed off power, also slipped easily into patterns of thought and behavior modeled by their recent masters.[91] So comfortable were they governing at the behest of the Americans that during the 1920s and 1930s the *caciques* in some respects lost interest in independence; they found it hard to imagine a life better suited to themselves than the one provided by US occupation, which allowed them a significant measure of political and social autonomy and access to an American market unfettered by the tariffs imposed by Washington on independent nations. Besides, as Benedict Anderson has observed, the *caciques* had by this time "switched from Spanish to English, and their children were going to school in Manhattan and Boston." Nor did they, unlike Indians or fellow Southeast Asian nationalists, inherit a monarchical tradition.[92] They agreed with the Americans on the difficulties presented by the need to incorporate into the state the pagans living upcountry, and they largely accepted, and even promulgated, stereotypes concerning the shiftlessness and indolence of small farmers and the poor.[93] Upper-class Indians came more often to British hill stations; so too did wealthy Filipinos join in the development of Baguio as part of an American strategy to keep Filipino politicians sufficiently interested in the place that they would not obstruct plans for its improvement.[94]

Like their Indian counterparts, the *ilustrados* embraced sensory refinement, and thus their own civilization, as their occupiers defined it. This was true for virtually all of them: Sergio Osmeña, speaker of the House of Representatives, senator, vice president, then president in 1944–1946; Elipdio Quirino, six years a senator, then member of both the Philippine Commission to the United States in 1934–1935 and the Constitutional Commission; and Manuel Roxas, twelve years speaker of the house, then the first president of the republic, in 1946—a man of "fiery oratory" in the Philippines oral/aural style, but one who, like the others, wore suits or jackets and ties, spoke English, and cooperated closely with the Americans through the transitions to Commonwealth then independent status.[95] Manuel Quezon was the central figure in the Philippines government during the first half of the twentieth century. The Americans regarded him as a *roué*, a diva, and a rascal whose extravagances included a yacht on which he cruised Manila Bay. "He must be kept constantly under good paternal management," cautioned H. H. Bandholtz in 1906.[96] Yet they also admired his patriotism and, most of all, his willingness to behave in ways that they recognized as versions of themselves. Quezon had a healthy disrespect for the arbitrary assertion of authority, especially that of the Catholic Church. He was direct in conversation and action, traits born of "an aggressive practicality" that proved effective in his dealings with the US Congress. At first a reluctant speaker of English, Quezon learned it quickly when he was appointed commissioner to Washington in 1909. Like Nehru, he was a sartorial hybrid, wearing Tagalog clothes at home but western-style polo shirts for informal meetings and suits for important occasions, and a gustatorial hybrid too, favoring steaks and beef adobos, and drinking more alcohol than most Filipinos. His official vehicle during the 1930s was an enormous Chrysler Airflow.[97] For all of his flamboyance, Quezon nevertheless demonstrated to American officials that he could be serious about the business of governing. Governor Murphy reported that during the first month of the commonwealth, "the relations between the President and myself have been harmonious." Quezon had shown a sincere desire "to avoid having the Commonwealth Government take any action which might be in any way embarrassing" to the US government, "or which might not meet with the approval of the administration."[98] All the sensory cues—gestural, sonic, gustatory and the rest—seemed right.

So were the senses put in order on the days of independence, during the vital ceremonies and rituals that characterized the victories of nationalism and the handovers of power. In the Philippines on July 4, 1946, people seemed inclined to contain their emotions, to show reserve, as if to prove to the Americans one last time their capacity for sensory politesse and self-restraint. The visual indicators of the transfer were solemn: the American flag was "gently lowered" and replaced by the Philippine flag—red, white, and blue, with the sun and three stars in its triangular white field. The Statue of Liberty featured prominently on the cover of the inauguration's official program. At night fireworks erupted over Manila, visual and sonic indicators of freedom, identical to the American practice on the same day each year. The thousands gathered in the Luneta for the ceremony heard from Senator Millard Tydings, Douglas MacArthur, and President Roxas—all, of course, speaking in English. With the declaration of independence, sirens went off in Manila and church bells pealed across the archipelago.[99] At the birth of the Commonwealth in 1935, the Filipino band had played "The Star Spangled Banner" and "Hail to the Chief." On Independence Day, the band played both the US and Philippine anthems. The latter, "Lupang Hinirang" ("Chosen Land"), had been commissioned by Emilio Aguinaldo in 1898 to accompany the declaration of independence from Spain, but the Americans had previously banned its performance.[100] There are no reports concerning the odor of independence, though the front end of the float piloted in the day's parade by the Manila Department of Public Works and Communication bore a slight resemblance to an angled toilet seat, no doubt unintentionally. Haptic courtesies were observed despite the crowds—there is little sign of jostling in video footage of the events—and MacArthur and Roxas warmly shook hands, though they stood apart from each other at a distance requiring that each incline his upper body toward the other in order that they might connect. *Life* magazine noted that the United States "still keeps some silken strings of influence threaded to the infant republic," most likely referring to the passage, two days before the ceremony, of the Bell Act, which pegged the Philippine peso to the dollar, opened the Philippines' territory and resources to special access by American companies and investors, and set quotas on Philippine exports to the United States.[101] Throughout the islands, people celebrated by eating traditional foods. That November, the Thanksgiving holiday passed without notice, turkey, or stuffing.[102]

Just over a year later, and with considerably more drama, the British handed over power to the governments of Pakistan and India. Ceremonies in the first, held August 14, 1947, were austere, as Jinnah greeted Mountbatten at the Sind Provincial Government House, the Pakistani leader's new official residence, and with a minimum of fanfare accepted leadership of the Muslim nation.[103] India, by contrast, offered British observers a last chance to reflect on South Asian exuberance and sensory unruliness, even if they were able to reassure themselves, in the end, that there was beauty in what remained of the Indian sensorium, and that the bodily constraints they had introduced to India were at least to some extent in effect. In Mewar, Mary Chenevix Trench and her family saw the Indian flag flying outside houses and admired the lights of the bazaar and the colorful saris of the women on their way to temple. There was little "shouting or fuss," only a single, halfhearted "Jai Hind!" ["Long Live India!"] whispered at them.[104] Delhi was visually transformed, "bedecking itself to usher in another chapter in its hoary history," wrote a correspondent for the *Times of India*. Throughout the capital city workers repainted the facades of buildings, mounted banners and archways over the processional routes, and strung wires for illumination, as India would officially become free at the stroke of midnight on the fifteenth.[105] In the evening an auspicious rainbow appeared. There was a good deal more noise in the capital than in Mewar: the crowds shouted "slogans of joy" honoring Gandhi, Nehru, and Mountbatten in what M. J. Akbar described as "a great and beautiful roar of spontaneous rejoicing." Inside the chamber of the Council of State building, where the legislature was to declare independence, a member blew a conch shell to summon the gods, then Assembly President Rajendra Prasad read an oath, first in Hindi, then in English, heralding the end of British control. Leaving the building, Mountbatten was engulfed by crowds and unable to return to his coach. It took Nehru climbing onto the roof and waving the crowd off to stop the press of bodies and allow Mountbatten to continue on his way.[106] Orders for sweets to celebrate independence had driven up prices for scarce sugar, though without any apparent deterrent effect.[107]

Thus did formal empires end. Yet empire left behind a residue of strategic concerns, economic interests, and emotional bonds not easily dismissed or denied.[108] The British did not leave South Asia altogether. "The great thing was," wrote Lord Gladwyn, the British undersecretary of state, "to try to establish a new and, if possible, an intimate relationship with old dependencies which, in our weakened state, it was impossible to hold down by force, even if that was desirable."[109] Pakistan and India remained Commonwealth states, retaining for a time British military advisers, trading extensively with Britain and within the Commonwealth and, perhaps above all, clinging tenaciously to affective ties that proved remarkably durable. The Americans stayed even more heavily involved in the Philippines. Thousands of US soldiers and sailors remained on bases—Clark Field and Subic Bay—in the archipelago, spending a good deal of money but engendering no end of ill will for their behavior. Postwar US aid allowed the new nation to import lavishly, running up an enormous trade deficit as it did so, and in the process enriching a handful of Filipino businessmen and landowners. Emotionally, Filipinos were at best ambivalent about the persistent American presence in their lives. American nostalgia for insular empire was consumed by

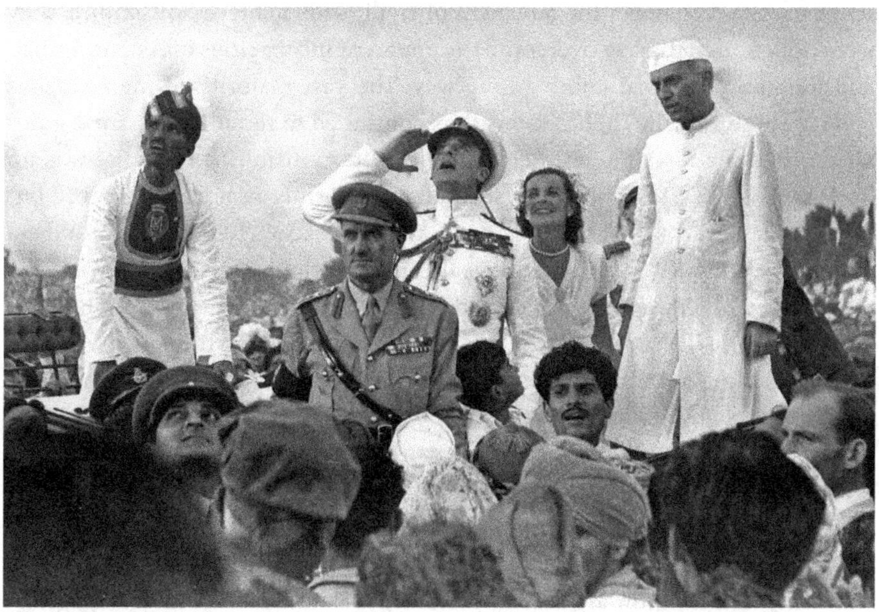

Figure C.3 Viceroy Mountbatten salutes the Indian flag, Delhi, Independence Day 1947. His wife, Edwina, is behind him; prime minister Nehru looks on. Nehru Memorial Museum and Library.

paternalism. Robert Taft, senator from Ohio and the son of the first US governor of the Philippines, conceded that Philippine independence was "I think, a good thing. But," he went on, "certainly we shall always be a big brother, if you please, to the Philippines."[110]

What of civilization, the moral rationale for empire, according to its architects? So central to the rhetoric of imperial origins in the nineteenth and early twentieth centuries, the word was mostly gone from the professions of friendship, whether magnanimous or strained, offered the new states at the time of their independence. In part, this was because the British and Americans had satisfied themselves that they had achieved some measure of civilization in their colonies, as the sights, sounds, smells, feel, and tastes of India and the Philippines now reflected the behavior of refined men and women. To a greater extent, the word went missing for a time because it was no longer fashionable, reeking as it did of racism, a too-fresh reminder of the deadly hubris of Hitler's Germany and Hirohito's Japan. That did not mean that imperial thinking had ended. Instead, "civilization" appeared more often in the plural, reflecting the relativism of postwar social science.[111] The task once called "civilization" was more often described as "development" (or "modernization"), terms that were never circumscribed by economics alone.[112] The communist threat during the Cold War required the continued involvement of the western powers, or so they reasoned, in the affairs of the newly independent states of Asia. Whatever the advances of civilization achieved by empire, they were not enough to have overcome the apparent incapacities of Asians. Indian and Filipino elites had come a long way. The vast majority of their citizens had not done as well. Their nations thus continued to require assistance, guidance, and direction to meet their new global responsibilities. Empire was no longer viable. Yet its imperatives seemed to its former practitioners more important than ever. And, as it turned out, the civilization concept was not dead but only resting. It gained ideological (and emotional) meaning during the Cold War, when it became associated with "western" institutions, such as the North Atlantic Treaty Organization, that embodied and promised to defend values resistant to communism.[113] Following the end of the Cold War, political scientists and politicians posited the supremacy of civilization, based on culture, as the most serious cause of world conflict. It meant "the broadest level of identification with which [a world citizen] intensely identifies," according to Samuel P. Huntington; religion was its most important component.[114] A clash of civilizations, particularly between "the West" and Islam, was likely, Huntington argued. Imperialism was not a word in Huntington's vocabulary, nor did he suggest that "civilizing" be deployed as a project aimed at nonwestern people. Huntington's civilization of values had little in common with Norbert Elias's civilization of manners—except insofar as both terms conveyed a powerful sense of difference between people, and in each case conferred on one group confidence in its own superiority.

The end of empire in India and the Philippines brought changes to the metropoles that were in their own ways as profound as those felt by its subjects. "The impact of colonialism on India was deep," Ashis Nandy has written. Yet because "the country was culturally fragmented and politically heterogeneous," it was able in part to "confine the cultural impact of imperialism to its urban centres, to its Westernized and semi-Westernized upper and middle classes, and to some sections of its traditional élites." But "that was not the case for the rulers from a relatively more homogeneous small island. They were overwhelmed by the experience of being colonial rulers. As a result, the long-term cultural damage colonialism did to the British society was greater" than that done to Indian—and while the Philippines was not nearly as large as India, nor the United States a small island, Nandy's point has relevance to the American situation as well.[115] In this way colonialism did not end in 1946 and 1947, and in its reverberations—its presence in the minds of men, as Nandy has put it—continues down to the present. The empire came home to Britain and the United States, in the form of immigrants from South Asia and the Philippines: in 2011 there were over three million South Asians living in the United Kingdom; in 2010 nearly 3.4 million Filipinos lived in the United States. They have contributed to a hybridization of cultures, and an encounter of bodies that has changed British and American sensoria more fully than was possible through the introduction of relative handfuls of Britons and Americans to India and the Philippines in the nineteenth and twentieth centuries. The sight of South Asians—women in saris, men in kurtas—in the United Kingdom, and Filipinos in the United States, is a common one; the sound of Hindi (and soundtracks from Bollywood musicals) or Tagalog (and Bruno Mars) is part of urban life too. Campaigns against foul odors had begun at home in the nineteenth century, and they continue there—the Filipina Gloria worries about the smell of her shrimp paste *binagoongan*, and in England young whites vent their hostility toward South Asians: "I just don't like Pakis," said one, using slang for all South Asians. "They stink. Pakis really reek. You can tell one in the street a mile away."[116] Still, chicken tikka masala has become Britain's national dish, bowdlerized to suit British tastes, while Filipino food, long a sleeper in the American restaurant scene, has made a greater impression recently with destinations like Bad Saint in Washington, DC and Maharlika in New York City.

None of this is to imply that empire is a happy thing that always ends well or that its subjects inevitably get the upper hand eventually. Psychoanalyst O. Mannoni wrote that "a colonial situation is created . . . the very instant a white man, even if he is alone, appears in the midst of a tribe so long as he is thought to be rich or powerful or merely immune to the local forces of magic, and so long as he derives from his position, even though only in his most secret self, a feeling of his own superiority."[117] Is it the case that whites, in Britain and the United States, continue to harbor such feelings of superiority regarding Indians and Filipinos as permanent abusers of the five senses, and therefore less than civilized? Do the sound of a Philippine accent or the odor of a "Paki" continue to offend in their adopted countries? Does colonialism thus remain in the minds of men and women? Fully two generations after formal empire ended in South Asia and the Philippines, these questions linger.

NOTES

Introduction

1. Mark M. Smith, *Sensing the Past: Seeing, Hearing, Smelling, Tasting, and Touching in History* (Berkeley, 2007), 18.
2. Laura Otis, *Membranes: Metaphors of Invasion in Nineteenth-Century Literature, Science, and Politics* (Baltimore, 1999).
3. Jon E. Wilson, *The Chaos of Empire: The British Raj and the Conquest of India* (New York, 2016), 6.
4. Representative titles on the history of the senses include Marshall McLuhan, *The Gutenberg Galaxy* (Toronto, 1962); Alain Corbin, *The Foul and the Fragrant: Odor and the French Social Imagination* (Cambridge, MA, 1986); J. Douglas Porteous, *Landscapes of the Mind: Worlds of Sense and Metaphor* (Toronto, 1990); David Howes, *The Varieties of Sensory Experience: A Sourcebook on the Anthropology of the Senses* (Toronto, 1991); Constance Classen, *Worlds of Sense: Exploring the Senses in History and Across Cultures* (London, 1993); Constance Classen, David Howes, and Anthony Synnott, *Aroma: The Cultural History of Smell* (New York, 1994); Alain Corbin, *Village Bells: Sound and Meaning in the 19th-Century French Countryside*, transl. by Martin Thom (New York, 1998); Leigh Eric Schmidt, *Hearing Things: Religion, Illusion, and American Enlightenment* (Cambridge, MA, 2000); Richard Cullen Rath, *How Early America Sounded* (Ithaca, NY, 2003); Michael Bull and Les Back, eds., *The Auditory Culture Reader* (Oxford, 2003); Carolyn Korsmeyer, ed., *The Taste Culture Reader: Experiencing Food and Drink* (Oxford, 2005); Constance Classen, ed., *The Book of Touch* (Oxford, 2005); Robert Jütte, *A History of the Senses from Antiquity to Cyberspace*, trans. James Lynn (Cambridge, 2005); David Howes, ed., *Empire of the Senses: The Sensual Culture Reader* (Oxford, 2005); Jim Drobnick, ed., *The Smell Culture Reader* (Oxford, 2006); Mark M. Smith, *How Race Is Made: Slavery, Segregation, and the Senses* (Chapel Hill, 2006); Smith, *Sensing the Past*; Elizabeth Edwards and Kaushik Bhaumik, eds., *Visual Sense: A Cultural Reader* (Oxford, 2008); "The Senses in American History: A Roundtable," *Journal of American History* 95, no. 2 (September 2008), 378–451; Andrew J. Rotter, "Empires of the Senses: How Seeing, Hearing, Smelling, Tasting, and Touching Shaped Imperial Encounters," *Diplomatic History* 35, no. 1 (January 2011), 2–19; "AHR Forum: The Senses in History," *American Historical Review* 116, no. 2 (April 2011), 307–400; Constance Classen, *The Deepest Sense: A Cultural History of Touch* (Urbana, 2012); Jonathan Reinarz, *Past Scents: Historical Perspectives on Smell* (Urbana, 2014); Andrew J. Rotter, "The Senses," in Costigliola and Hogan, eds., *Explaining the History of American Foreign Relations*, 317–33.
5. Seeger quoted in David Howes, "To Summon All the Senses," in Howes, ed., *The Varieties of Sensory Experience*, 3. Or, as Robert Jütte has written, "There can be no such thing as a natural history of the senses, only a social history of human sense perception." Jütte, *History of the Senses*, 9.

6. Norbert Elias, *The Civilizing Process: The History of Manners*, trans. Edmund Jephcott (New York, 1978).
7. McLuhan, *The Gutenberg Galaxy*.
8. Mark S. R. Jenner, "Tasting Lichfield, Touching China: Sir John Floyer's Senses," *The Historical Journal* 53, no. 3 (2010), 669.
9. This point is made by David Howes and Marc Lalonde in "The History of Sensibilities: Of the Standard of Taste in Mid-Eighteenth Century England and the Circulation of Smells in Post-Revolutionary France," *Dialectical Anthropology* 16, no. 2 (1991), 125–35.
10. Walter J. Ong, *The Presence of the Word* (New Haven, CT, 1967); David Howes, "Can These Dry Bones Live? An Anthropological Approach to the History of the Senses," *Journal of American History* 95, no. 2 (September 2008), 448; Smith, *Sensing the Past*, 1–18; David Howes and Constance Classen, "Conclusion: Sounding Sensory Profiles," in Howes, ed., *Varieties of Sensory Experience*, 257–88.
11. Julian Go, *Patterns of Empire: The British and American Empires, 1688 to the Present* (New York, 2011), 4–5.
12. Julian Go, "Introduction: Global Perspectives on the U.S. Colonial State in the Philippines," in Go and Foster, eds., *Colonial State in the Philippines*, 22.
13. See, for example, Peter Stanley, *A Nation in the Making: The Philippines and the United States, 1899–1921* (Cambridge, MA, 1974), 99–100.
14. William H. Anderson, *The Philippine Problem* (New York, 1939), 146. In this way, I heed Ann Laura Stoler's call "for more reflection on the history and politics of comparison . . . doing a certain kind of comparative colonial history," including paying "attention to practices of colonial comparison by colonial governments themselves." Ann Laura Stoler, "Tense and Tender Ties: The Politics of Comparison in North American History and (Post) Colonial Studies," in Stoler, ed., *Haunted By Empire*, 23.
15. Paul A. Kramer, "Empires, Exceptions, and Anglo-Saxons: Race and Rule between the British and United States Empires, 1880–1910," *Journal of American History* 88, no. 4 (March 2002), 1324; Stuart Anderson, *Race and Rapprochement: Anglo-Saxonism and Anglo-American Relations, 1895–1904* (East Brunswick, NJ, 1981), 11–12, 20, 119.
16. Anderson, *Race and Rapprochement*, 57–58.
17. Kramer, "Empires," 1334.
18. David Gilmour, *The Ruling Caste: Imperial Lives in the Victorian Raj* (New York, 2005), xiii.
19. Leonard Wood, Diary, January 1–December 31, 1926, entry for May 8, Leonard Wood Papers, Box 23, MD, LC. Willingdon also told Wood that he thought "the Gandhi Movement in India is about at an end."
20. Price Collier, *The West in the East* (New York, 1911), 44, 253–54; John Bancroft Devins, *An Observer in the Philippines, or, Life in Our New Possessions* (Boston, 1905), 118. Other comparisons are possible, of course: the Philippines and South Africa are more closely matched in scale and timing than the Philippines and India. Yet the common tropicality of the latter two and the centrality of India to the British Empire, coupled with my own longstanding interest in India, tipped the balance here. I also considered adding French Indochina to the comparison, but found the prospect of another vast set of variables frankly daunting.
21. Patricio N. Abinales, "Progressive-Machine Conflict in Early-Twentieth-Century U.S. Politics and Colonial-State Building in the Philippines," in Go and Foster, eds., *Colonial State in the Philippines*, 161, 166.
22. See, for example, Rozina Visram, *Ayahs, Lascars and Princes: Indians in Britain 1700–1947* (London, 1986), 182–83.
23. James C. Scott, *Seeing Like a State: How Certain Schemes to Improve the Human Condition Have Failed* (New Haven, CT, 1998), 183.
24. E. M. Collingham, *Imperial Bodies: The Physical Experience of the Raj, c. 1800–1947* (Cambridge, 2001), 10.
25. Edward Said, "Criticism/ Self Criticism," *Lingua Franca*, February–March 1992, 39–40; Sander L. Gilman, *Difference and Pathology: Stereotypes of Sexuality, Race, and Madness* (Ithaca, NY, 1995), 12, 19–25.

26. Francis G. Hutchins, *The Illusion of Permanence: British Imperialism in India* (Princeton, NJ, 1967), 59; Rudyard Kipling, "The White Man's Burden," reprinted in Rudyard Kipling, *100 Poems, Old and New*, Thomas Pinney, ed. (New York, 2013), 111–13.
27. Clifford Geertz, *After the Fact: Two Centuries, Four Decades, One Anthropologist* (Cambridge, MA, 1995), 43.

Chapter 1

1. Recollections of Anne Bremner, MSS Eur 226/4, Private Papers, IOR, BL.
2. Margery Hall, "Autobiography: 'And the Nights Were More Terrible Than the Days,'" MSS Eur 226/11, Private Papers, IOR, BL.
3. Major G. Horne, "Breakfast in Bangalore," J. M. Bourne Papers, CSAS.
4. Recollections of Anne Bremner.
5. Margery Hall, "Autobiography."
6. Mary Chenevix Trench, memoir "A Child's Experience of Gilgit, 1934–37," MSS Eur F226/33, Mary Chenevix Trench Papers, IOR, Private Papers, BL.
7. Viola Bayley, memoir "Hangu in 1934," Viola Bayley Papers, Small Collections, Box 2, CSAS.
8. Erica Farquharson, memoir "Indian Idyll," J. M. Bourne Papers, CSAS.
9. Tim Edensor, "The Social Life of the Senses: Ordering and Disordering the Modern Sensorium," in Howes, ed., *A Cultural History of the Senses in the Modern Age*, 38–39.
10. Allen, *Plain Tales from the Raj*, 13.
11. Census data show that there were approximately 155,500 Britons in India in 1931, and 19,800 "whites" (not "yellow" or "brown" or "negro") in the Philippines in 1939. Of course, not all Americans were white, nor were all whites Americans.
12. Mary H. Fee, *A Woman's Impressions of the Philippines* (Chicago, 1910), 46–50.
13. Grace Paulding Memoir, William and Grace Paulding Papers, 1873–1956, Box 1, USMHI.
14. Victor G. Heiser, *Annual Report of the Bureau of Health for the Fiscal Year ended June 30, 1912* (Manila, 1913), 63–64.
15. William H. Brown, Paul F. Russell, and Clara Palafox Cariño, *Health Through Knowledge and Habits* (Boston, 1933), 95.
16. Elias, *The Civilizing Process*, 53–54, 53–59, 126–27, 131, 135, 146.
17. Raymond Williams, *Keywords: A Vocabulary of Culture and Society* (New York, 1983), 57–58. See also Margrit Pernau, "Teaching Emotions: The Encounter between Victorian Values and Indo-Persian Concepts of Civility in Nineteenth-Century Delhi," in Sengupta and Ali, eds., *Knowledge Production, Pedagogy, and Institutions in Colonial India*, 227–47.
18. *Webster's American Dictionary of the English Language* (New York, 1841), 148.
19. G. C. Merriam to Taft, February 12, 1904, William Howard Taft Papers, Cornell University Library (microfilm), Reel 42.
20. McGee was in charge of the ethnological exhibits at the 1904 St. Louis World Fair. See Rebecca Edwards, *New Spirits: Americans in the "Gilded Age," 1865–1905* (New York, 2015), 239.
21. Ronald Inden, *Imagining India* (Oxford, 1990), 44; Thomas R. Metcalf, *Ideologies of the Raj* (Cambridge, 1995), 10–15; Edward Said, *Orientalism* (New York, 1978).
22. Metcalf, *Ideologies of the Raj*, 30; Inden, *Imagining India*, 45; Lawrence James, *Raj: The Making and Unmaking of British India* (London, 1997), 180; Adam Knowles, "Conjecturing Rudeness: James Mill's Utilitarian Philosophy of History and the British Civilizing Mission," in Watt and Mann, eds., *Civilizing Missions in Colonial and Postcolonial South Asia*, 37–63; Sabyasachi Bhattacharya, *Talking Back: The Idea of Civilization in the Indian Nationalist Discourse* (New Delhi, 2011), 16.
23. Metcalf, *Ideologies of the Raj*, 32–34, 39, 66; John Darwin, *Unfinished Empire: The Global Expansion of Britain* (New York, 2012), 103; Mark Tunick, "Tolerant Imperialism: John Stuart Mill's Defense of British Rule in India," *Review of Politics* 68 (2006), 1–26; Lynn Zastoupil, *John Stuart Mill and India* (Stanford, 1994), 175.
24. Gail Bederman, *Manliness and Civilization: A Cultural History of Gender and Race in the United States, 1880–1917* (Chicago, 1995), 23.
25. McKinley to Dewey and Otis, January 8, 1899, Quotations from Speeches and Statements by the President of the U.S. Concerning the Philippines Islands, 1900–1904, and

Correspondence of the Philippine Commission (compiled 1900–1906), [R]ecord [G]roup 350: Records of the War Department, BIA Box 1, NAII.

26. *Report of the Philippine Commission to the President*, Vol. I (Washington, DC, 1900), 3–4. The First Commission included Admiral George Dewey, General Elwell Otis, Jacob Gould Schurman, Charles Denby, and Dean C. Worcester.
27. McKinley speech, Dubuque, October 16, 1899, Quotations from Speeches and Statements by the President of the U.S. Concerning the Philippines Islands, 1900–1904, and Correspondence of the Philippine Commission (compiled 1900–1906), RG 350, Box 1, NAII. See also speeches in Sioux Falls IA, Madison WI, Racine WI, and Warren, OH.
28. Theodore Roosevelt, extract from Annual Message to Congress, December 6, 1904, "Compilation: Brief Extracts from well-considered opinions expressed by officials, ex-officials, etc.," Confidential File, 1914–1935, RG 350, Box 9, NA II.
29. Inden, *Imagining India*, 54.
30. James, *Raj*, 57.
31. Roderick Cavaliero, *Strangers in the Land: The Rise and Decline of the British Indian Empire* (London, 2002), 84–85.
32. Allen, *Plain Tales from the Raj*, 200.
33. Nigel Yates, *Anglican Ritualism in Victorian Britain 1830–1910* (Oxford, 1999), 95, 103, 163, 217, 277–78; James Bentley, *Ritualism and Politics in Victorian Britain: The Attempt to Legislate for Belief* (Oxford, 1978), 23.
34. Bentley, *Ritualism and Politics*, 43.
35. Charles Henry Brent Diary, September 6, 1902, Charles Henry Brent Papers, Box 1, MD, LC.
36. Brent Diary, January 17, 1903, Box 2.
37. Charles Henry Brent, "Religious Conditions in the Philippine Islands," nd [1904], Brent Papers, Box 6.
38. Igorrote, or Igorot, was a term used by the Spaniards to identify the people living in northern Luzon. Along with "Negritos," the Spaniards regarded them as distinct from the lowland Tagalogs and other upcountry folk, including Ilocanos and Cagayans. The Americans adopted this taxonomy, though its use in retrospect is problematic. See Paul Barclay, "'They Have for the Coast Dwellers a Traditional Hatred': Governing Igorots in Northern Luzon and Central Taiwan, 1895–1915," in Go and Foster, eds., *Colonial State in the Philippines*, 218, 223; and Rebecca Tinio McKenna, *American Imperial Pastoral: The Architecture of US Colonialism in the Philippines* (Chicago, 2017), 8.
39. Brent to Mrs. Monks, February 16, 1903, Brent Papers, Box 6.
40. Brent Diary, June 29, 1905, Box 1.
41. Leonard Wood, diary entry, August 13, 1923, Leonard Wood Papers, Box 21, MD, LC.
42. Constance Classen, "The Witch's Senses: Sensory Ideologies and Transgressive Femininities from the Renaissance to Modernity," in Howes, ed., *Empire of the Senses*, 70.
43. Margaret MacMillan, *Women of the Raj* (London, 1988), 13.
44. Stanley Karnow, *In Our Image: America's Empire in the Philippines* (New York, 1989), 213.
45. David Arnold, *Colonizing the Body: State Medicine and Epidemic Disease in Nineteenth-Century India* (Berkeley, 1993), 255.
46. Ernest R. Tilton to Julia S. Tilton, March 16, 1900, Rollin N. Tilton Papers, Box 43, USMHI.
47. G. Morris Carstairs, *The Twice-Born: A Study of a Community of High-Caste Hindus* (London, 1957), 164; Alan Roland, *In Search of Self in India and Japan: Toward a Cross-Cultural Psychology* (Princeton, NJ, 1988), 267; Lloyd I. Rudolph and Susanne Hoeber Rudolph, *The Modernity of Tradition: Political Development in India* (Chicago, 1967), 215–16; Mrinalini Sinha, *Colonial Masculinity: The "Manly Englishman" and the "Effeminate Bengali" in the Late Nineteenth Century* (Manchester, 1995).
48. James, *Raj*, 435.
49. Theodore Friend, *Between Two Empires: The Ordeal of the Philippines 1929–1946* (New Haven, CT, 1965), 29.
50. Zohreh T. Sullivan, *Narratives of the Empire: The Fictions of Rudyard Kipling* (New York, 1993), 3.
51. Chota Mem (Mrs. C. Lang), *The English Bride in India* (London, 1909), 32.
52. Edith Moses, *Unofficial Letters of an Official's Wife* (New York, 1908), 16.

53. Brent to Bishop Hall, May 5, 1904, Brent Papers, Box 6; William Howard Taft to Howard C. Hollister, October 15, 1900, Taft Papers, Reel 31.
54. Rudyard Kipling, "His Chance in Life," *Plain Tales from the Hills* (Oxford, 1987), 61; Rene Ontal, "Fagen and Other Ghosts: African-Americans and the Philippine-American War," in Shaw and Francia, eds., *Vestiges of War*, 122.
55. Ashis Nandy, *The Intimate Enemy: Loss and Recovery of Self under Colonialism* (New Delhi, 1983), 15–16.
56. Bederman, *Manliness and Civilization*, 30.
57. Nancy Tomes, *The Gospel of Germs: Men, Women and the Microbe in American Life* (Cambridge, MA, 1998), 132, emphasis in original.
58. George Orwell, *The Road to Wigan Pier* (San Diego, 1958), 128, emphasis in original.
59. Virginia Smith, *Clean: A History of Personal Hygiene and Purity* (Oxford, 2007), 280.
60. Iris Macfarlane, *Daughters of the Empire: A Memoir of Life and Times in the British Raj* (Oxford, 2006), 125.
61. The best example of this was Homer Plessy, classified as black, who rode in a whites-only section of a New Orleans streetcar in 1892. See Smith, *How Race Is Made*, 66–76. Antoinette Burton notes that during the Victorian period, "most English people formed their views about 'Negroes' from stage representations and other caricatures. " Antoinette Burton, *Empire in Question: Reading, Writing, and Teaching British Imperialism* (London, 2011), 224.
62. "Scientific taxonomies of race stress the 'concrete' measures of racial membership," writes Ann Laura Stoler, "but they, like social taxonomies, depend implicitly on a belief in the different sensibilities and sensory regimes imagined to distinguish human kinds." Ann Laura Stoler, "Intimidations of Empire: Predicaments of the Tactile and Unseen," in her *Haunted By Empire*, 2.
63. William A. Cohen, "Introduction: Locating Filth," in Cohen and Johnson, eds., *Filth*, vii–xxxvii; Gilman, *Difference and Pathology*, 22–25; Otis, *Membranes*.
64. Allen, *Plain Tales from the Raj*, 184–85, 199.
65. Rudyard Kipling, "Beyond the Pale," in his *Plain Tales from the Hills*, 127–32.
66. Quoted in Friend, *Between Two Empires*, 35.
67. Brent Diary 1914, Brent Papers, Box 2; Wood Diary, October 2, 1924, Wood Papers, Box 22.
68. Macfarlane, *Daughters of the Empire*, 146.
69. Lady Chapman, memoir "British India Recollected" [1931–1933], Lady Chapman Papers, CSAS.
70. Allen, *Plain Tales from the Raj*, 99.
71. George Orwell, *Burmese Days* (Orlando, 1934), 23–24.
72. Karnow, *In Our Image*, 212–13. The exception to this rule was the country club in Baguio, the American version of a British hill station. By 1911, twenty members of the Filipino political elite were members. See McKenna, *American Imperial Pastoral*, 150.
73. Frank Murphy, "Education," address given in Manila, January 31, 1934, Frank Murphy Papers, Bentley Historical Library, University of Michigan (microfilm), Reel 99. See also Bederman, *Manliness and Civilization*, 25.
74. Metcalf, *Ideologies of the Raj*, 66–87.
75. Nicholas Roosevelt, *The Philippines: A Treasure and a Problem* (New York, 1926), 325.
76. Frank C. Laubach to his mother, August 11, 1918, Frank C. Laubach Collection, Special Collection, Syracuse University Library, Box 1.
77. Taft to Justice John Harlan, June 30, 1900, Taft Papers, Reel 30.
78. Allen, *Plain Tales from the Raj*, 41–42.
79. Winifred Denison to Grandmother, July 13, 1914, David P. Barrows Papers, Box 34, Bancroft Library, University of California-Berkeley.
80. Moses, *Unofficial Letters*, 5, 14, 39.
81. Roosevelt, *The Philippines*, 13–14.
82. Martin V. Melosi, *Garbage in the Cities: Refuse, Reform, and the Environment* (Pittsburgh, 2005), 33; Peter Stallybrass and Allon White, *The Politics and Poetics of Transgression* (Ithaca, NY, 1986), 51.
83. David Howes, "Empires of the Senses," in his *Empire of the Senses*, 11.
84. Bederman, *Manliness and Civilization*, 63.

85. Carol Hyde to her parents, December 9, 1932, Carol Hyde Papers, CSAS.
86. Farquharson, "Indian Idyll."
87. Warwick Anderson, *Colonial Pathologies: American Tropical Medicine, Race, and Hygiene in the Philippines* (Durham, NC, 2006), 59, 91, 94.
88. Classen, Howes, and Synnott, *Aroma*, 165; Gunnar Myrdal, *An American Dilemma: The Negro Problem and Modern Democracy*, Vol. I (New York,1944), 107.
89. Andrew J. Rotter, *Comrades at Odds: The United States and India, 1947–1964*, (Ithaca, NY, 2000), 150; Kathleen M. Brown, *Foul Bodies: Cleanliness in Early America* (New Haven, CT, 2009), 237, 362; Andrew J. Rotter, "William Howard Taft's Drawers," in Blower and Bradley, eds., *The Familiar Made Strange*, 46–58.
90. Lizzie Collingham, *Curry: A Tale of Cooks and Conquerors* (Oxford, 2006), 158–59, 163–64, 167–68; Emily Bronson Conger, *An Ohio Woman in the Philippines* (Akron, 1904), 56, 75, 83, 96–97; Paul A. Kramer, *The Blood of Government: Race, Empire, the United States and the Philippines* (Chapel Hill, 2006), 266.
91. Quoted in Walsh, *Domesticity in Colonial India*, 120.
92. David Arnold has described this idea as "tropicality," representing "Asia as an area of heat and humidity which possessed distinctive vegetation, flora and fauna, a distinctive epidemiology, and produced distinctive (distinctively undesirable) human and social characteristics." David Arnold, *The Tropics and the Traveling Gaze: India, Landscape, and Science, 1800–1856* (Seattle, 2006), 37. Quotation is from Sunil Amrith, "Health and Sovereignty in the New Asia: The Decline and Rise of the Tropics," in Kumar and Basu, eds., *Medical Encounters in British India*, 98.
93. Benjamin Kidd, *The Control of the Tropics* (New York, 1898), 50–51, 63.
94. Elizabeth Buettner, *Empire Families: Britons and Late Imperial India* (Oxford, 2004), 32; Wilson, *The Chaos of Empire*, 389.
95. McKenna, *American Imperial Pastoral*, 21–22.
96. Bishop Brent, "Religious Conditions in the Philippine Islands," nd [1904], Brent Papers, Box 6.
97. Letter, Charles Routt to *The Daily Scioto Gazette*, October 20, 1902, Richie Routt Papers, Box 1, USMHI.
98. Anderson, *The Philippine Problem*, 305.
99. Anne McClintock, *Imperial Leather: Race, Gender, and Sexuality in the Colonial Contest* (London, 1995), 32, 223.
100. David Howes, "Forming Perceptions," in Howes, ed., *Empire of the Senses*, 399.
101. Darwin, *Unfinished Empire*, 205.
102. Daniel R. Williams, *The Odyssey of the Philippines Commission* (Chicago, 1913), 249–50.
103. William Ian Miller, *The Anatomy of Disgust* (Cambridge, MA, 1977), 6, 9, 33, 36, 50–51, 65. See also Erving Goffman, *Relations in Public* (New York, 1971).
104. Milton Walter Meyer, *Letters Home: The Meyers & Capiz 1919–1943* (Claremont, CA, 2003), 353.
105. Indira Ghose, *Memsahibs Abroad: Writings By Women Travellers in Nineteenth-Century India* (Delhi, 1998), 5.
106. Metcalf, *Ideologies of the Raj*, 160–61, 177–78; Alan Bewell, *Romanticism and Colonial Disease* (Baltimore, 1999), 19.
107. Warwick Anderson, "Excremental Colonialism: Public Health and the Poetics of Pollution," *Critical Inquiry* 12, no. 3 (Spring 1995), 657; Victor Heiser, M. D., *An American Doctor's Odyssey: Adventures in Forty-Five Countries* (New York, 1936), 112–13; Victor G. Heiser, "Unsolved Health Problems Peculiar to the Philippines," *Philippine Journal of Science* 5B, no. 2 (July 1910), 171–78.
108. Moses, *Unofficial Letters*, 233.
109. Philippa Levine, *Prostitution, Race, and Politics: Policing Venereal Disease in the British Empire* (New York, 2003), 7; Paul A. Kramer, "The Darkness That Enters the Home: The Politics of Prostitution during the Philippine-American War," in Stoler, ed., *Haunted By Empire*, 373; C. H. Brent, "Suggestions for Statement Regarding Moral Conditions in the Philippine Islands," October 17, 1904, Brent Papers, Box 6. It should be said that there remained in these empires an element of romance concerning the primitivism of Indians and Filipinos

the Anglo-Americans sought to extinguish. Kipling's India and Theodore Roosevelt's Philippines were places to establish one's manhood through hunting, fighting, and playing games: theaters of fantasy in which to enact what Roosevelt called the "barbarian virtues." See Metcalf, *Ideologies of the Raj*, 161–66; and Matthew Frye Jacobson, *Barbarian Virtues: The United States Encounters Foreign Peoples at Home and Abroad, 1876–1917* (New York, 2000).

110. Quoted in Sinha, *Colonial Masculinity*, 15.
111. Gilmour, *The Ruling Caste*, 13–14.
112. Cavaliero, *Strangers in the Land*, 202.
113. *Report of the Philippine Commission to the President*, Vol. III (Washington, DC, 1901), 377–78.
114. David P. Barrows, "Testimony before the Insular Affairs Committee, U.S. Senate, March 12–13, 1902," Barrows Papers, Box 2.
115. Taft to Bishop William Lawrence, February 14, 1904, Taft Papers, Reel 42.
116. Moses, *Unofficial Letters*, 119, 253.
117. Eli Lundy Huggins to his sisters, May 5, 1901, Eli Lundy Huggins Papers, Bancroft Library, University of California-Berkeley.
118. *Report of the Philippine Commission*, Vol. III, 343–44.
119. Wilson, *The Chaos of Empire*, 498.
120. Pernau, "Teaching Emotions," 227.
121. Walsh, *Domesticity in Colonial India*, 8.
122. Satyacaraṇ Mithra, *A Husband's Advice to His Wife*, reprinted in Walsh, *Colonial Domesticity*, 177–80.
123. James, *Raj*, 507.
124. S. Iftikhar Hussain, *Hints on Indian Etiquette, Specially Designed for the Use of Europeans* (Lucknow, 1911), 2–3, 11, 24; Syed Fakhruddin Aboobaker El Edroos, *Modern Indian Etiquette* (Surat, 1922), 12–13.
125. El Edroos, *Modern Indian Etiquette*, 21–22, 49.
126. Evelyn Dagmar Bogle, "India in the 1920s," V. M. L. Bogle Papers, CSAS.
127. Ghose, *Memsahibs Abroad*, 285–86, emphasis in original.
128. Salil Tripathi, "Meanwhile: Gandhi, for One, Would Have Found It Funny," *New York Times*, January 21, 2004.
129. Bhattacharya, *Talking Back*, 60.
130. Ibid., 71, 82.
131. Karnow, *In Our Image*, 68–72; José Rizal, *Noli Me Tangere*, transl. Harold Augenbaum (New York, 2006 [1887]).
132. *Heraldo Filipino*, February 24, 1899, reprinted in Dean C. Worcester, *The Philippines Past and Present* (New York, 1930), 213.
133. Canning Eyot, ed., *The Story of the Lopez Family: A Page from the History of the War in the Philippines* (Boston, 1904), 172–74.
134. Arthur W. Ferguson to Taft, January 16, 1902, Taft Papers, Reel 34.
135. Quoted in Stanley, *A Nation in the Making*, 166–67.

Chapter 2

1. Darwin, *Unfinished Empire*, 77–79.
2. *Times of London*, quoted in Go, *Patterns of Empire*, 73.
3. James, *Raj*, 52.
4. Mark M. Smith, *The Smell of Battle, the Taste of Siege: A Sensory History of the Civil War* (New York, 2015).
5. Shak Hedayut Ali and T. Rattray, "The Causes of the Indian Mutiny," *Times of London*, April 1, 1858.
6. "Mohun Lol's Letter on the Mutiny—its cause—Rise & Progress. Delhie—Nov. 1857," Home Miscellaneous Series, IOR/H/725: Mutiny Papers of Sir J[ohn]. W. Kaye, part I, BL.
7. Syed Ahmed Khan, *The Causes of the Indian Revolt* (Oxford, 2000 [1858]), 42–43.
8. Christopher Hibbert, *The Great Mutiny: India 1957* (New York, 1978), 48.
9. Khan, *Causes of the Indian Revolt*, 52.

10. Hibbert, *The Great Mutiny*, 59; James, *Raj*, 234–35.
11. Kim A. Wagner, *The Great Fear of 1857: Rumours, Conspiracies and the Making of the Indian Uprising* (Oxford, 2010), 64; Elizabeth Sneyd, "Reminiscences of the Dreadful Mutiny in India in 1857," Photo MSS Eur 044, BL.
12. James, *Raj*, 235.
13. Ghose, *Memsahibs Abroad*, 200.
14. Wagner, *The Great Fear*, 68.
15. Parama Roy, *Alimentary Tracts: Appetites, Aversions, and the Postcolonial* (Durham, NC, 2010), 41; Wagner, *The Great Fear*, 69–71, 80.
16. Saul David, "Greased Cartridges and the Great Mutiny of 1857: A Pretext to Rebel or the Final Straw?," in Roy, ed., *War and Society in Colonial India*, 82–113.
17. Hibbert, *The Great Mutiny*, 64–65.
18. "The Crisis in the Punjab, from the 10th of May until the Fall of Delhi by a Punjab Employé. For the Benefit of the 'Lawrence Asylum'" (Lahore, 1858), MSS Eur D 1019, Robert Montgomery Papers, Vol. II, 1849–56, BL.
19. A. Taylor to Montgomery, n.d., "Selections from the Public Correspondence of the Administration for the Affairs of the Punjab, 'Punjab Mutiny Report'" (Lahore, 1859), Montgomery Papers, Vol. III: Indian Mutiny 1857.
20. Wagner, *The Great Fear*, 95, 101–02; David, "Greased Cartridges," 87; Tapti Roy, *The Politics of a Popular Uprising: Bundelkhand in 1857* (New Delhi, 1994), 50–51.
21. Wagner, *The Great Fear*, 126.
22. Hibbert, *The Great Mutiny*, 32.
23. Ghose, *Memsahibs Abroad*, 200.
24. Hibbert, *The Great Mutiny*, 33–34.
25. Sneyd, "Reminiscences of the Dreadful Mutiny."
26. Mrs. Amy Haines' Narrative [of the rebellion], Add MS 41488, BL.
27. "The Story of Miss Sutherland," Add MS 41488, BL.
28. David Arnold, "Salutation and Subversion: Gestural Politics in Nineteenth-Century India," *Past and Present* (2009), Supplement 4: *The Politics of Gesture: Historical Persepctives*, ed. Michael J. Braddick, 191–211 (quotations 203, 204, 205).
29. General Innes, Ferozepore, to Robert Montgomery, May 16, 1857, "Selections from the Public Correspondence of the Administration for the Affairs of the Punjab, 'Punjab Mutiny Report'" (Lahore, 1859), Montgomery Papers, Vol. III.
30. "The Crisis in the Punjab."
31. Account by "Mr. Cooper" of the events of July 30, 1857, "Selections from the Public Correspondence."
32. "3 Letters dated Cawnpore May–June 1857 from Emma Sophia Ewart (d. 1857), wife of Lt.-Col. John Ewart (1803–1857), Bengal Army, written to her sister [Fanny] describing events of the Mutiny shortly before she and her family died; also a copy of a prayer of thanksgiving for the end of the Mutiny," MSS Eur B 267, BL.
33. Act No. XVII of 1857, Eur MSS 506, Norman Chevers Papers, BL.
34. Quoted in Arnold, "Salutation and Subversion," 206.
35. Robert Montgomery, "General Report on the Administration of the Punjab Territories for the Years 1856–57 and 1857–58," January 22, 1859, MSS Eur 1019, Montgomery Papers.
36. Sneyd, "Reminiscences."
37. Ghose, *Memsahibs Abroad*, 206.
38. The Journal of Chardin Johnson, entry for November 6, 1857, MSS Eur A 161, BL.
39. Robert Young, *Reminiscences of the Great and Good Sir Henry Lawrence, K.C.B., also of the Indian Sepoy Mutiny of 1857, Including the Siege and Recapture of Delhi; being Extracts from the Story of my Chequered Life* (Dehra Dun, 1893), MSS Eur F85/134, BL.
40. Journal of Chardin Johnson, entries for December 6, 1857, and January 13, 1858.
41. Letter from an officer in the camp before Delhi, June 24, 1857, "The Crisis in the Punjab."
42. "The Crisis in the Punjab."
43. S. H. Batson, "Delhi Massacre!!" (Lahore, September 15, 1857), Chevers Papers.
44. Mrs. Amy Haines, "Narrative."

45. Sir Penderel Moon, *The British Conquest and Dominion of India* (London, 1989), 709–16; James, *Raj*, 252–53.
46. Journal of Chardin Johnson, November 8, 1857.
47. Hibbert, *The Great Mutiny*, 33.
48. Philindus, "On the Study of Indian Languages," *Times of London*, December 31, 1857.
49. *The Indian News*, February 19, 1858.
50. Sneyd, "Reminiscences of the Dreadful Mutiny."
51. Hibbert, *The Great Mutiny*, 56.
52. "Crisis in the Punjab."
53. Journal of Chardin Johnson, November 29, 1857.
54. Robert Montgomery, "General Report on the Administration of the Punjab Territories for the Years 1856–57 and 1857–58," January 22, 1859, Montgomery Papers.
55. Chevers Papers.
56. "To the Chief Commander for the Punjab," nd., "The Crisis in the Punjab."
57. Montgomery, "General Report."
58. "The Crisis in the Punjab."
59. Ibid.
60. Ibid.
61. Ibid., Taylor to Montgomery, n.d.
62. Ghose, *Memsahibs Abroad*, 204; Mrs. Amy Haines' Narrative.
63. Brigadier Inglis to Secretary of the Government Military Department, Calcutta, 26th September 1857, Chevers Papers.
64. "Colonel Baynes' account of the proceedings of the Storming party of the 2nd column of attack—City of Delhi, September 14th 1857," Kaye Papers.
65. Young, "*Reminiscences*."
66. Chardin Johnson Journal, January 18, 1858.
67. "2 Years Experience during the Great Sepoy Mutiny of 1857–1858," by "Osborn," January 12, 1858, Kaye Papers.
68. "Memo"by Deputy Comm. Of Oudh ["Arudgy"?], audience with Rajah [illegible] "of Kali Kanker," September 21, 1858, Montgomery Papers.
69. Wagner, *The Great Fear*, 138.
70. "India: The British Army," *Times of London*, May 29, 1858.
71. Roy, *Alimentary Tracts*, 64.
72. Sneyd, "Reminiscences of the Deadly Mutiny."
73. Quoted in Zahid R. Chaudhary, *Afterimage of Empire: Photography in Nineteenth-Century India* (Minneapolis, 2012), 19.
74. Letter from an officer of the garrison, *Glasgow Herald*, August 24, 1857.
75. Young, "*Reminiscences*."
76. Chardin Johnson Journal, November 21, 1857.
77. "Mortality in the Army," *Times of India*, March 27, 1858.
78. Chardin Johnson Journal, December 1, 1857; Amy Haines's Narrative.
79. Young, "*Reminiscences*."
80. F. O. Mayne, Magistrate of Banda, to E. C. Bayley, "Narrative of Events Attending the Outbreak of Disturbances and the Restoration of Authority in the District of Banda, in 1857–1858," Kaye Papers.
81. Young, "*Reminiscences*."
82. Our Special Correspondent, "India," May 29, 1858, *Times of London*.
83. James, *Raj*, 225.
84. Amy Haines' Narrative; Emma Ewart to Fanny, "3 Letters dated Cawnpore."
85. Chardin Johnson Journal, October 24, November 24, 1857.
86. Letter from an officer late of the garrison of Delhi, June 18, 1857, *Glasgow Herald*.
87. Mayne to Bayley, "Narrative of Events."
88. "Osborn," extracts from "2 Years Experience."
89. Letter from Williamson Bros and Co (Calcutta) to "correspondents in London," July 20, 1857, Chevers Papers.

90. "Memorandum, containing the results of enquiries made by desire of the Governor General into the rumours of European females having been dishonoured during the late rebellion," December 30, 1857, collected and commented on by W. Muir," Kaye Papers.
91. Arthur Roberts, Goordaspoor, to Robert Montgomery, July 17, 1857, Montgomery Papers.
92. James, *Raj*, 259.
93. Cavaliero, *Strangers in the Land*, 144.
94. Taylor to Montgomery, "Punjab Mutiny Report."
95. Chardin Johnson Journal, April 12, 1858.
96. Young, "*Reminiscences*"; letter from Kavanaugh, Lucknow, to Montgomery, July 8, 1958, Montgomery Papers.
97. Chardin Johnson Journal, November 28, December 20, 1857.
98. "Indian Luxuries," in *Comus, or the Indian Charivari*, May 23, 1857, Chevers Papers.
99. Mrs. Amy Haines Narrative.
100. Sir John Kaye, *Kaye's and Mallenson's History of the Indian Mutiny of 1857–8*, ed. by Colonel Mallenson, Vol. II (London, 1889), 250.
101. Roy, *Alimentary Tracts*, 67.
102. Walter LaFeber, *The New Empire: An Interpretation of American Expansion, 1860–1898* (Ithaca, NY, 1963), 333–51; Karnow, *In Our Image*, 102.
103. Karnow, *In Our Image*, 75–77; Stuart Creighton Miller, *"Benevolent Assimilation": The American Conquest of the Philippines, 1899–1903* (New Haven, CT, 1982), 35–39; Michael E. Shay, ed., *A Civilian in Lawton's 1899 Philippine Campaign: The Letters of Robert D. Carter*(Columbia, MO, 2013), 32; Brian McAllister Linn, *The Philippine War 1899–1902* (Lawrence, KS, 2000), 42.
104. Karnow, *In Our Image*, 130–31, 139–40; Miller, *"Benevolent Assimilation,"* 58–61; Linn, *Philippine War*, 26, 31–32, 44–46. Miller finds only one example of an American shot to death during this period, and notes that Aguinaldo, who investigated the incident, told his counterpart, General Elwell Otis, that the soldier had been shot accidentally by a fellow American.
105. Isabel Anderson, *The Spell of the Hawaiian Islands and the Philippines* (Boston, 1916), 181.
106. Linn, *Philippine War*, 147.
107. Ibid., 275; Karnow, *In Our Image*, 194.
108. Samuel B. M. Young, "Our Soldiers in the Philippines," address to the Men's Club of the Church of the Epiphany, Washington, DC, November 13, 1902, Samuel B. M. Young Papers, Box 10, USMHI.
109. Matthew A. Batson to Flossie, November 9, 1900, Matthew A. Batson Papers, Box 2, USMHI.
110. William C. Brown diary, entries for June 1 and August 14, 1900, William C. Brown Papers, Box 2, USMHI.
111. "The Personal Journal of Lieutenant Dana True Merrill, Philippine Islands, 1898–1901," entry for June 5, 1900, Box 1, Dana True Merrill Papers, USMHI.
112. William Howard Taft to Henry Cabot Lodge, October 22, 1901, William Howard Taft Papers, Cornell University Library (microfilm), Reel 33.
113. Cornelius Gardener to Taft, December 16, 1901, Taft Papers, Reel 34.
114. Henry C. Rowland, "Fighting Life in the Philippines," *McClure's* 19 (May–October 1902), 241–47.
115. George K. Hunter to Taft, May 16, 1900, and June 4, 1900, Taft Papers, Reel 30.
116. Linn, *Philippine War*, 12.
117. Shay, *A Civilian*, 63.
118. Capt. Ernest R. Tilton to Julia S. Tilton, December 31, 1899, Rollin N. Tilton Papers, Box 43, USMHI.
119. Pearl K. Rice to his parents, November 26, 1899, Richie Routt Papers, Box 1; Merrill Journal, entry for May 13, 1900, Box 1; Walter L. Cutter, "Wearing the Khaki: The Diary of a High Private," Walter L. Cutter Papers, Box 1, USMHI.
120. Letter, Charles Fischback to *Daily Scioto Gazette*, November 24, 1899, Routt Papers, Box 1.
121. Robert Carter to his father, September 28, 1899, in Shay, *A Civilian*, 154.

122. Albert Sonnichsen, *Ten Months a Captive Among Filipinos: Being a Narrative of Adventure and Observation During Imprisonment on the Island of Luzon* (New York, 1901), 127.
123. Conger, *An Ohio Woman*, 131.
124. Kramer, *Blood of Government*, 127.
125. Ernest R. Tilton to Julia S. Tilton, February 6, 1900, Box 43, Tilton Papers.
126. Ernest R. Tilton to Julia S. Tilton, February 18, 1900, Box 43, Tilton Papers.
127. Frederick Funston, *Memories of Two Wars: Cuban and Philippine Experiences* (New York, 1911), 232.
128. Joseph P. McCallus, *Gentleman Soldier: John Clifford Brown and the Philippine-American War* (College Station, TX, 2004), 84; John F. Bass, "Cemetery Ridge," February 9, 1899, reprinted in Marrion Wilcox, ed., *Harper's History of the War in the Philippines* (New York, 1900), 113.
129. Interview with Clenard McLaughlin, by Don Rickey Jr., October 27, 1971, Clenard McLaughlin Papers, Box 1, USMHI.
130. William Howard Taft to William R. Day, August 16, 1900, Taft Papers, Reel 31.
131. Letter from Lt. Lee McCoy to *Daily Scioto Gazette*, January 28, 1900, Routt Papers, Box 1; Letter from John Holmes to *Daily Scioto Gazette*, January 25, 1900, Routt Papers, Box 1.
132. Linn, *Philippine War*, 127.
133. Henry F. Hoyt, *A Frontier Doctor* (New York, 1929), 230.
134. George Telfer to Lottie, February 19, 1899, in Sara Bunnett, ed., *Manila Envelopes: Oregon Volunteer Lt. George F. Telfer's Spanish-American War Letters* (Portland, 1987), 131.
135. Bass, "Cemetery Ridge," 118; Linn, *Philippine War*, 100.
136. Bass, "With Wheaton's Flying Column," March 20, 1899, in Wilcox, *Harper's History*, 149.
137. Bass, "The Santa Cruz Raid," April 29, 1899, in Wilcox, *Harper's History*, 169.
138. Funston, *Memories*, 183.
139. Merrill, "Personal Journal," entry for May 13, 1900; Guy V. Henry Jr., to his mother, March 25, 1901, Guy V. Henry Papers, Box 3, USMHI.
140. Samuel Young Diary, entry for November 5, 1899, Box 9, Young Papers.
141. Bass, "The Malolos Campaign," April 4, 1899, Wilcox, *Harper's History*, 163; A. L. Dade to Adjutant, May 7, 1900, Young Papers, Box 12.
142. "The Odd Side of Things," *Manila Times*, November 9, 1899.
143. Laurence Halstead Memoir, Halstead-Maus Family Papers, Box 1, USMHI.
144. Merrill, "Personal Journal," April 29, 1899.
145. Cutter, "Diary of a High Private."
146. Bass, "Battle-Scenes Described," February 5, 1899, Wilcox, *Harper's History*, 110–12.
147. Bass, "In the Trenches—A Night on the Gunboat *Laguna de Bay*.—With the 'Flying Column,'" Wilcox, *Harper's History*, 146–48.
148. Ernest Tilton to Julia Tilton, January 29, 1900, Tilton Papers, Box 43.
149. Merrill, "Personal Journal," September 5, 1899.
150. Funston, *Memories*, 191–92.
151. Cutter, "Diary of a High Private."
152. Bass, "Letter Written from Los Banos," Wilcox, *Harper's History*, 228.
153. Anna Page Russell Maus, "Old Army Days: Reminiscences by the Wife of an Army Surgeon," nd., Halstead-Maus Family Papers, Box 2, USMHI.
154. Pearl K. Rice to his parents, November 26, 1899, Routt Papers, Box 1; Benjamin E. Neal Diaries, entry for February 28, 1902, Benjamin Neal Papers, Box 1, Syracuse University Library; Conger, *An Ohio Woman*, 107, 151.
155. George Brandle to *Daily Scioto Gazette*, May 29, 1902, Routt Papers, Box 1.
156. "The Slums of Manila," *Manila Times*, July 11, 1899.
157. Miller, *"Benevolent Assimilation,"* 243.
158. William Paulding Memoir, Grace and William Paulding Papers, Box 1, USMHI; Lee McCoy to *Daily Scioto Gazette*, January 28, 1900, Routt Papers, Box 1.
159. "The Belle of Jolo," *The Jolo Howler*, January 1, 1902, Cutter Papers, Box 1.
160. Bunnett, *Manila Envelopes*, 33, 40, 43, 74, 110, 151.
161. Linn, *Philippine War*, 40–41.
162. James M. Smith to *Daily Scioto Gazette*, February 2, 1900, Routt Papers, Box 1.

163. Bunnett, *Manila Envelopes*, 68; Ernest to Julia Tilton, April 19, 1900, Tilton Papers; *Merriam-Webster Online Dictionary*. https://www.merriam-webster.com/
164. Bunnett, *Manila Envelopes*, 55.
165. Sonnichsen, *Ten Months a Captive*, 187.
166. Carter to his father, May 13, 1899, in Shay, *A Civilian*, 74.
167. Linn, *Philippine War*, 142; Willis Bliss Wilcox, *Through Luzon on Highways and Byways* (Philadelphia, 1901), 191.
168. Bass, "Cemetery Ridge," Wilcox, *Harper's History*, 113–15; Henry C. Logan, "The Davao River Expedition," nd, Routt Papers, Box 1; Linn, *Philippine War*, 147.
169. James M. Phalen, "An Experiment with Orange-Red Underwear," *Philippine Journal of Science* 5B, no. 6 (December 1910), 525–47.
170. Andrew J. Rotter, "William Howard Taft's Drawers," 46–58.
171. *Dhobi* itch is a condition caused by the fungus *tinea cruris* and largely affecting the crotch; it is also called "crotch rot" or "jock itch." It is a type of ringworm, which is itself fungal and not a worm at all, and it is aggravated by the inability to stay cool and dry between the legs.
172. Cutter, "Diary of a High Private."
173. Robert Carter to his father, June 1, July 22, August 1, 1899, Shay, *A Civilian*, 88, 105, 116.
174. Hoyt, *Frontier Doctor*, 248.
175. Bunnett, *Manila Envelopes*, 34, 70.
176. Bass, "Along the Shores of the Laguna de Bay in a Dugout," December 30, 1898, Wilcox, *Harper's History*, 79.
177. Samuel Young Diary, entry for November 25, 1899; Young letter to his daughters, December 18, 1899, Young Papers, Box 9.
178. F. A. Fenn, "Idaho's Part in the Battle," Wilcox, *Harper's History*, 124; Funston, *Memories*, 196.
179. Sonnichsen, *Ten Months a Captive*, 85, 88.
180. Carter to his father, September 28, 1899, Shay, *A Civilian*, 154.
181. McCoy to *Daily Scioto Gazette*, January 28, 1900.
182. Ernest Tilton to Lottie Tilton, May 1900, Tilton Papers, Box 43.
183. Linn, *Philippine War*, 238.
184. Christopher J. Einolf, *America in the Philippines, 1899–1902: The First Torture Scandal* (New York, 2014), 181; Kenneth De Bevoise, *Agents of Apocalypse: Epidemic Disease in the Colonial Philippines* (Princeton, NJ, 1995), 84–87; Kramer, "The Darkness That Enters the Home," 366–404; Taft to Secretary of War, January 17, 1901, Taft Papers, Reel 31; Taft to Dr. David D. Thompson, April 12, 1902, Taft Papers, Reel 35.
185. Juliana to Clemencia Lopez, February 14, 1902, in Eyot, *Story of the Lopez Family*, 121.
186. Hoyt, *Frontier Doctor*, 209.
187. Linn, *Philippine War*, 210–12; Miller, *"Benevolent Assimilation,"* 200–04.
188. *Report of the Philippine Commission to the President*, Vol. 2, (Washington, DC, 1900), 240.
189. William C. Brown Diary, entry for September 12, 1900, Box 2, William C. Brown Papers, USMHI.
190. Guy V. Henry, "Brief Narrative of the Life of Guy V. Henry, Jr.," Box 4, Henry Papers; Ernest Tilton to Julia Tilton, March 16, 1900, Tilton Papers, Box 43.
191. John F. Bass and John McCutcheon, "The Malolos Campaign," April 4, 1899, Wilcox, *Harper's History*, 165.
192. George Brandle to *Daily Scioto Gazette*, December 12, 1900, Routt Papers, Box 1.
193. Ernest Tilton to Julia Tilton, June 14, 1900, Tilton Papers, Box 43.
194. Cutter, "Diary of a High Private."
195. Anderson, *Colonial Pathologies*, 43.
196. Young, "Our Soldiers in the Philippines."
197. George Brandle to *Daily Scioto Gazette*, May 29, 1902, Routt Papers, Box 1; Linn, *Philippine War*, 147; Ernest Tilton to Julia Tilton, April 11, 1900, Tilton Papers, Box 43.
198. George Telfer to Lottie Telfer, September 19, 1898, Bunnett, *Manila Envelopes*, 54.
199. Letter from John Doyle to *Chillicothe Daily Gazette*, February 15, 1899, Routt Papers, Box 1.
200. George Brandle to *Daily Scioto Gazette*, December 12, 1900, Routt Papers, Box 1.
201. Conger, *An Ohio Woman*, 75; Cutter, "Diary of a High Private."
202. Juliana to Clemencia Lopez, January 21, 1902, Eyot, *Story of the Lopez Family*, 94.

203. Ernest Tilton to Julia Tilton, January 29, 1900, Tilton Papers, Box 43.
204. Simeon A. Villa, "The Flight and Wanderings of Emilio Aguinaldo, From His Abandonment of Bagambang until His Capture in Palanan," transl. by J. C. Hixson, Simeon A. Villa Papers, Box 1, USMHI.
205. William C. Brown, "Incidents in Aguinaldo's Capture," *Infantry Journal* (June 1925), Brown Papers, Box 2.
206. Henry Bixby Luard Diary, MSS Eur C262, BL.
207. "Life in Lucknow," *Times of London*, March 24, 1859.
208. Collingham, *Imperial Bodies*, 6–10.
209. "Scenes from the Camp, Pictures of War from Northern Lines. Sights and Scenes from the Soldiers Who are Chasing Aggie," *Freedom: The Giant of the Orient*, May 17, 1899.

Chapter 3

1. Martin Jay, *Downcast Eyes: The Denigration of Vision in Twentieth-Century French Thought* (Berkeley, 1993), 10.
2. Such are the arguments of Smith, *Sensing the Past*, 19–21, and Howes, "Empires of the Senses," 1–2. For a perceptive summary and gentle critique, see James W. Cook, "Seeing the Visual in U.S. History," *Journal of American History* 95, no. 2 (September 2008), 432–41.
3. Donald M. Lowe, *History of Bourgeois Perception* (Chicago, 1982), 8, 21.
4. Jütte, *History of the Senses*, 186–90, 200–02; Constance Classen, "Introduction: The Transformation of Perception," in Classen, ed., *A Cultural History of the Senses in the Age of Empire*, 7–8. The *flâneur* was not solely a visual observer: "It is through all of their senses that *flâneurs* make sense of the city." Estelle Murail, "A Body Passes By: The Flâneur and the Senses in Nineteenth-Century London and Paris," *The Senses and Society* 12, no. 2 (2017), 164.
5. Jay, *Downcast Eyes*, 10.
6. John F. Kasson, *Rudeness and Civility: Manners in Nineteenth-Century Urban America* (New York, 1993), 44; Simon Gunn, *The Public Culture of the Victorian Middle Class: Ritual and Authority in the English Industrial City 1840–1914* (Manchester, 2000), 66–67.
7. Quoted in Kasson, *Rudeness and Civility*, 167.
8. Sharrona Pearl, *About Faces: Physiognomy in Nineteenth-Century Britain* (Cambridge, MA, 2010), 1, 16, 22.
9. Anne C. Wilson, *Hints for the First Years of Residence in India* (Oxford, 1904), 33, 52.
10. McCullock et. al., *India: Geographical, Statistical, and Historical*, quoted in Hutchins, *Illusion of Permanence*, 68.
11. Quoted in David Brody, *Visualizing American Empire: Orientalism and Imperialism in the Philippines* (Chicago, 2010), 118.
12. "Funston's Nerve Too Wily; Filipinos Off Their Guard," *New York Evening Journal*, March 28, 1901.
13. Kipling's *Kim* does this. See Hutchins, *Illusion of Permanence*, 156.
14. Hilda Bourne Memoir, "It Was Like This," J. M. Bourne Papers, CSAS.
15. Dane Kennedy, *The Magic Mountains: Hill Stations in the British Raj* (Berkeley, 1996), 6.
16. Sir Frank Pearson Memoir, Private Papers, IOR, MSS Eur F226/21, Sir Frank Pearson Papers, BL.
17. Wrenn, Bennett and Co. catalogue, Madras, ca. 1900, Private Papers, IOR, MSS Eur C950, BL.
18. Kasson, *Rudeness and Civility*, 115.
19. Williams, *Odyssey*, 63–64.
20. Shay, ed., *A Civilian*, 145.
21. T. H. Pardo de Tavera to William Howard Taft, February 9, 1904, William Howard Taft Papers, Cornell University Library (microfilm), Reel 42.
22. Quoted in Christopher Pinney, *Camera Indica: The Social Life of Indian Photographs* (Chicago, 1997), 41–42.
23. Quoted in Visram, *Ayahs, Lascars and Princes*, 57–58.
24. Nora Scott, *An Indian Journal* (London, 1994), 116.
25. Ghose, *Memsahibs Abroad*, 129; Pinney, *Camera Indica*, 20. British jurists found Indians contemptuous of copyright law and all too willing to practice deceptive advertising that

abused it. See H. D. H. Rance memoir, IOR, Private Papers, MSS Eur F226/23, Major H. D. H. Rance Papers, BL.

26. Arnold, *Colonizing the Body*, 88–89.
27. James, *Raj*, 196.
28. Janaki Nair, "Uncovering the *Zenana*: Visions of Indian Womanhood in Englishwomen's Writings, 1813–1940," in Hall, ed., *Cultures of Empire*, 226–27; Gilmour, *The Ruling Caste*, 257.
29. Piya Pal-Lapinski, "Infection as Resistance: Medical Discourse, Indian Courtesans, and Flawed Memsahibs in Flora Steel's Colonial Fiction," *Ariel: A Review of International English Literature* 30, no. 3 (July 1999), 141–61.
30. Krishnalal Shridharani, *My India, My America* (Garden City, NY, 1943), 94; Andrew J. Rotter, *Comrades at Odds: The United States and India, 1947-1964* (Ithaca, 2000), 8.
31. Mrs. Robert Moss King, *The Diary of a Civilian's Wife in India 1877–1882*, Vol. I (London, 1884), 243–44.
32. Peter Lamont, *The Rise of the Indian Rope Trick: How a Spectacular Hoax Became History* (New York, 2004), 98–99.
33. Ruth H. B. Hunt Diaries, entry for May 22, 1929, Ruth H. B. Hunt Papers, Box 1, Syracuse University Library.
34. Karen Halttunen, *Confidence Men and Painted Women* (Cambridge, MA, 1982).
35. Charles E. Griffith, "The Music of the Philippine Islands," *Philippine Education Magazine*, November 1928, 327.
36. George Telfer to Willis Telfer, October 7, 1898, in Bunnett, *Manila Envelopes*, 67.
37. Mrs. William Howard [Helen] Taft, *Recollections of Full Years* (New York, 1914), 162.
38. W. H. Taft, address at Union Reading College, Manila, December 17, 1903, reprinted in John Devins, *An Observer in the Philippines*, 397.
39. Roosevelt, *The Philippines*, 5.
40. Fernando Feliu, ""Science, Sight and the Ordering of Colonial Societies," in Edwards and Bhaumik, eds. *Visual Sense*, 122, 124.
41. Frank Laubach to Miss Lamson, May 28, 1918, Frank C. Laubach Papers, Box 1, Syracuse University Library.
42. John P. McAdams, Brig. Gen., Retired, to Capt. George W. Jean, November 24, 1950, George W. Jean Papers, Box 1, USMHI.
43. Carol Hyde letter to her parents, March 15, 1933, Hyde Papers, CSAS.
44. Wilson, *Hints for the First Years*, 36.
45. Rianne Siebenga, "Colonial India's 'Fanatical Fakirs' and Their Popular Representations," *History and Anthropology* 23, no. 4 (December 2012), 445–66; Evelyn Beeton Memoir, Beeton Papers, CSAS.
46. James, *Raj*, 515.
47. Carol Hyde letter to her parents, December 12, 1932, Hyde Papers.
48. R. C. C. Hunt Memoir "Innocents in India," Hunt Papers, CSAS; Allen, *Plain Tales from the Raj*, 16; Hyde to her parents, March 15, 1933, Hyde Papers.
49. Benito M. Vergara Jr., *Displaying Filipinos: Photography and Colonialism in Early 20th Century Philippines* (Quezon City, 1995), 116.
50. Williams, *Odyssey*, 49, 52–53.
51. *Report of the Philippine Commission to the President*, Vol. I (Washington, DC, 1900), 11–12, 183–84.
52. Moses, *Unofficial Letters*, 345.
53. *Report of the Philippine Commission*, Vol. II (Washington, DC, 1900), 68–69, 180, 222–23.
54. Wilcox, *Through Luzon*, viii.
55. Katherine Mayo, *The Isles of Fear: The Truth about the Philippines* (New York, 1924), 196.
56. Eli Lundy Huggins to "Cousin," December 12, 1900, Eli Lundy Huggins Papers, Box 1, Bancroft Library, University of California-Berkeley; Lt. Laurence Halstead Memoir, 1901, Halstead-Maus Family Papers, Box 1, USMHI.
57. Moses, *Unofficial Letters*, 127.
58. Sonnichsen, *Ten Months a Captive*, 13, 127.
59. W. C. Forbes Journal, Vol. IV, entry for May 2, 1910, W. C. Forbes Papers, Houghton Library, Harvard University.

60. Alice M. Kelly, "The Bua School: A Few Personal Notes," in Pecson and Racelis, eds., *Tales of the American Teachers in the Philippines*, 79.
61. Devins, *An Observer in the Philippines*, 181.
62. William B. Freer, *The Philippine Experiences of an American Teacher: A Narrative of Work and Travel in the Philippine Islands* (New York, 1906), 202.
63. Conger, *An Ohio Woman*, 72, 159.
64. Ibid., 72.
65. Alice M. Fuller, *Housekeeping and Household Arts* (Manila, 1911), 12–13, 53.
66. Philippa Levine, "Naked Natives and Noble Savages: The Cultural Work of Nakedness in Imperial Britain," in Crosbie and Hampton, eds., *The Cultural Construction of the British World*, 28, 37.
67. Ibid., 23; James, *Raj*, 217.
68. Ghose, *Memsahibs Abroad*, 43.
69. MacMillan, *Women of the Raj*, 104.
70. Gilmour, *The Ruling Caste*, 173.
71. Bernard Cohn, "Cloth, Clothes, and Colonialism: India in the Nineteenth Century," in Weiner and Schneider, eds., *Cloth and Human Experience*, 331.
72. Carol Hyde to her parents, January 24, 1933, Hyde Papers.
73. Devins, *An Observer in the Philippines*, 56.
74. Frank C. Laubach, "Notes taken in the Dansalan Market," September 25, 1933, Laubach Papers, Box 130.
75. *Report of the Philippine Commission to the President*, Vol. III (Manila, 1901), 389.
76. Charles Henry Brent Diary, entries for February 6–7, 1903, Charles Henry Brent Papers, Box 2, MD, LC.
77. Ralph Kent Buckland, *In the Land of the Filipino* (New York, 1912), 78–79.
78. Heiser, *American Doctor's Odyssey*, 194.
79. Frank Laubach to his father, February 22, 1915, Laubach Papers, Box 1.
80. Constance Classen and David Howes, "The Museum as Sensescape: Western Sensibilities and Indigenous Artifacts," in Edwards, Gosden, and Phillips, eds., *Sensible Objects*, 207.
81. Arnold, *Colonizing the Body*, 116.
82. Lt. Gen. Sir Ernest Bradfield, "Unimportant Story," Bradfield Papers, CSAS.
83. Margery Hall, "Autobiography: 'And the Nights Were More Terrible Than the Days,'" IOR, Private Papers, MSS Eur F226/11, Margery Hall Papers, BL.
84. Allen, *Plain Tales from the Raj*, 37.
85. Flora Annie Steel and Grace Gardiner, *The Complete Indian Housekeeper and Cook*. Ed. Ralph Crane and Anna Johnston (Oxford, 2010 [1888]), 170–71.
86. Allen, *Plain Tales from the Raj*, 123.
87. Macfarlane, *Daughters of Empire*, 138.
88. Forbes Journal, Vol. IV, entry for April 16, 1910.
89. Anna Page Russell, Maus, "Old Army Days: Reminiscences by the Wife of an Army Surgeon," Halstead-Maus Family Papers, USMHI.
90. Worcester, *The Philippines Past and Present*, 139.
91. Buckland, *Land of the Filipino*, 75.
92. Roosevelt, *The Philippines*, 78.
93. Mayo, *Isles of Fear*, 207.
94. Hunt Diaries, entry for August 8, 1929, Hunt Papers, Box 1.
95. Karnow, *In Our Image*, 233; Williams, *Odyssey*, 97–98.
96. Arnold, *The Tropics and the Travelling Gaze*, 25.
97. Chaudhary, *Afterimage of Empire* , 112.
98. Ghose, *Memsahibs Abroad*, 47–48.
99. King, *Diary of a Civilian's Wife*, Vol. I, 124–25.
100. Kate Platt, *The Home and Health in India and the Tropical Countries* (London, 1923), 29.
101. Erica Farquharson, "Indian Idyll," J. M. Bourne Papers, CSAS. See also Jack Gibson, "As I Saw It," Jack Gibson Papers, Box 3, CSAS, and King, *Diary of a Civilian's Wife*, Vol. I, 183.
102. Platt, *Home and Health In India*, 29.
103. Moses, *Unofficial Letters*, 147.

104. Ibid., 100.
105. Taft, *Recollections*, 97.
106. Moses, *Unofficial Letters*, 96; Frank C. Laubach, "Notes taken in the Dansalan Market," September 25, 1933, Laubach Papers, Box 1.
107. Freer, *Philippine Experiences*, 66, 201–02.
108. Scott, *Seeing Like a State*, 78, 82, 183.
109. Benedict Anderson, *Imagined Communities: Reflections on the Origins and Spread of Nationalism* (London, 1991), 184.
110. James, *Raj*, 63; Nicholas Dirks, "Foreword" to Bernard S. Cohn, *Colonialism and its Forms of Knowledge: The British in India* (Princeton, NJ, 1996), xvi.
111. Cavaliero, *Strangers in the Land*, 154–55.
112. Gilmour, *The Ruling Caste*, 176.
113. Metcalf, *Ideologies of the Raj*, 200–01.
114. Gilmour, *The Ruling Caste*, 176–77.
115. Richard Saumarez Smith, *Rule by Records: Land Registration and Village Custom in Early British Panjab* (Delhi, 1996), 3.
116. Taft to John C. Spooner, September 3, 1900, Taft Papers, Reel 31. He had not changed his mind a year later: the "natives are a curious people and as absolutely unable to govern themselves, even if all the people were as well educated as those who have had education, as children. They do not know how to begin anything; they are absolutely lacking in the initiative and entirely wanting in those virtues of self-restraint and honesty in public administration without which any government becomes a farce." Taft to Howard Hollister, August 27, 1901, Taft Papers, Reel 33.
117. *Report of the Philippine Commission*, Vol. I, 183.
118. Stanley, *A Nation in the Making*, 73–74. For an excellent overview, see also Michael Cullinane, *Ilustrado Politics: Filipino Elite Responses to American Rule, 1898–1908* (Manila, 2003).
119. Taft to Secretary of War, December 23, 1903, Taft Papers, Reel 41.
120. Stanley, *A Nation in the Making*, 74–75, 132–33; Worcester, *The Philippines Past and Present*, 414, 554; Williams, *Odyssey*, 140–42; W. H. Taft, "Civil Government in the Philippines," 86–87; Taft to Mr. Bishop, April 25, 1901, Taft Papers, Reel 32.
121. Bernard S. Cohn, "The Census: Social Structure and Objectification in South Asia," in his *An Anthropologist Among the Historians and Other Essays*, 232; see also "Representing Authority in Victorian India," in his *An Anthropologist Among the Historians*, 652; Arnold, *Tropics and the Travelling Gaze*, 34.
122. Bernard S. Cohn, "Notes on the History of the Study of Indian Society and Culture," in Singer and Cohn, eds., *Structure and Change in Indian Society*, 15.
123. David Arnold, "'An Ancient Race Outworn': Malaria and Race in Colonial India, 1860–1930," in Ernst and Harris, eds., *Race, Science and Medicine*, 129–30.
124. Kramer, *Blood of Government*, 220.
125. *Census of the Philippine Islands*, Vol. I (Washington, DC, 1905), 11.
126. Ibid., 22–23.
127. Ibid., 39–42.
128. Martin Jay and Sumathi Ramaswamy, "The Imperial Optic," in Jay and Ramaswamy, eds., *Empires of Vision*, 33.
129. Ian Barrow, *Making History, Drawing Territory: British Mapping in India, c. 1756–1905* (New Delhi, 2003), 23.
130. Memoir of Sir Herbert Thompson, IOR, Private Papers, MSS Eur F226/29, Sir Herbert Thompson Papers, BL.
131. Arnold, *Tropics and the Travelling Gaze*, 84.
132. J. L. H. Williams Memoir, IOR, Private Papers, MSS Eur C796/3, J. L. H. Williams Papers, BL.
133. *Census of the Philippine Islands*, Vol. I, 14.
134. Brody, *Visualizing American Empire*, 89–90, 97.
135. M. L. Stewart to Fred W. Carpenter, April 28, 1903, Taft Papers, Reel 39.

136. Charles Mead to Taft, November 2, 1900, Taft Papers, Reel 31; B[enito] Legarde to Taft, May 15, 1902, Taft Papers, Reel 36; Worcester, *The Philippines Past and Present*, 547.
137. Worcester, *The Philippines Past and Present*, 548.
138. Meyer, *Letters Home*, 33.
139. McKenna, *American Imperial Pastoral*, 98, 105, 156–57.
140. James, *Raj*, 330, 338.
141. Metcalf, *Ideologies of the Raj*, 149–50.
142. Kennedy, *Magic Mountains*, 82.
143. See, for example, Brian Stoddart, *A People's Collector in the British Raj: Arthur Galletti* (New Delhi, 2011).
144. Brody, *Visualizing American Empire*, 145; Victor G. Heiser Diary, entry for January 10, 1912, Victor G. Heiser Papers, Box 73, APS.
145. Williams, *Odyssey*, 101, 151.
146. Taft to Mr. Bishop, April 25, 1901, Taft Papers, Reel 32.
147. Taft to Señor Dumaguila, January 23, 1903, Taft Papers, Reel 38.
148. Forbes Journal, Vol. III, entry for July 17, 1909, Forbes Papers.
149. Roosevelt, *The Philippines*, 41.
150. Queen Victoria commissioned from the Austrian painter Rudolf Swoboda a series of head portraits of her Indian subjects to hang in her summer residence. Saloni Mathur, *India By Design: Colonial History and Cultural Display* (Berkeley, 2007), 80.
151. Pinney, *Camera Indica*, 17.
152. John Falconer, "'A Pure Labor of Love,'" in Hight and Sampson, eds., *Colonialist Photography*, 57; Gael Newton, "South-East Asia: Malaya, Singapore, Philippines," in Hannavy, ed., *Encyclopedia of Nineteenth-Century Photography*, 1313–16.
153. Pinney, *Camera Indica*, 23–24.
154. Gary D. Sampson, "Unmasking the Colonial Picturesque," in Hight and Sampson, *Colonialist Photography*, 89–90.
155. James R. Ryan, *Picturing Empire: Photography and the Visualization of the British Empire* (Chicago, 1997), 51–52.
156. Ibid., 195–97; Chaudhary, *Afterimage of Empire*, 40.
157. Pinney, *Camera Indica*, 57; Mathur, *India By Design*, 116–17.
158. Metcalf, *Ideologies of the Raj*, 117.
159. Falconer, "A Pure Labor of Love," 52–55, 71–72, 79.
160. Ryan, *Picturing Empire*, 156, 158.
161. Pinney, *Camera Indica*, 44.
162. Nerissa S. Balce, *Body Parts of Empire: Visual Abjection, Filipino Images, and the American Archive* (Ann Arbor, 2016), 50–51, 80.
163. Sonnichsen, *Ten Months a Captive*, 385.
164. Vergara, *Displaying Filipinos*, 26.
165. Kramer, *Blood of Government*, 282–83.
166. Heiser Diary, April 28, 1912, Heiser Papers.
167. Heiser, *American Doctor's Odyssey*, 165.
168. G. D. Rice, "Art in the Philippines," *The Art Amateur* (February 1902), 68.
169. Freer, *Philippine Experiences*, 266.
170. Vergara, *Displaying Filipinos*, 123.
171. Roosevelt, *The Philippines*, 79–81.
172. *Our Islands and Their People as Seen with Camera and Pencil*, intro. by Major-General Joseph Wheeler, with special descriptive matter and narratives by José de Olivares (St. Louis, 1899), Vol. II, 551, 553, 555, 558.
173. Vergara, *Displaying Filipinos*, 4, 58.
174. Kramer, *Blood of Government*, 229–30, 366–69; McKenna, *American Imperial Pastoral*, 132.
175. James, *Raj*, 493–94. See also Peter H. Hoffenberg, *An Empire on Display: English, Indian, and Australian Exhibitions from the Crystal Palace to the Great War* (Berkeley, 2001).
176. Quoted in John M. Mackenzie, "Exhibiting Empire and the Delhi Durbar of 1911: Imperial and Cultural Contexts," in McAleer and Mackenzie, eds., *Exhibiting the Empire*, 194.

177. Bernard S. Cohn, "Representing Authority," 632, 635, 648–49, 660–61.
178. Ibid, 667, 671–72.
179. Mackenzie, "Exhibiting Empire," 202.
180. Leonard Wood Diary, entry for November 8, 1921, Wood Papers, MD, LC.
181. Robert W. Rydell, *All the World's a Fair: Visions of Empire at American International Expositions, 1876–1916* (Chicago, 1984), 160.
182. Kramer, *Blood of Government*, 265.
183. Rydell, *All the World's a Fair*, 173–74.
184. Nancy J. Parezo and Don D. Fowler, *Anthropology Goes to the Fair: The 1904 Louisiana Purchase Exposition* (Lincoln, 2007), 178–88; Devins, *An Observer in the Philippines*, 366.
185. Kramer, *Blood of Government*, 276.
186. Ibid., 258, 274.
187. Parezo and Fowler, *Anthropology Goes to the Fair*, 177, 185.
188. Kramer, *Blood of Government*, 280–81.
189. Rishi Kumar Agarwal, "Origin of Spectacles in India," *British Journal of Opthalmology* 55, 2 (1971), 128–29.
190. King, *Diary of a Civilian's Wife*, Vol. I, 115; MacMillan, *Women of the Raj*, 64.
191. Ghose, *Memsahibs Abroad*, 292–93.
192. King, *Diary of a Civilian's Wife*, Vol. II, 157, 198.
193. Allen, *Plain Tales from the Raj*, 202; MacMillan, *Women of the Raj*, 176; Michael H. Fisher, *Counterflows to Colonialism: Indian Travellers and Settlers in Britain, 1600–1857* (Delhi, 2004), 11; Mrs. B. Bayley, "Memoir of Life in India 1929–1939," Bayley Papers, Box 2, CSAS.
194. Sanjay Subramanyam, "On the Hat-Wearers, Their Toilet Practices, and Other Curious Usages," in Chatterjee and Hawes, *Europe Observed*, 65.
195. Hilda Bourne, "It Was Like This," J. M. Bourne Papers, CSAS.
196. Irene Bose, "Unwoven Carpet of Hindustan," Bose Papers, Box 1, CSAS.
197. Lady Reynolds Memoir, IOR, Private Papers, MSS Eur 226/25, Reynolds Papers, BL.
198. Susanne Hoeber Rudolph and Lloyd I. Rudolph, with Mohan Singh Kanota, eds., *Reversing the Gaze: Amar Singh's Diary, A Colonial Subject's Narrative of Imperial India* (Boulder, CO, 2002), 10.
199. Diana Eck, *Darśan: Seeing the Divine Image in India* (Chambersburg, PA, 1985), 3–7. See also Lawrence Babb, "Glancing: Visual Interaction in Hinduism," *Journal of Anthropological Research* 37 , 4 (1981), 387–401.
200. Cohn, "Cloth, Clothes, and Colonialism," 346.
201. M. L. Darling, "Diary of a Tour, 1930," Darling Papers, Box 2, CSAS. See also Rotter, *Comrades at Odds*, 225–27.
202. Buckland, *Land of the Filipino*, 109–10; Moses, *Unofficial Letters*, 134.
203. Kelly, "The Bua School," 79.
204. James E. McColl to Captain Gallman, January 16, 1914, Burton Harrison Papers, Box 41, MD, LC.
205. Philippine Constabulary, "Confidential Report," June 13, 194, Harrison Papers, Box 38.
206. Report from Pro Libertad, December 3, 1923, Correspondence of the Philippine Commission (compiled 1900–1906), Box 3, NAII.
207. Fenella Cannell, *Power and Intimacy in the Christian Philippines* (Cambridge, 1999), 85.
208. "Aguinaldo to Brother Filipinos, Asking a Christmas Present from Brother Filipinos," December 1899, *Report of the Philippine Commission*, Vol. II, 430.
209. Sonnichsen, *Ten Months a Captive*, 386.
210. Freer, *Philippine Experiences*, 280–81.
211. Speech by Manuel Quezon, Cleveland, April 14, 1914, Harrison Papers, Box 42.
212. Friend, *Between Two Empires*, 24.
213. Anderson, *The Philippine Problem*, 321.
214. Roosevelt, *The Philippines*, 240–41.
215. Taft to "Hol" Hollister, May 26, 1901, Taft Papers, Reel 32.
216. Buckland, *Land of the Filipino*, 216–18.
217. Vicente Rama, "Murphy is a Murderer," *Bag-Ong*, December 14, 1934, Frank Murphy Papers, Bentley Historical Library, University of Michigan (microfilm), Reel 99.

Chapter 4

1. Emily Thompson, *The Soundscape of Modernity: Architectural Acoustics and the Culture of Listening in America, 1900–1933* (Cambridge, MA, 2002), 1; R. Murray Schafer, *The Tuning of the World* (New York, 1977), 274–75.
2. Hillel Schwartz, "The Indefensible Ear: A History," in Bull and Back, eds., *Auditory Culture Reader*, 490–91.
3. Ibid., 491.
4. Karin Bijsterveld, "The Diabolical Symphony of the Mechanical Age: Technology and Symbolism of Sound in European and North American Noise Abatement Campaigns, 1900–1940," in Bull and Back, eds., *Auditory Culture Reader*, 182.
5. Peter Bailey, *Popular Culture and Performance in the Victorian City* (Cambridge, 1998), 204.
6. Sophia Rosenfeld, "On Being Heard: A Case for Paying Attention to the Historical Ear," *American Historical Review* 116, no. 2 (April 2011), 323.
7. Thompson, *Soundscape of Modernity*, 131.
8. Dan McKenzie, *A City of Din: A Tirade Against Noise* (London, 1916), 63.
9. Kathleen A. Feeley and Jennifer Frost, eds., "Introduction," in Feeley and Frost, eds., *When Private Talk Goes Public*, 4.
10. Smith, *How Race Is Made*, 79.
11. Jonathan Sterne, "Medicine's Acoustic Culture: Mediate Auscultation, the Stethoscope and the 'Autopsy of the Living,'" in Bull and Back, eds., *Auditory Culture Reader*, 192, 204.
12. Bailey, *Popular Culture and Performance*, 196. Other important historical studies of sound include Rath, *How Early America Sounded*; Sarah Keyes, "'Like a Roaring Lion': The Overland Trail as a Sonic Conquest," *Journal of American History* 96, no. 1 (June 2009), 19–43; and the essays collected in Mark M. Smith, ed., *Hearing History: A Reader* (Athens, GA, 2004).
13. Darwin, *Unfinished Empire*, 300–01.
14. John M. Picker, *Victorian Soundscapes* (New York, 2003), 4.
15. Kate Flint, "The Social Life of the Senses: The Assaults and Seductions of Modernity," in Classen, ed., *A Cultural History of the Senses in the Age of Empire*, 30.
16. Picker, *Victorian Soundscapes*, 42–43.
17. Bailey, *Popular Culture and Performance*, 205.
18. Picker, *Victorian Soundscapes*, 51, 57, 59, 66.
19. Bijsterveld, "The Diabolical Symphony," in Bull and Back, eds., *Auditory Culture Reader*, 178.
20. David Stradling, *Smokestacks and Progressives: Environmentalists, Engineers, and Air Quality in America, 1881–1951* (Baltimore, 1999); Thompson, *Soundscape of Modernity*, 122.
21. Raymond Smilor, "Cacophony at 34th and 6th: The Noise Problem in America, 1900–1930," *American Studies*, 18 (1977), 24.
22. Quoted in Thompson, *Soundscape of Modernity*, 119.
23. Kasson, *Rudeness and Civility*, 126.
24. Quoted in Smilor, "Cacophony at 34th and 6th," 27.
25. Thompson, *Soundscape of Modernity*, 121, 126.
26. Smilor, "Cacophony at 34th and 6th," 31–32.
27. Allen, *Plain Tales from the Raj*, 127.
28. Arnold, *The Tropics and the Travelling Gaze*, 202.
29. MacMillan, *Women of the Raj*, 137.
30. Ibid., 81; Anne Bremner Memoir, Anne Bremner Papers, Private Papers, I[ndia] O[ffice] R[ecords], MSS Eur F226/4, BL; King, *Diary of a Civilian's Wife*, Vol. I, 93–94.
31. Ghose, *Memsahibs Abroad*, 228.
32. Allen, *Plain Tales from the Raj*, 95.
33. Ghose, *Memsahibs Abroad*, 70–71.
34. Erica Farquharson, "Indian Idyll," J. M. Bourne Papers, CSAS.
35. Collingham, *Imperial Bodies*, 169.
36. Letter to the Editor, "Noises in Bombay," *Times of India*, July 28, 1919.
37. F[rank]. L[ugard]. Brayne, *Village Uplift in India* (Allahabad, n.d. [1927]), 135.
38. Collingham, *Imperial Bodies*, 16.
39. Ghose, *Memsahibs Abroad*, 68–69.

40. King, *Diary of a Civilian's Wife*, Vol. I, 278–79.
41. King, *Diary of a Civilian's Wife*, Vol. II, 130.
42. Alice Dorothea Teale Memoir, Papers of Anglican Missions of India, Small Collections, Box 1, CSAS.
43. Evelyn Beeton Memoir, Beeton Papers, CSAS.
44. Hilda Bourne, "It Was Like This," J. M. Bourne Papers, CSAS.
45. R. C. C. Hunt, "Innocents in India," Hunt Papers, CSAS.
46. Miss L. Stevenson, "Notes of a Visit to India," *Times of India*, August 24, 1888.
47. Viola Bayley, "Hangyu in 1934," Small Collections, Box 2, CSAS.
48. Ghose, *Memsahibs Abroad*, 40–41.
49. Evelyn Beeton Memoir, Beeton Papers, CSAS.
50. "India," *Times of London*, December 22, 1858.
51. Bourne, "It Was Like This."
52. M. L. Darling, "Diary of Tour," Darling Papers, Box 2, CSAS.
53. George F. Atkinson, *Curry and Rice: The Ingredients of Social Life at "Our Station" in India* (Chennai, 2001 [1889]), 119.
54. Allen, *Plain Tales from the Raj*, 75.
55. Bourne, "It Was Like This."
56. Buettner, *Empire Families*, 31.
57. Ghose, *Memsahibs Abroad*, 232; King, *Diary of a Civilian's Wife*, Vol. I, 153.
58. Beeton Memoir.
59. King, *Diary of a Civilian's Wife*, Vol. II, 148.
60. Buettner, *Empire Families*, 42, 85–86.
61. Fee, *A Woman's Impressions*, 46–47.
62. Moses, *Unofficial Letters*, 241, 286–87.
63. Jeremi Suri, *Liberty's Surest Guardian: American Nation-Building from the Founders to Obama* (New York, 2011), 98.
64. Taft, address at Union Reading College, Manila, December 17, 1903, reprinted in John Bancroft Devins, *An Observer in the Philippines*, 394.
65. William Cameron Forbes Journal, Vol. I, note 22, William Cameron Forbes Papers, Harvard University Library; J. G. Harbord to Nicholas Roosevelt, January 31, 1927, Nicholas Roosevelt Papers, Box 10, Syracuse University Library; Taft to William Day, August 16, 1900, William Howard Taft Papers, Cornell University Library (microfilm), Reel 31.
66. Robert Bennett Bean, "Filipino Ears—A Classification of Ear Types," *Philippine Journal of Science* 4A (January 1909), 50. See also his *The Racial Anatomy of the Philippine Islanders* (Philadelphia, 1910).
67. Worcester, *The Philippines Past and Present*, facing page 426.
68. Devins, *An Observer in the Philippines*, 77–78.
69. Memoirs of Grace Paulding, William and Grace Paulding Papers, Box 1, USMHI.
70. Ruth H. B. Hunt diaries, entry for May 20, 1929, Hunt Papers, Box 1, Syracuse University Library.
71. C. H. Brent to Edith, February 26, 1903, Charles Henry Brent Papers, Box 63, MD, LC; Freer, *Philippine Experiences*, 8–9.
72. Josephine Craig and Austin Craig, *Farthest Westing: A Philippine Footnote* (Philadelphia, 1940), 106.
73. Forbes Journal, Vol. IV, entry for May 5, 1910, Forbes Papers.
74. Moses, *Unofficial Letters*, 94; C. H. Brent diary, entry for August 15, 1905, Brent Papers.
75. Griffith, "The Music of the Philippine Islands," 327.
76. Testimony of Manuel Xerez y Burgos, September 7, 1899, *Report of the Philippine Commission*, Vol. II (Washington, DC, 1900), 411.
77. C. H. Brent to Edith Brent, February 26, 1903, Box 2, Brent Papers; Taft, *Recollections*, 125; Stevens quoted in Vergara, *Displaying Filipinos*, 134, 136.
78. David P. Barrows, "Fourth Lecture, October 5, 1927, Barrows Papers, Box 6, Bancroft Library, University of California-Berkeley.
79. Moses, *Unofficial Letters*, 78.
80. Anderson, *The Philippine Problem*, 310.

81. Benjamin E. Neal Diaries, entry for February 28, 1902, Neal Papers, Box 1, Syracuse University Library. See also Conger, *An Ohio Woman*, 107, 151; and Freer, *Philippine Experiences*, 94.
82. Craig and Craig, *Farthest Westing*, 25.
83. James, *Raj*, 320–21.
84. George H. Dern to the President, November 23, 1935, Confidential File 1914–1935, R[ecord] G[roup] 350, BIA, NA II, College Park, MD.
85. Paula Richman, "Introduction: The Diversity of the Râmâyana Tradition," in Richman, ed., *Many Ramayanas*, 3–21.
86. Sir Herbert Thompson Memoir, Private Papers, IOR, MSS Eur F226/29, BL.
87. George Percival Scriven, "An American in Bohol, The Philippines, 1899–1901." Online Archival Collection, Special Collections Library, Duke University. https://library.duke.edu/rubenstein/scriptorium/scriven/
88. Sir Herbert Thompson Memoir.
89. Freer, *Philippine Experiences*, 142–43; De Bevoise, *Agents of Apocalypse*, 97.
90. As could an accusatory silence. At Curzon's Delhi durbar in 1903, according to Jon Wilson, "Indian participation occurred in silent ritual," and when the nationalist Lala Lajpat Rai died less than three weeks after being beaten by government police in 1928, his funeral was attended by 100,000 silent mourners. Wilson, *The Chaos of Empire*, 371, 428.
91. Constance Maude Memoir, Maude Papers, CSAS.
92. Proceedings of the Government of India in the Home Department (Education), Simla, July 15, 1885 (Calcutta, 1913), 553.
93. Burton Stein, *A History of India* (Malden, MA, 1998), 293.
94. Bernard Bate, "'To Persuade Them Into Speech and Action': Oratory and the Tamil Political, Madras, 1905–1919," *Comparative Studies in Society and History* 55, no. 1 (2013), 142–66.
95. Henry Woodd Nevinson, *The New Spirit of India* (London, 1908), 217–18.
96. W. H. Taft to Bellamy Storer, May 18, 1901, Taft Papers, Reel 32; Roosevelt, *The Philippines*, 70.
97. Mayo, *Isles of Fear*, 208.
98. Hunt Diaries, July 29, 1929.
99. Friend, *Between Two Empires*, 30.
100. Karnow, *In Our Image*, 202.
101. Cipriano Cid, "Wide Interest Shown in Debate Between Roxas and Judge de Joya," *Manila Daily Bulletin*, February 9, 1931.
102. Gonzalo Cue Malay, *Frases Usuales Para La Conversación* (Manila, 1904), 15, 29.
103. Williams, *Odyssey*, 254.
104. Sonnichsen, *Ten Months a Captive*, 289.
105. Taft to Wilfley, May 16, 1903; A. G. Harvey to Taft, May 16, 1903; Wilfley to Taft, May 18, 1903; all Taft Papers, Reel 39.
106. Sir Herbert Thompson Memoir.
107. Javed Majeed, "What's in a (Proper) Name? Particulars, Individuals, and Authorship in the Linguistic Survey of India and Colonial Scholarship," in Sengupta and Ali, eds., *Knowledge Production*, 23.
108. Gloria Goodwin Reheja, "Caste, Colonialism, and the Speech of the Colonized: Entextualization and Disciplinary Control in India," *American Ethnologist* 23, no. 3 (August 1996), 494–513.
109. Karnow, *In Our Image*, 212.
110. Amparo Santamaria Lardizabal, "Pioneer American Teachers and Philippine Education," in Pecson and Racelis, eds., *Tales*, 107. General Douglas MacArthur's Filipina mistress was called Dimples.
111. Corbin, *Village Bells*, 79–80, 97, 101–02.
112. Ibid, 299, 305.
113. James, *Raj*, 229.
114. Tim Barringer, "Sonic Spectacles of Empire: The Audio-Visual Nexus, Delhi-London 1911–12," in Edwards, Gosden, and Phillips, eds., *Sensible Objects*, 189.
115. "An Indian Village from a Sanitation Point of View," *Times of India*, August 23, 1888.

116. For the evidently more successful deployment of bells at missions in Cape Colony, see Giordano Nanni, *The Colonisation of Time: Ritual, Routine and Resistance in the British Empire* (Manchester, 2012), 164–70.
117. Freer, *Philippine Experiences*, 191; Buckland, *Land of the Filipino*, 124, 240–43.
118. Affidavit of Eugenio Diaz, printed in Augusto V. De Viana, ed. *The I Stories: The Events in the Philippine Revolution and the Filipino-American War as told by Its Eyewitnesses and Participants* (Manila, 2006), 142.
119. Miller, "*Benevolent Assimilation,*" 201–04.
120. Heiser, *American Doctor's Odyssey*, 110–11.
121. Buckland, *Land of the Filipino*, 124; Williams, *Odyssey*, 125.
122. Laurence Halstead Memoir, Halstead-Maus Family Papers, Box 1, USMHI.
123. Barringer, "Sonic Spectacles," 177–78.
124. Alfred Edward Zealley and J. Ord Hume, *Famous Bands of the British Empire: Brief Historical Records of the recognised leading Military Bands and Brass Bands in the Empire* (London, 1926), 52.
125. Trevor Herbert and Margaret Sarkissian, "Victorian Bands and Their Dissemination in the Colonies," *Popular Music* 16, no. 2 (1997), 166, 169–70.
126. Allen, *Plain Tales from the Raj*, 142.
127. Sir Fraser Noble, "Something in India: A Memoir of Service in the Northwest Frontier," Private Papers, IOR, MSS Eur F226/18, BL.
128. Lt. Gen. Sir Ernest Bradfield, "Unimportant Story," Bradfield Papers, CSAS.
129. Anne Bremner Memoir, Anne Bremner Papers, Private Papers, IOR, MSS Eur F226/4, BL.
130. Hilda Bourne, Letter to "Tittipu" (daughter), December 28, 1013, J. M. Bourne Papers, CSAS.
131. Terence O. Ranger, *Dance and Society in Eastern Africa 1890–1970: The Beni Ngoma* (Berkeley, 1975), 13; Terence Ranger, "The Invention of Tradition in Colonial Africa," in Hobsbawm and Ranger, eds., *The Invention of Tradition*, 221–62.
132. Herbert and Sarkissian, "Victorian Bands," 172.
133. Mary Talusan, "Music, Race, and Imperialism: The Philippines Constabulary Band at the 1904 St. Louis World's Fair," *Philippine Studies* 52, no. 4 (2004), 506–07.
134. "Use Bands to Lure Locusts," *Manila Times*, October 11, 1913.
135. Talusan, "Music, Race, and Imperialism," 500; Anna Page Russell Maus, "Old Army Days: Reminiscences by the Wife of an Army Surgeon," Halstead-Maus Family Papers, USMHI; Neal diaries, entry for February 28, 1902.
136. Taft, *Recollections*, 163–64.
137. *Report of the Philippines Commission*, Vol. III, 380–81.
138. W. C. Forbes, Journal, Vol. II (1904).
139. Taft, *Recollections*, 162; Theodore Roosevelt Jr., Diary, February–July, 1932, entry for March 22, Theodore Roosevelt Jr. Papers, Box 2, MD, LC.
140. Talusan, "Music, Race, and Imperialism," 504.
141. W. H. Taft to Martin Ocampo, October 2, 1902, Taft Papers, Reel 37; Manila Symphony Orchestra programs, 1911–1914, American Collection, Rizal Library, Ataneo de Manila University, Manila, PI.
142. David P. Barrows to the Secretary to the Military Governor, "Preliminary Term of Manila Normal School April 10–May 10, 1901, May 22, 1901, Barrows Papers, Box 1.
143. Quoted in Bijsteveldt, "Noise Abatement," 170.
144. Cohn, *Colonialism and Its Forms of Knowledge*, 40–41.
145. Anil Kumar, *Medicine and the Raj: British Medical Policy in India 1835–1911* (Walnut Creek, CA, 1998), 75.
146. Darwin, *Unfinished Empire*, 210.
147. Cohn, *Colonialism and Its Forms of Knowledge*, 41.
148. Visram, *Ayahs, Lascars and Princes*, 31.
149. Steel and Gardiner, *Complete Indian Housekeeper*, 12.
150. Allen, *Plain Tales from the Raj*, 72.
151. James, *Raj*, 159.

152. Kate Teltscher, "The Floating Lexicon: *Hobson-Jobson* and the *OED*," in Sengupta and Ali, eds., *Knowledge Production*, 41.
153. Buettner, *Empire Families*, 41–42; Edmund C. P. Hull, *The European in India; or, India's Vade Mecum* (London, 1878), 141–42; Lady Chapman, "British India Recollected," Lady Chapman Papers, CSAS.
154. Ghose, *Memsahibs Abroad*, 87.
155. David, "Greased Cartridges," 94.
156. Gauri Viswanathan, *Masks of Conquest: Literary Study and British Rule in India* (New York, 1989), 44.
157. Gerald Hare to Jack Gibson, May 13, 1937, Jack Gibson Papers, Box 2, CSAS.
158. W. A. Barnes Diary, entries for January 8, 9, 23, 1933, Box 2; notes, "Reasons for Learning English," nd, Box 5; *Principles of the International Phonetic Association*, n.d., Box 5, W. A. Barnes Papers, CSAS.
159. Scott, *An Indian Journal*, 119.
160. Benedict Anderson, "Cacique Democracy in the Philippines: Origins and Dreams," in Rafael, ed., *Discrepant Histories*, 6.
161. Conger, *An Ohio Woman*, 61.
162. Quoted in Glenn Anthony May, *Social Engineering in the Philippines: The Aims, Execution, and Impact of American Colonial Policy, 1900–1913* (Westport, CT, 1980), 94.
163. David P. Barrows, "Report Upon the Public Schools of Manila," December 1, 1900, Barrows Papers, Box 6.
164. Anderson, *Colonial Pathologies*, 117.
165. Renato Constantino, "The Miseducation of the Filipino," in Shaw and Francia, eds., *Vestiges of War*, 181.
166. Linn, *Philippine War*, 203, 258.
167. Karnow, *In Our Image*, 201. Schools did not have as their only purpose revision of the sonic environment of the islands. As Taft wrote in late 1903, "The erection of handsome, permanent, airy and healthy school houses would have an excellent effect both in enlarging school capacity and in giving ocular demonstration of the importance which the Government attaches to the general system of education." Taft to The Secretary of War, December 23, 1903, Taft Papers, Reel 41.
168. Taft, "Civil Government in the Philippines," 49–50.
169. *Report of the Philippine Commission*, Vol. I, 32.
170. "Manners and Morals," *The Philippine Teacher* 2, no. 2 (July 1905), 17.
171. Barrows, "Report of a Visit to the Provinces of Bataan and Pampanga," January 31, 1901, Barrows Papers, Box 6; "Report of the Bureau of Education," November 1935, Frank Murphy Papers, University of Michigan Library (microfilm), Reel 102; P. F. Jernegan, "Our Philippines," *The Philippine Teacher* 1, no. 2 (January 15, 1905), 23.
172. May, *Social Engineering*, 92–93; W. H. Taft to Fred Atkinson, April 24, 1900, Taft Papers, Reel 30.
173. Barrows, "Eighth Annual Report of the Director of Education, July 1, 1907, to June 30, 1908," Barrows Papers, Box 6.
174. Barrows to Charles P. G. Scott, September 29, 1906, Barrows Papers, Box 1.
175. Buckland, *Land of the Filipino*, 91–92.
176. Leonard Wood Diary, May 1–June 25, 1921, Leonard Wood Papers, Box 19, MD, LC; Paul Monroe et al., *A Survey of the Educational System of the Philippine Islands* (Manila, 1925), 39–43. See also Commonwealth of the Philippines, *Graded Exercises in Sentence Rhythm and Emphasis Through Inflection* (Manila, 1940).
177. Government of the Philippine Islands, Department of Public Instruction, Bureau of Education, *Course of Study in Phonics for Primary Grades* (Manila, 1932), iii, 11, 16–17, 43, 45–46, 48, 52–53, 81–83.
178. Barrows, testimony before the Insular Affairs Committee, U.S. Senate, March 12–13, 1902, 694–95, 699.
179. "The New India," *Times of London*, May 9, 1924.
180. James, *Raj*, 346–47.

Chapter 5

1. Patrick Süskind, *Perfume: The Story of a Murderer*. Transl. John E. Woods (New York, 1986), 82.
2. Rachel Herz, "I Know What I Like: Understanding Odor Preferences," in Drobnick, ed., *The Smell Culture Reader*, 190–91.
3. Classen, Howes, and Synnott, *Aroma*, 51–52, 69–70; Miller, *Anatomy of Disgust*, 75; Reinarz, *Past Scents*, 25, 114.
4. Elias, *The Civilizing Process*, 111.
5. Gale Largey and Rod Watson, "The Sociology of Odors," in Drobnick, ed., *Smell Culture Reader*, 29.
6. Katherine Ashenburg, *The Dirt on Clean: An Unsanitized History* (New York, 2007), 10–11. Note, however, Andrew Kettler's argument that French Jesuits campaigning for souls among Native Americans during the seventeenth century had some success because of both parties' "olfactory inclusive spiritual sensoriums." Andrew Kettler, "'Ravishing Odors of Paradise': Jesuits, Olfaction, and Seventeenth-Century North America," *Journal of North American Studies* 50, no. 4 (November 2016), 827.
7. McLuhan, *The Gutenberg Galaxy*.
8. Reinarz, *Past Scents*, 208.
9. Classen, Howes, and Synnott, *Aroma*, 3–4. In 1898, a group of Cambridge University researchers went to Melanesia to study the "primitives." They found that, while the Melanesian sense of smell was no stronger than that of Europeans, the "natives" did seem "to attach more meaning" to odors." Constance Classen, "Introduction," 19.
10. Jim Drobnick, "Preface," in his *Smell Culture Reader*, 14–15. Like Drobnick, Mark S. R. Jenner cautions that odorlessness was not always considered possible or desirable: it was "the removal of *particular* scents," or the replacement of foul smells by sweet ones, that "civilized" men and women sought. Mark S. R. Jenner, "Follow Your Nose? Smell, Smelling, and Their Histories," *American Historical Review* 116, no. 2 (April 2011), 341.
11. Allen, *Plain Tales from the Raj*, 37.
12. MacMillan, *Women of the Raj*, 33.
13. Erica Farquharson, "Indian Idyll," J. M. Bourne Papers, CSAS.
14. Reminiscence of Major T. E. Browsdon, MSS Eur 226/5, BL.
15. Rudyard Kipling, *The City of Dreadful Night* (New York, 1899), 8–9. Another Briton remarked that Calcutta was "the abscess on the anus of the Empire." J. L. H. Williams Memoir, MSS Eur C796/3, Private Papers, IOR, BL.
16. Fee, *A Woman's Impressions*, 46–50; Craig and Craig, *Farthest Westing*, 33, 68; Government of the Philippine Islands, Department of the Interior, Bureau of Public Health, *Annual Report of the Commissioner of Public Health*, September 1, 1903–August 31, 1904 (Manila, 1905), 15–16.
17. Arnold, *The Tropics and the Traveling Gaze*, 37. See also Amrith, "Health and Sovereignty in the New Asia," 98.
18. Melanie A. Kiechle, *The Smell Detectives: An Olfactory History of Nineteenth-Century Urban America* (Seattle, 2017), 33–39.
19. The primacy of smell to distinguish tropical others from civilized selves was by no means reserved to India and the Philippines. When British and French explorers arrived in Tasmania in the late eighteenth century, they recoiled at the stench of fish oil, used by the Aboriginals as insect repellent; the Aboriginals, on the other hand, reacted "with strong marks of distaste" to the smell of pork eaten by the Europeans. Shino Konishi, "Discovering the Savage Senses: French and British Explorers' Encounters with Aboriginal People," in West-Sooby, ed., *Discovery and Empire*, 106. Xuelei Huang has described British efforts to deodorize Shanghai within and beyond their concession in the city, much as they tried to do in India. See Xuelei Huang, "Deodorising China: Odour, Ordure, and Colonial (Dis)order in Shanghai, 1840s–1940s," *Modern Asian Studies* 50, no. 3 (2016), 1092–112. Nor, for that matter, was such thinking confined to Oceania and Asia. "It is by its scent that the New World first makes itself known to the traveler," wrote Claude Lévi-Strauss, "and it is difficult to describe that scent to anyone who has not experienced it." Claude Lévi-Strauss, *Tristes Tropiques* (Paris, 1955), 82.

20. Classen, "Introduction," 2.
21. Hector Gavin, *Sketches and Illustrations, of Bethnal Green. A Type of the Condition of the Metropolis and Other Large Towns* (London, 1848), 4, 9–10, 19–20, 50.
22. Jacob A. Riis, *How the Other Half Lives*. Ed. with Intro. by David Leviatin (Boston, 1996 [1890]), 88, 90, 93, 108, 121, 141, 157, 166. (Riis found "the negro" to be "the cleanest of the new tenants.")
23. Melanie Kiechle, "The Smell Detectives," *Chemical Heritage* (Summer 2011), 32–36. Air conditioning was introduced in American theaters in the 1910s, in part because the odor in them on summer days was said to be unbearable. Before its advent, at least one theater hired an attendant to walk to aisles spraying patrons with an atomizer of perfume. Gail Cooper, *Air-Conditioning America: Engineers and the Controlled Environment, 1900–1960* (Baltimore, 1998), 83.
24. Martin V. Melosi, *The Sanitary City: Urban Infrastructure in America from Colonial Times to the Present* (Baltimore, 2000), 103; Eileen Cleere, *The Sanitary Arts: Aesthetic Culture and the Victorian Cleanliness Campaigns* (Columbus, OH, 2014).
25. Arnold, *Colonizing the Body*, 97–98.
26. I am grateful to Paul Kramer for this insight, and I quote from his personal communication, July 24, 2015.
27. Corbin, *The Foul and the Fragrant*, 39, 68, 210–11; Jütte, *A History of the Senses*, 269.
28. Classen, Howes, and Synnott, *Aroma*, 84; Classen, *Worlds of Sense*, 31.
29. Corbin, *The Foul and the Fragrant*, 76, 214.
30. Classen, Howes, and Synnott, *Aroma*, 26, 230; Smith, *Clean*, 280.
31. Quoted in Ashenburg, *The Dirt on Clean*, 170.
32. Kasson, *Rudeness and Civility*, 124–25.
33. Corbin, *The Foul and the Fragrant*, 39; Alan Hyde, "Offensive Bodies," in Drobnick, ed., *Smell Culture Reader*, 53–58.
34. Smith, *How Race Is Made*, 24, emphasis in original.
35. Corbin, *The Foul and the Fragrant*, 274.
36. Myrdal, *An American Dilemma*, 107. Georg Simmel wrote in *Soziologie* (1908): "The exclusion of the Negro from high society in North America appears to be due to his body odor." Quoted in Hyde, "Offensive Bodies," 56.
37. Margery Hall, "Autobiography: 'And the Nights Were More Terrible Than the Days," Private Papers, IOR, MSS Eur 226/11, BL.
38. "India," *Times of London*, December 14, 1874.
39. Sir Herbert Thompson Memoir, Private Papers, IOR, MSS Eur F226/29, BL.
40. Hudson quoted in Classen, Howes, and Synnott, *Aroma*, 168–69.
41. Devins, *An Observer in the Philippines*, 51; Letter from Lt. Lee McCoy in *Daily Scioto Gazette*, January 28, 1900, Richie Routt Papers, Box 1, USMHI.
42. Craig and Craig, *Farthest Westing*, 74.
43. Ruth Hunt, Travel Journals, Box 1, Hunt Papers, Special Collections, Syracuse University Library.
44. Anderson, *The Spell of the Hawaiian Islands*, 129, 225–26.
45. Thomas Gallwey to William Gallwey, December 17, 1877, Gallwey Papers, CSAS; J. A. Jones, *Manual of Hygiene, Sanitation, and Sanitary Engineering, with Special Reference to Indian Conditions* (Madras, 1896), 98–99.
46. Quoted in Collingham, *Imperial Bodies*, 147.
47. "Editorial," *Times of India*, August 18, 1888.
48. Commonwealth of The Philippines, *Graded Exercises in Sentence Rhythm*, 60–61, 66–67; William Paulding Memoir, Box 1, William and Grace Paulding Papers, USMHI; Dr. Heiser's Diary, Manila, entry for January 8, 1931, Heiser Papers, Series IV, Box 100, APS; Brown, Russell, and Cariño, *Health Through Knowledge and Habits*, 158.
49. Corbin, *The Foul and the Fragrant*, 64–65.
50. Reinarz, *Past Scents*, 188; Stephen Halliday, *The Great Stink of London: Sir Joseph Bazalgette and the Cleansing of the Victorian Metropolis* (Phoenix Mill, UK, 1999), 127.
51. Classen, Howes, and Synnott, *Aroma*, 59; Halliday, *Great Stink*, 135.

52. Melanie Kiechle, "Navigating by Nose: Fresh Air, Stench Nuisance, and the Urban Environment, 1840–1880," *Journal of Urban History* (March, 2015), 5; John Duffy, *The Sanitarians: A History of American Public Health* (Urbana, 1990), 187.
53. David S. Barnes, "Cargo, 'Infection,' and the Logic of Quarantine in the Nineteenth Century," *Bulletin of the History of Medicine* 88, no. 1 (Spring 2014), 76, 88.
54. Eleanor Margolies, "Vagueness Gridlocked: A Map of the Smells of New York," in Drobnick, ed., *Smell Culture Reader*, 112. Recently, scientists have speculated that ovarian cancer may have a detectable odor before it shows up in other tests, and have suggested that dogs, with their keen senses of smell, might be able to sniff out cancer at an early stage. Veronique Greenwood, "What Does Cancer Smell Like?," *New York Times*, November 19, 2013.
55. David S. Barnes, "Confronting Sensory Crisis in the Great Stinks of London and Paris," in Cohen and Johnson, eds., *Filth*, 106–07, 115–16.
56. David S. Barnes, *The Great Stink of Paris and the Nineteenth-Century Struggle against Filth and Germs* (Baltimore, 2006), 3, 12, 44, 138, 211. See also Corbin, *The Foul and the Fragrant*, 223–24, 227.
57. Tomes, *Gospel of Germs*, 238; Barnes, *Great Stink*, 237.
58. Classen, Howes, and Synnott, *Aroma*, 124; James McHugh, *Sandalwood and Carrion: Smell in Indian Religion and Culture* (New York, 2012); Sir Fraser Noble, "Something in India: A Memoir of Service in the Frontier Province," Private Papers, IOR, MSS Eur F226/18, BL; MacMillan, *Women of the Raj*, 33; Gilmour, *The Ruling Caste*, 269; Ghose, *Memsahibs Abroad*, 165.
59. Sydney Greenbie, *The Romantic East* (New York, 1930), 40–41; Allen, *Plain Tales from the Raj*, 55–56; Reminiscence of Anne Bremner, Private Papers, IOR, MSS Eur 226/4, BL; Thomas Gallwey to William Gallwey, December 17, 1877, Gallwey Papers; Steel and Gardiner, *Complete Indian Housekeeper*, 194–95; TS Memoir by Evelyn Beeton, Beeton Papers, CSAS; Hall, "Autobiography."
60. Devins, *An Observer in the Philippines*, 107; Journal of William Cameron Forbes, Vol. II, entry for May 4, 1906, William Cameron Forbes Papers, Houghton Library, Harvard University.
61. Brown, Russell, and Cariño, *Health Through Knowledge and Habits*, 148, 152, 223, 267; Diary of Charles Henry Brent, entry for April 29, 1902, Brent Papers, MD, LC; Buckland, *Land of the Filipino*, 160–61.
62. Heiser, *American Doctor's Odyssey*, 138.
63. Florence Horn, *Orphans of the Pacific* (New York, 1941), 29.
64. MacMillan, *Women of the Raj*, 60; Scott, *An Indian Journal*, 51; Ghose, *Memsahibs Abroad*, 165.
65. Williams, *Odyssey*, 307.
66. Anne Bremner Memoir, Private Papers, IOR, MSS Eur 226/4, BL; Mrs. King, *Diary of a Civilian's Wife*, Vol. I, 39; Lady Reynolds Memoir, Private Papers, IOR, MSS Eur 226/25, BL.
67. Fuller, *Housekeeping and Household Arts*, 49.
68. James McHugh, "The Disputed Civets and the Complexion of the God: Secretions and History in India," *Journal of the American Oriental Society* 132, no. 2 (April–June 2012), 245–73.
69. "The Philippines. Professor Worcester's Account of His Observations and Experiences in the Islands—The Corrupt Spanish Government—The Friars and Their Influence," *Manila Times*, July 7, 1899.
70. Otis, *Membranes*. The average man produces some 2.4 pounds of feces and urine each day. See Dominiek Dendooven, "Trench Crap: Excremental Aspects of the First World War," in Saunders and Cornish, eds., *Modern Conflict and the Senses*, 188.
71. Miller, *Anatomy of Disgust*, 69.
72. See Brayne, *Village Uplift in India*, 22. Others found the odor of dung fires homely; see the Ruth Barton Memoir, Barton Papers, Box 2, Small Collections, CSAS; and Farquharson, "Indian Idyll."
73. Vijay Prashad, "The Technology of Sanitation in Colonial Delhi," *Modern Asian Studies* 35, no. 1 (February 2001), 119; T. G. Hewlett "Village Sanitation in Indian," 1896 (microfiche) IOR, 1/609, BL; T. G. Hewlett, "An Indian Village from a Sanitation Point of View," Part II, *Times of India*, August 24, 1888.
74. Steel and Gardiner, *Complete Indian Housekeeper*, 163–64.

75. From the Superintendent, Detention Barracks, Aden, to the Officer in Charge, Detention Barracks, Aden, August 7, 1922, IOR/R/20/A/2499, BL.
76. Hall, "'And the Nights Were More Terrible than the Days.'"
77. Conger, *An Ohio Woman*, 70.
78. Fuller, *Housekeeping and Household Arts*, 49.
79. "Our Filthy Canals," *Manila Times*, April 25, 1903.
80. Grace Paulding Memoir, Box 1, William and Grace Paulding Papers, USMHI.
81. Bunnett, *Manila Envelopes*, 110.
82. Hewlett, "Village Sanitation in India."
83. Anderson, *Colonial Pathologies*, 104.
84. W. F. Bynum, "In Retrospect: *On the Mode of Communication of Cholera*—John Snow," *Nature*, March 14, 2013, 169–70; Rodney Sullivan, "Cholera and Colonialism in the Philippines," in Macleod and Lewis, eds., *Disease, Medicine, and Empire*, 284–300.
85. J. B. Harrison, "Allahabad: A Sanitary History," in Ballhatchet and Harrison, eds., *The City in South Asia*, 174.
86. Memorandum by the Army Sanitary Commission on the Report of the Sanitary Commissioner of Bengal for 1897, July 20, 1899, Proceedings of the Home Department—Sanitary (Calcutta, 1900), NAI.
87. Sir Leonard Rogers, "The Conditions Influencing the Incidence and Spread of Cholera in India," paper in Major General Sir Leonard Rogers Collection (GB 0809 Rogers), London School of Hygiene and Tropical Medicine.
88. Collingham, *Imperial Bodies*, 87–90.
89. Comment by Sir Michael F. O'Dwyer, on Sir Leonard Rogers, "The Forecasting and Control of Cholera Epidemics in India," *Journal of the Royal Society of Arts* LXXV, no. 3874 (February 18, 1927), 354, Rogers Collection.
90. Mr. Justice Cunningham, "The Public Health in India," *Times of London*, January 30, 1888.
91. Rogers, "Conditions Influencing" and "The Forecasting and Control."
92. Radhika Ramasubban, "Imperial Health in British India, 1857–1900," in MacLeod and Lewis, eds., *Disease, Medicine, and Empire*, 54; comments on Rogers, "The Forecasting and Control," by Lt. Col. T. R. Mulroney (351) and Lt. Col. C. C. S. Barry (352), Rogers Collection.
93. Arnold, *Tropics and the Travelling Gaze*, 46.
94. Irene Bose, "Unwoven Carpet of Hindustan," Bose Papers, CSAS.
95. De Bevoise, *Agents of Apocalypse*, 174. The epidemic returned in 1888–89.
96. Worcester, *The Philippines Past and Present*, 331.
97. Benjamin Neal Diary, entry for August 28 [24], 1901, Neal Papers, Box 1, Special Collections, Syracuse University Library.
98. Ralph T. Edwards, "A Biological Study of the Water Supply of the Philippine Islands, with a Description of a New Pathogenic Organism," *Philippine Journal of Science* 3B, no. 1 (January 1908), 125; Victor G. Heiser, "Some Considerations with Regard to the Cause of the Frequent Reappearance of Cholera in the Philippine Islands, with Statistics Beginning with the Outbreak in 1902 to January 1, 1908," *Philippine Journal of Science* 3B, no. 1 (January 1908), 95; Allan McLaughlin, "The Suppression of a Cholera Epidemic in Manila," *Philippine Journal of Science* 4B, no. 1 (February 1909), 54.
99. Edwin C. Shattuck to the Director of Health, November 20, 1906; Richard P. Strong to the Director of the Bureau of Health, November 22, 1906; both Heiser Papers, Series IV, Box 73; Comment on Dr. McLaughlin's paper by Dr. R. P. Strong, *Philippine Journal of Science* 4B, no. 1 (February 1909), 65; Brent Diary, November 23, 1906, Box 53.
100. De Bevoise, *Agents of Apocalypse*, 177.
101. Reynaldo C. Ileto, "Cholera and the Origins of the American Sanitary Order in the Philippines," in Rafael, ed., *Discrepant Histories*, 59; Worcester, *The Philippines Past and Present*, 333–39; Sullivan, "Cholera and Colonialism," 291.
102. De Bevoise, *Agents of Apocalypse*, 181.
103. Anna Page Russell Maus, "Old Army Days: Reminiscences by the Wife of an Army Surgeon," Halstead-Maus Family Papers, USMHI; Ileto, "Cholera and the Origins," 63–64; De Bevoise, *Agents of Apocalypse*, 166.
104. Heiser, *American Doctor's Odyssey*, 106.

105. Dean Worcester to W. H. Taft, April 5, 1902, William Howard Taft Papers, Cornell University (microfilm), Reel 35.
106. Bureau of Public Health, *Annual Report of the Commissioner of Public Health, September 1, 1903–August 31, 1904* (Manila, 1905), 49.
107. Ileto, "Cholera and the Origins," 53–54.
108. Quoted in Jharna Gourlay, *Florence Nightingale and the Health of the Raj* (Aldershot, 2003), 260–61.
109. Richard L. Bushman and Claudia L. Bushman, "The Early History of Cleanliness in America," *Journal of American History* 74, no. 4 (March 1988), 1231; Mary Ting Yi Lui, *The Chinatown Trunk Mystery: Murder, Miscegenation, and Other Dangerous Encounters in Turn-of-the-Century New York City* (Princeton, NJ, 2005), 27–28.
110. Anderson, *The Spell of the Hawaiian Islands*, 224.
111. Duffy, *The Sanitarians*, 175–77.
112. Quoted in Melosi, *The Sanitary City*, 143.
113. Extract from the Proceedings of the Council of the Governor of Bombay, 18th March 1889, IOR/L/PJ/6/278, file 924, BL.
114. Office of the Civil Administrative Medical Officer, Aden, to the First Assistant Resident, 17th July 1928, IOR/R/20/A/2499, BL; "Bombay Drainage," *Times of India*, September 8, 1905; "Bombay Municipal Corporation," *Times of India*, December 12, 1905.
115. "Lord Dufferin in the Calcutta Slums," *Times of India*, May 23, 1888.
116. "Sanitation in Belgaum," letter to the editor by K. R. Gopalaha Aiyer, *Times of India*, September 25, 1919.
117. Memorandum by the Army Sanitary Commission on the Report of the Sanitary Commission for Bombay for 1897, June 9, 1899, *Proceedings of the Home Department—Sanitary*, NAI; Extracts from Proceedings of the Government of Bengal Municipal Department—Sanitary Report, June 30, 1903, in *Proceedings of the Home Department—Sanitary*, NAI; Memorandum by the Army Sanitary Commission on the Report of the Sanitary Commissioner of Madras for 1897, June 9, 1899, in *Proceedings of the Home Department—Sanitary*, NAI; Papers of J. L. H. Williams, MSS Eur C796/12, BL.
118. Kennedy, *Magic Mountains*, 191.
119. Hewlett, "Village Sanitation in India"; T. G. Hewlett, "An Indian Village from a Sanitation Point of View," Part I, *Times of India*, August 23, 1888.
120. Brayne, *Village Uplift*, 11, 29, 107.
121. Harrison, "Allahabad."
122. Prashad, "Technology of Sanitation."
123. Moses, *Unofficial Letters*, 233.
124. Anderson, *Colonial Pathologies*, 104.
125. Thomas W. Jackson, "Sanitary Conditions and Needs in Provincial Towns," *Philippine Journal of Science* 3B, 5 (November 1908), 431–37.
126. Paul Clements, "Medical Survey of the Town of Taytay," *Philippine Journal of Science* 4B, 4 (August 1909), 247–55.
127. Anderson, *Colonial Pathologies*, 18.
128. Government of the Philippine Islands, *Annual Report of the Commissioner of Public Health, September 1, 1903—August 31, 1904* (Manila, 1905), 15–16, 76.
129. "The Slums of Manila," *Manila Times*, July 11, 1899.
130. Daniel F. Doeppers, *Feeding Manila in Peace and War, 1850–1945* (Madison, WI, 2016), 254.
131. Taft to William A. Edwards, July 10, 1900, Taft Papers, Reel 31.
132. Taft to Secretary of War, December 23, 1903, Taft Papers, Reel 41.
133. "Sewer System Badly Needed," *Manila Times*, August 27, 1903.
134. Heiser, *American Doctor's Odyssey*, 35; Anderson, *Colonial Pathologies*, 68–69.
135. Victor G. Heiser, M. D., *Annual Report of the Bureau of Health for the Philippine Islands, July 1, 1908–June 30, 1909* (Manila, 1909), 6, 19–22; Victor G. Heiser, M. D., *Annual Report of the Bureau of Health for the Philippine Islands, July 1, 1912–June 30, 1913* (Manila, 1913).
136. De Bevoise, *Agents of Apocalypse*, 53–55; Anderson, "Excremental Colonialism," 647.
137. Anderson, *Colonial Pathologies*, 120; Dr. Heiser's Diary, March 25, 1929, January 6, 1931, Heiser Papers, Series IV, Box 98.

138. Dr. Heiser's Diary, March 25, 1929, Heiser Papers, Series IV, Box 98.
139. Ibid., January 6, 1931.
140. Anderson, *Colonial Pathologies*, 228.
141. David Shulman, "The Scent of Memory in Hindu South India," in Drobnick, ed., *Smell Culture Reader*, 415; McHugh, *Sandalwood and Carrion*, 27, 30, 77, 80, 90, 218, 245.
142. Classen, Howes, and Synnott, *Aroma*, 113–14.
143. Darwin, *Unfinished Empire*, 53; Memo, undated [August 1921], unsigned, IOR/R/20/A/2499, BL.
144. Bourne, "It Was Like This."
145. Visram, *Ayahs, Lascars and Princes*, 65–66, 184–85.
146. Orwell, *Burmese Days*, 145.
147. Quoted in Reheja, "Caste, Colonialism, and the Speech of the Colonized," 498. Some years ago, I had the discomfiting experience in Varanasi of being sniffed audibly by an Indian scholar, a vegetarian, who then wrinkled his nose, sighed, and said, "I can always smell meat in the sweat of Americans."
148. Ambeth R. Ocampo, "The Smell of Philippines History," *Philippine Daily Inquirer*, April 11, 2013.
149. Frank C. Laubach, "Notes taken in the Dansalan Market," September 25, 1933, Laubach Papers, Special Collections, Syracuse University Library.
150. Devins, *An Observer in the Philippines*, 51.
151. Ambeth R. Ocampo, "Smell and the Filipino Identity," *Philippine Daily Inquirer*, April 8, 2016.
152. Taft, *Recollections*, 123; Dr. Heiser's Diary, December 1, 1912, Heiser Papers, Series IV, Box 73.
153. Rep. Vicente Rama, "Murphy is a Murderer," *Bag-Ong*, December 14, 1934, Frank Murphy Papers, University of Michigan Library (microfilm), Reel 99.

Chapter 6

1. David Howes, "Sensorial Anthropology," in Howes, ed., *Varieties of Sensory Experience*, 169.
2. Yi-Fu Tuan, *Passing Strange and Wonderful: Aesthetics, Nature, and Culture* (Washington, DC, 1993), 45.
3. Classen, *The Deepest Sense*, 3, 9, 137, 182, 190.
4. Allen, *Plain Tales from the Raj*, 213.
5. Ralph Crane and Anna Johnston, "Introduction," in Steel and Gardiner, *Complete Indian Housekeeper*, xxiv.
6. Abraham Eraly, *The Mughal World: Life in India's Last Golden Age* (London, 2007), 203; Taft, *Recollections*, 104.
7. Quoted in Stanley, *A Nation in the Making*, 104.
8. Ibid, 227; Jesse R. Wilson, *Through Shining Archway* (New York, 1953), 13; Allen, *Plain Tales from the Raj*, 72; Meyer, *Letters Home*, 27.
9. King, *Diary of a Civilian's Wife* Vol. II, 72–73.
10. Heiser, *American Doctor's Odyssey*, 69–70.
11. *Report of the Philippine Commission to the President*, Vol. IV (Washington, DC, 1901), 24.
12. Anne Bremner Memoir, MSS Eur 226/4, Private Papers, IOR, BL.
13. Macfarlane, *Daughters of Empire*, 32.
14. MacMillan, *Women of the Raj*, 71.
15. Moon, *British Conquest*, 660–62.
16. Atkinson, *Curry and Rice*, 13–14; King, *Diary of a Civilian's Wife*, Vol. I, 257–58.
17. Michael Snow and Ray Desmond, *Railways of the Raj* (New York, 1980), 37; Ravi Ahuja, "'The Bridge Builders': Some Notes on Railways, Pilgrimage and the British 'Civilizing Mission' in Colonial India," in Fischer-Tiné and Mann, eds., *Colonialism as Civilizing Mission*, 96.
18. King, *Diary of a Civilian's Wife*, Vol. I, 71.
19. J. L. H. Williams Memoir, MSS Eur 796/3, Private Papers, IOR, BL.
20. Carol Hyde to her parents, January 16, 1933, Hyde Papers, CSAS.
21. Jack Gibson, "As I Saw It," entry for November 7, 1938, Jack Gibson Papers, Box 3, CSAS.

22. King, *Diary of a Civilian's Wife*, Vol. I, 171–72.
23. Devins, *An Observer in the Philippines*, 50.
24. James W. Beardsley, "The Progress of Public Works in the Philippine Islands," *Journal of Race Development* 1, no. 2 (October 1910), 171.
25. Heiser, *American Doctor's Odyssey*, 43.
26. William Howard Taft, "Civil Government," 37.
27. Charles Henry Brent Diary, entry for November 2, 1902, C. H. Brent Papers, Box 1, MD, LC.
28. Heiser, *American Doctor's Odyssey*, 43; W. H. Taft to "Hol" Hollister, September 21, 1903, William Howard Taft Papers, Cornell University Library (microfilm), Reel 40.
29. David P. Barrows to Mr. Beardslee, July 24, 1909, David P. Barrows Papers, Box 1, Bancroft Library, University of California-Berkeley.
30. May, *Social Engineering*, 146, 165.
31. Karnow, *In Our Image*, 215; McKenna, *American Imperial Pastoral*, 50–51.
32. Heiser, *American Doctor's Odyssey*, 51; William Cameron Forbes Journal, Vol. III, entry for June 21, 1909, W. C. Forbes Papers, Harvard University Library.
33. Forbes Journal, Vol. III, May 31, 1909.
34. Forbes Journal, Vol. III, April 22, 1909.
35. May, *Social Engineering*, 146; Karnow, *In Our Image*, 218.
36. Forbes Journal, Vol. II, April 17, 1908 (footnote).
37. Allen, *Plain Tales from the Raj*, 327.
38. *Report of the Philippine Commission to the President*, Vol. II (Washington, DC, 1900), 238.
39. Bewell, *Romanticism and Colonial Disease*, 16; Scott, *An Indian Journal*, 20; Ghose, *Memsahibs Abroad*, 221.
40. Quoted in Collingham, *Imperial Bodies*, 178.
41. Joseph Fayrer, *European Child-Life in Bengal* (London, 1873), 30.
42. William Howard Taft to Sally S. Shaffer, October 24, 1901, Taft Papers, Reel 33; Francis Burton Harrison to Lindley M. Garrison, July 6, 1914, Harrison Papers, Box 40, MD, LC.
43. Williams, *Odyssey*, 139.
44. George F. Telfer to Lottie, August 24, 1898, August 27, 1898, in Bunnett, *Manila Envelopes*, 40, 43; Leonard Wood Diary, entry for May 26, 1921, Wood Papers, Box 19, MD, LC.
45. Worcester, *The Philippines Past and Present*, 282.
46. James Johnson, *The influence of tropical climates, more especially the climate of India, on European constitutions; the principal effects and diseases thereby induced* (London, 1813), 59, 169; Arnold, *The Tropics and the Traveling Gaze*, 48.
47. *Report of the Philippines Commission to the President*, Vol. I (1900), 161.
48. Quoted in Miller, "*Benevolent Assimilation*," 240.
49. Steel and Gardiner, *Complete Indian Housekeeper*, 197.
50. Taft, *Recollections*, 102–03.
51. Cooper, *Air Conditioning America*.
52. Freer, *Philippine Experiences*, 141; Moses, *Unofficial Letters*, 229.
53. Freer, *Philippine Experiences*, 237; Margery Hall, "Autobiography: 'And the Nights Were More Terrible than the Days,'" MSS Eur F226/11, Private Papers, IOR, BL.
54. Freer, *Philippine Experiences*, 237.
55. Sir Herbert Thompson memoirs, MSS Eur F226/29, Private Papers, IOR, BL.
56. Ibid; Carol Hyde to her parents, January 24, 1933, Hyde Papers; Hall, "Autobiography"; Evelyn Beeton Memoir, Beeton Papers, CSAS; Heiser, *American Doctor's Odyssey*, 42; Victor Heiser, Log of Leper Collecting Trip, January 1915, Series IV, Box 98, Victor C. Heiser Papers, APS; Anderson, "Excremental Colonialism," 654.
57. Hall, "Autobiography"; Bunnett, *Manila Envelopes*, 55.
58. Hyde to parents, January 24, 1933.
59. J. L. H. Williams Memoir; Allen, *Plain Tales from the Raj*, 120.
60. Grace Paulding Memoir, William and Grace Paulding Papers, Box 1, USMHI; Gilmour, *The Ruling Caste*, 295; Scott, *An Indian Journal*, 19, 34–35.
61. Rudyard Kipling, "Rikki-Tikki-Tavi," in his *The Jungle Book* (New York, 1894), 60.
62. Smith, *Clean*, 300.
63. Metcalf, *Ideologies of the Raj*, 177; Collingham, *Imperial Bodies*, 171.

64. Anderson, "Excremental Colonialism," 640–41.
65. Gustave Le Bon, *The Crowd: A Study of the Popular Mind* (London, 1903 [1895]), 19; Stephen Kern, *The Culture of Time and Space* (Cambridge, MA, 1983), 221–22.
66. Smith, *How Race Is Made*, 54.
67. Cohn, *Colonialism and Its Forms of Knowledge*, 10.
68. Wilson, *The Chaos of Empire*, 395.
69. Williams, *Odyssey*, 54.
70. On the last point, see Harold R. Isaacs, *Scratches on Our Minds: American Views of China and India* (New York, 1958), 101–04.
71. Macfarlane, *Daughters of Empire*, 125.
72. King, *Diary of a Civilian's Wife*, Vol. I, 26–27.
73. Johnson, *The influence of tropical climates*, 420–21.
74. Ghose, *Memsahibs Abroad*, 131; Gilmour, *The Ruling Caste*, 474; D. H. Biscoe Memoir, MSS Eur F226/3, Private Papers, IOR, BL.
75. Beeton Memoir.
76. Collingham, *Imperial Bodies*, 144.
77. Williams, *Odyssey*, 163; Anderson, *The Spell of the Hawaiian Islands*, 127; Grace Paulding Memoir.
78. A. G. Greenwood to W. H. Taft, February 25, 1902, Taft Papers, Reel 35.
79. W. H. Taft to H. C. Lodge, October 10, 1903, Taft Papers, Reel 40.
80. Conger, *An Ohio Woman*, 68; Sonnichsen, *Ten Months a Captive*, 88; McCallus, *Gentleman Soldier*, 85.
81. Juan Miciano, Ariston Bautista, Mariano Martin, and Manuel Gomez, "The Care of Infants," *Annual Report of the Commissioner of Public Health, September 1, 1903—August 31, 1904* (Manila, 1904), 269; Mrs. Samuel Francis Gaches, *Good Cooking and Health in the Tropics* (Manila, 1922), 334.
82. Grace Paulding Memoir.
83. Weston P. Chamberlain, "Observations on the Influence of the Philippine Climate on White Men of the Blond and of the Brunette Type," *Philippine Journal of Science* 6, no. 6 (December 1911), 427–66; H. D. Gibbs, "A Study of the Effect of Tropical Sunlight Upon Men, Monkeys, and Rabbits and a Discussion of the Proper Clothing for the Tropical Climate," *Philippine Journal of Science* 2B, no. 2 (April 1912), 91–114.
84. Hans Aron, "Investigation of the Action of the Tropical Sun on Men and Animals," *Philippine Journal of Science* 6, no. 2 (April 1911), 101–32.
85. William A. Cohen, "Introduction," in Cohen and Johnson, eds., *Filth*, ix.
86. Bushman and Bushman, "The Early History of Cleanliness in America," 1213–38.
87. McClintock, *Imperial Leather*, 214.
88. Buettner, *Empire Families*, 59.
89. Macfarlane, *Daughters of Empire*, 51.
90. Servando D. Halili Jr., *Iconography of the New Empire: Race and Gender Images in the American Colonization of the Philippines* (Manila, 2006), 61–63.
91. C. H. Brent letter to Edith, February 26, 1903, Brent Papers, Box 63.
92. Robert B. Minturn Jr., *From New York to Delhi by Way of Rio de Janeiro, Australia, and China* (New York, 1858), 105.
93. MacMillan, *Women of the Raj*, 7.
94. Evelyn Beeton Memoir, Beeton Papers, CSAS; Irene Bose, "Unwoven Carpet of Hindustan," Bose Papers, CSAS.
95. Hall, "Autobiography."
96. H. H. Risley, Secretary, Government of India, to multiple parties, August 21, 1905, *Proceedings of the Home Department—Sanitary*, August 1905, no. 299.
97. Conger, *An Ohio Woman*, 51.
98. Robert Carter to Father, September 28, 1899, in Shay, *A Civilian*, 154.
99. Karnow, *In Our Image*, 205.
100. George Telfer to Hazel, October 9, 1898, Bunnett, *Manila Envelopes*, 70.
101. Kasson, *Rudeness and Civility*, 142.
102. Stanley, *A Nation in the Making*, 202–03.

103. Forbes Journal, Vol. IV, May 4, 1910.
104. Bureau of Public Health, *Annual Report of the Commissioner of Public Health* [E. C. Carter], September 1, 1903–August 31, 1904 (Manila, 1905), 14.
105. Heiser, *American Doctor's Odyssey*, 35, 59, 111–13, 117, 201; Heiser, "Diary of leper-collecting trip beginning November 20, 1912," Heiser Papers, Series IV, Box 99.
106. Brown, Russell, and Cariño, *Health Through Knowledge and Habits*, 139–44; Fuller, *Housekeeping and Household Arts*, 51.
107. Edward J. Murphy to David Barrows, February 4 and August 21, 1909, Barrows Papers, Box 25.
108. Carol Hyde to her parents, December 12, 1932, Hyde Papers; J. L. H. Williams Memoir.
109. Taft, *Recollections*, 87, 145–46; Brown, *Foul Bodies*, 30.
110. If they wore underwear. In the United States, "gentlemen" apparently eschewed underwear during the summer, and some soldiers, whose access to underwear might be limited and who quickly soiled it, went without. C. Willett and Phillis Cunnington, *The History of Underclothes* (London, 1951), 131.
111. Alain Corbin, *Time, Desire, and Horror: Towards a History of the Senses*, transl. Jean Birrell (Cambridge, 1995), 14–16; Johnson, *The influence of tropical climates*, 423.
112. Platt, *Home and Health in India*, 58; Steel and Gardiner, *Complete Indian Housekeeper*, 208–09.
113. Wilson, *Hints for the First Years*, 12, Collingham, *Imperial Bodies*, 87.
114. W. H. Taft to The John Shillito Co., January 10, 1901, Taft Papers, Reel 31; Taft to Shillito, October 23, 1902, Taft Papers, Reel 37.
115. Shaun Cole, *The Story of Men's Underwear* (New York, 2010), 55.
116. "Have You Got Your Balbriggans On?" *Irish Times*, February 2, 2010; Daniel Delis Hill, *American Menswear: From the Civil War to the Twenty-First Century* (Lubbock, TX, 2011), 63–64, 99–100.
117. Telfer to Lottie, October 2, 1898, in Bunnett, *Manila Envelopes*, 58.
118. David Arnold, "Introduction: Disease, Medicine and Empire," in Arnold, ed., *Imperial Medicine and Indigenous Societies*, 3–6; De Bevoise, *Agents of Apocalypse*, 42.
119. Heiser, *American Doctor's Odyssey*, 34.
120. Arnold, "Introduction," 12; Weston P. Chamberlain, "The Study of Tropical Diseases in the Philippine Islands," *Journal of the American Medical Association* 58, no. 14 (1912), 998–1002.
121. Melosi, *Garbage in the Cities*, 21–22; and his *The Sanitary City*, 111; Major General Sir Leonard Rogers, "Climate and Disease Incidence in India. With Special Reference to Leprosy, Phthsis, Pneumonia and Small Pox," 1925, Rogers Collection, London School of Hygiene and Tropical Medicine, London.
122. Arnold, "Introduction," 7; Ramasubban, "Imperial Health in British India, 1857–1900," 55; Sanjoy Bhattacharya, Mark Harrison, and Michael Worboys, *Fractured States: Smallpox, Public Health, and Vaccination Policy in British India 1800–1947* (New Delhi, 2005), 76; *Report of the Commission*, Vol. IV, 32.
123. Metcalf, *Ideologies of the Raj*, 177.
124. Allen, *Plain Tales from the Raj*, 157.
125. Metcalf, *Ideologies of the Raj*, 177–78.
126. Kennedy, *Magic Mountains*, 29.
127. MacMillan, *Women of the Raj*, 83; Collingham, *Imperial Bodies*, 88.
128. Hibbert, *The Great Mutiny*, 28.
129. Wilson, *Hints for the First Years*, 15; Lady Chapman, "British India Recollected," Lady Chapman Papers, CSAS; Collingham, *Imperial Bodies*, 88.
130. Karnow, *In Our Image*, 211.
131. McKenna, *American Imperial Pastoral*, 157.
132. W. H. Taft to H. C. Lodge, June 14, 1903, Taft Papers, Reel 39.
133. Worcester, *The Philippines Past and Present*, 381–82.
134. Heiser, *American Doctor's Odyssey*, 75.
135. Benjamin Neal Diary, entry for August 28 [24], 1901, Neal Papers, Syracuse University Library.
136. Kennedy, *Magic Mountains*, 36.

137. Macfarlane, *Daughters of Empire*, 165.
138. Allen, *Plain Tales from the Raj*, 125.
139. Johnson, *The influence of tropical climates*, 26, 28.
140. Gilmour, *The Ruling Caste*, 81; Allen, *Plain Tales from the Raj*, 125; Heiser, "Diary of Leper-collecting Trip . . . November 20, 1912"; Platt, *Home and Health in India*, 146; Grace Paulding Memoir.
141. Biscoe Memoir; Sonnichsen, *Ten Months a Captive*, 235.
142. W. H. Taft to Jacob J. Schmidlapp, July 19, 1901, Taft Papers, Reel 33.
143. Copy of cable for newspapers, December 17, 1901, Taft Papers, Reel 34; W. H. Taft to Henry Hoyt, March 16, 1903, Taft Papers, Reel 38; Jonathan Lurie, *William Howard Taft: The Travails of a Progressive Conservative* (New York, 2012), 55; Taft, *Recollections*, 229, 234; Heiser, *American Doctor's Odyssey*, 49.
144. Sir Joseph Fayrer, *Tropical Dysentery and Chronic Diarrhea: Liver Abcess [sic]—Malarial Cachexia—Insolation of Other Forms of Tropical Disease* (London, 1881), 31, 34.
145. See, for example, Wilcox, *Through Luzon*, 59–60.
146. Victor G. Heiser, "Annual Report of the Bureau of Health for the Philippine Islands for the Fiscal Year Ended June 30, 1912" (Manila, 1913), 13.
147. Doeppers, *Feeding Manila in Peace and War*, 257.
148. W. H. Taft to Henry Hoyt, March 16, 1903, Taft Papers, Reel 38.
149. Kamya Raman and Anantanarayanan Raman, "Amoebic Dysentery and Introduction of Ementine Source *Carapichea ipecacuanha* in Indian Subcontinent," *Indian Journal of History of Science* 52, no. 1 (2017), 54–65.
150. De Bevoise, *Agents of Apocalypse*, 53.
151. James Stevens Simmons, Tom F. Whayne, Gaylord West Anderson, and Harold Maclachlan Horack, *Global Epidemiology: A Geography of Disease and Sanitation* (London, 1944), 118.
152. Helen Bynum, *Spitting Blood: The History of Tuberculosis* (Oxford, 2012), 110, 182.
153. Dr. C. Muthu, "Tuberculosis in India," *Proceedings of the First National Congress on Tuberculosis*, Manila, December 13–18, 1926 (Manila, 1927), 85.
154. Arnold, *Colonizing the Body*, 106–07.
155. Dr. Rodney H. True, "Betel Chewing," *Pharmaceutical Review* 14, no. 1 (January 1896), 130–33.
156. Kramer, *Blood of Government*, 103.
157. Dr. Leoncio Lopez-Rizal and Dr. Proceso Gabriel, "Some Factors in the Causation of Tuberculosis in the Philippines," *Proceedings of the First National Congress on Tuberculosis*, 132–34.
158. Ursula D. Donato, "Modern Health Crusade in Schools," *Proceedings of the First National Congress on Tuberculosis*, 553–55.
159. Emilia Lantin, "Care of a Tuberculosis in the Home," *Proceedings of the First National Congress on Tuberculosis*, 569–73.
160. Brown, Russell, and Cariño, *Health Through Knowledge and Habits*, 37–38.
161. Duffy, *The Sanitarians*, 200; Tomes, *Gospel of Germs*, 124; Fernando Calderon, "Tuberculosis in the Philippine Islands," *Proceedings of the First National Congress on Tuberculosis*, 36–37.
162. Arnold, *Colonizing the Body*, 200.
163. J. C. Perry, M. D., "Plague; Mode of Dissemination and Methods for Control," *Medical Record* 74, no. 9 (August 29, 1908), 345–51.
164. Arnold, *Colonizing the Body*, 203–04.
165. James, *Raj*, 357.
166. I. J. Catanach, "Plague and the Tensions of Empire," in Arnold, ed., *Imperial Medicine and Indigenous Societies*, 162.
167. "Report of the Indian Plague Commission," *Proceedings of the Home Department—Sanitary*, July 1900 (Calcutta, 1901), 14, 19–20, 42.
168. Catanach, "Plague and the Tensions of Empire," 162.
169. W. B. Bannerman to General [Home] Department, October 10, 1899, *Proceedings of the Home Department—Sanitary* (Calcutta, 1900), 31–33; J. K. Condon to the Secretary of the Government of India, Home Department, January 10, 1902, *Proceedings of the Home Department—Sanitary* (Calcutta, 1902), 615.

170. L. P. Shirres to the Secretary of the Government of India, Home Department, November 10, 1904, *Proceedings of the Home Department—Sanitary* (Calcutta, 1905), 413, and reply by J. C. Fergusson, March 14, 1905, 419.
171. "Report of the Indian Plague Commission," 16.
172. Ibid., 132.
173. J. L. H. Williams Memoir.
174. Arnold, *Colonizing the Body*, 221.
175. Catanach, "Plague and the Tensions of Empire," 160.
176. "Proceedings of the Hon'ble the Lieutenant-Governor of the Punjab in the Home (Medical and Sanitary) Department, March 9, 1904, in *Proceedings of the Home Department—Sanitary* (Calcutta, 1904), 770–74.
177. Heiser, *American Doctor's Odyssey*, 89, 91.
178. Anna Page Russell Maus, "Old Army Days: Reminiscences by the Wife of an Army Surgeon," Halstead-Maus Family Papers, USMHI.
179. "The Army's Fight with Plague and Cholera in Manila," *San Francisco Chronicle*, October 19, 1902.
180. W. H. Taft to John W. Harlan, May 19, 1901, Taft Papers, Reel 32; *Report of the Philippine Commission to the Secretary of War, 1907*, Part 2 (Washington, DC, 1908), 12.
181. David Arnold, "Smallpox and Colonial Medicine in Nineteenth-Century India," in Arnold, ed., *Imperial Medicine*, 46, 49.
182. Bhattacharya, Harrison, and Worboys, *Fractured States*, 2.
183. Donald R. Hopkins, *The Greatest Killer: Smallpox in History* (Chicago, 1983), 151.
184. Arnold, "Smallpox and Colonial Medicine," 47.
185. Bhattacharya, Harrison, and Worboys, *Fractured States*, 4.
186. Arnold, "Smallpox and Colonial Medicine," 49–56; Memorandum by the Army Sanitary Commission on the Report of the Sanitary Commissioner of Burma for 1897, June 9, 1899, *Proceedings of the Home Department—Sanitary* (Calcutta, 1900), 127.
187. Arnold, "Smallpox and Colonial Medicine," 60.
188. Memorandum by the Army Sanitary Commission on the Report of the Sanitary Commissioner of Bengal for 1898, May 29, 1900, *Proceedings of the Home Department—Sanitary* (Calcutta, 1902), 319; "Report on Vaccination in Burma for the period 1896–97 to 1898–99," August 1, 1899, ibid, 510.
189. Arnold, "Smallpox and Colonial Medicine," 58.
190. Bhatttacharya, Harrison, and Worboys, *Fractured States*, 16.
191. De Bevoise, *Agents of Apocalypse*, 102.
192. George D. DeShon to Dr. J. R. Furst, February 15, 1913, George D. DeShon Papers, Box 1, USMHI.
193. Maus, "Old Army Days."
194. De Bevoise, *Agents of Apocalypse*, 117.
195. Ibid, 116–17; Maus, "Old Army Days."
196. Heiser, "Unsolved Health Problems," 171–78.
197. Steel and Gardiner, *Complete Indian Housekeeper*, 171–72.
198. Quoted in Kumar, *Medicine and the Raj*, 177.
199. David Arnold, "Malaria and Race," in Ernst and Harris, eds., *Race, Science, and Medicine*, 125.
200. Ronald Ross, *Mosquito Brigades and How to Organise Them* (New York, 1902), 21.
201. Rohan Deb Roy, "Quinine, Mosquitoes and Empire: Reassembling Malaria in British India, 1890–1910," *South Asian History and Culture* 4, no. 1 (January 2013), 65–86.
202. De Bevoise, *Agents of Apocalypse*, 143, 156–57; Walter L. Cutter, "Wearing the Khaki: The Diary of a High Private," Cutter Papers, Box 1, USMHI.
203. *7th Annual Report of the Philippine Commission, 1906*, Part II (Washington, DC, 1907), 14.
204. Heiser, "Unsolved Health Problems," 172.
205. Anderson, *Colonial Pathologies*, 91, 94.
206. Mary Douglas, *Leviticus as Literature* (Oxford, 2000), 190.
207. Classen, *The Deepest Sense*, 57.

208. Rod Edmond, *Leprosy and Empire: A Medical and Cultural History* (Cambridge, 2006), 10, 19–20, 72–73; "The Leper Problem," *Times of India,* September 10, 1919. Leprosy is officially known as Hansen's Disease.
209. Robert Sinclair Black, "Remarks on Leprosy in Cape Colony," *The Lancet,* April 28, 1906, 1167–72; Arthur Newsholme, ed., *Public Health: The Journal of the Incorporated Society of Medical Officers of Health,* Vol. V, October, 1892 to September, 1893 (London, 1893), 377–78.
210. Jane Buckingham, *Leprosy in Colonial South India: Medicine and Confinement* (London, 2002), 15.
211. Zachary Gussow, *Leprosy, Racism, and Public Health: Social Policy in Chronic Disease Control* (Boulder, CO, 1989), 204, 217.
212. Buckingham, *Leprosy in Colonial South India,* 32, 35.
213. "The Indian Village From a Sanitation Point of View," *Times of India,* August 23, 1888.
214. *Medical Record,* April 7, 1900, 591. The Secretary of the British Leprosy Commission told Leonard Wood in 1924 the British "certainly have 300,000 lepers in India and probably a million." Wood Diary, entry for October 12, 1924, Box 22, Wood Papers.
215. Buckingham, *Leprosy in Colonial South India,* 7, 31, 61–3, 68, 79, 82, 88–94.
216. Ibid, 159, 163, 171, 180–87; Lt. General Sir Ernest Bradfield, "Unimportant Story," Bradfield Papers, CSAS.
217. L. P. Shirres, Secretary to the Government of Bengal, to the Secretary of the Government of India, Home Department, March 10, 1906, *Proceedings of the Home Department—Medical,* April 1906, nos. 15–21, 5; Report of the Superintendent of St. John's Leper Asylum, Mandalay, n.d. [1906], in ibid, 16.
218. Heiser, *American Doctor's Odyssey,* 227.
219. Mayo, *The Isles of Fear,* 169.
220. Dr. Arlington Pond, "Special Report on Sanitary Work in the City of Cebu," *Annual Report of the Commissioner of Public Health, September 1, 1903—August 31, 1904* (Manila, 1905), 213.
221. Warwick Anderson, "States of Hygiene: Race 'Improvement' and Biomedical Citizenship in Australia and the Colonial Philippines," in Stoler, ed., *Haunted By Empire,* 99; Heiser, *American Doctor's Odyssey,* 220.
222. Testimony of Jose Luis de Luzuriaga, September 11, 1899, *Report of the Commission,* Vol. II, 418; Grace Paulding Memoir.
223. Rizal, *Noli Me Tangere,* 182.
224. Brody, *Visualizing American Empire,* 69–71.
225. Gussow, *Leprosy, Racism, and Public Health,* 11, 56. Leprosaria were built on Penikese Island, Massachusetts, in 1905, and in Carville, Louisiana, after World War I.
226. Victor G. Heiser, "Sanitation in the Philippines: With Special Reference to its Effect Upon Other Tropical Countries," *Journal of Race Development* 3, no. 2 (October 1912), 127.
227. Ronald Fettes Chapman, *Leonard Wood and Leprosy in the Philippines: The Culion Leper Colony* (Lanham, MD, 1982), 7–8.
228. Brown, Russell, and Cariño, *Health Through Knowledge and Habits,* 305.
229. Anderson, "States of Hygiene," 100–01; Victor G. Heiser, "Fighting Leprosy in the Philippines," *The World's Work* (January 1916), 310–20.
230. Heiser, *American Doctor's Odyssey,* 236; Heiser, Memorandum of Leper-Collecting Trip, Culion, June 30, 1913, Series IV, Box 99, Heiser Papers.
231. Chapman, *Leonard Wood and Leprosy,* 14–15; Heiser, "Fighting Leprosy," 311.
232. John Parascandola, "Chaulmoogra Oil and the Treatment of Leprosy," *Pharmaceutical History* 45, no. 2 (2003), 47–57.
233. Victor G. Heiser, "Suppression of Leprosy in the Philippines," Lake Mohonk Conference, October 14–16, 1914, Series III, Box 65, Heiser Papers.
234. See, for example, Heiser, "Leper-Collecting Trips," Series IV, Box 99, 1912, entries for February 28, May 10, May 22, December 8, Heiser Papers.
235. Harry F. Hawley, "Reminiscences of Life in the Philippines with David P. Barrows," ND, Box 17, Barrows Papers.
236. See, for example, Heiser, "Leper-Collecting Trips," Series IV, Box 99, 1912, May 23, 26; Heiser, Memorandum of Leper Collecting Trip, Calapan, June 29, 1913.

237. Dr. Heiser's Diary, December 1932, Heiser Papers, Series V, Box 81, December 21.
238. G. C. Dunham, "Memorandum for the Governor-General," September 21, 1935, Frank Murphy Papers, Bentley Historical Library, University of Michigan (microfilm), Reel 101.
239. Heiser, *American Doctor's Odyssey*, 243; Dr. Heiser's Diary, Series IV, Box 98, May 5, 1928.
240. Chapman, *Leonard Wood and Leprosy*, 92, 95.
241. J. Weldon Jones, "Weekly Report—Miscellaneous Topics," for week ending October 11, 1936, Murphy Papers, Reel 106.
242. Chapman, *Leonard Wood and Leprosy*, 87.
243. Guy V. Henry Jr., "Brief Narrative of the Life of Guy V. Henry, Jr.," Henry Papers, Box 4, USMHI.
244. Hutchins, *Illusion of Permanence*, 45–46.
245. Gilmour, *The Ruling Caste*, 263; MacMillan, *Women of the Raj*, 51; James Elfers, *The Tours to End All Tours: The Story of Major League Baseball's 1913–1914 World Tour* (Lincoln, NE, 2003), 143–44.
246. Allen, *Plain Tales from the Raj*, 107.
247. Rajani Sudan, *The Alchemy of Empire: Abject Materials and the Technologies of Colonialism* (New York, 2016), 3.
248. Louise P. Brown, "The Philippine Embroidery Industry," *Manila Daily Bulletin*, Anniversary Number 1919, 72; Wilcox, *Through Luzon*, 164, 208; Kristen Hoganson, *Consumers' Imperium: The Global Production of American Domesticity, 1865–1920* (Chapel Hill, 2007), 95–96.
249. Beeton Memoir.
250. Hoyt, *Frontier Doctor*, 248; Buckland, *Land of the Filipino*, 135; Freer, *Philippine Experiences*, 209.
251. Taft, *Recollections*, 71.
252. Chota Mem," *The English Bride*, 34–35.
253. Allen, *Plain Tales from the Raj*, 158, 160.
254. Beeton Memoir.
255. MacMillan, *Women of the Raj*, 105.
256. Ibid, 138; Macfarlane, *Daughters of Empire*, 41; Platt, *Home and Health in India*, 84; Roy, *Alimentary Tracts*, 15.
257. Kenneth Ballhatchet, *Race, Sex, and Class under the Raj: Imperial Attitudes and Policies and their Critics, 1793–1905* (New York, 1980), 10; Arnold, *Colonizing the Body*, 85; D. H. Biscoe Memoir, MSS Eur F226/3, Private Papers, IOR, BL.
258. Collingham, *Imperial Bodies*, 32; testimony of Dr. Barker, *Report of the Philippine Commission*, Vol. II, 235.
259. Johnson, *The influence of tropical climates*, 479.
260. Nandy, *The Intimate Enemy*, 10.
261. James, *Raj*, 218.
262. J. L. H. Williams Memoir.
263. Allen, *Plain Tales from the Raj*, 23.
264. Ibid., 31, 65.
265. Levine, *Prostitution, Race, and Politics*, 7.
266. Ballhatchet, *Race, Sex, and Class*, 44; Elizabeth B. Van Heyningen, "The Social Evil in the Cape Colony 1868–1902: Prostitution and the Contagious Diseases Acts," *Journal of Southern African Studies* 10, no. 2 (April 1984), 170–97.
267. Biscoe Memoir.
268. J. L. H. Williams Memoir.
269. Testimony of Dr. Barker, *Report of the Philippine Commission*, 235.
270. De Bevoise, *Agents of Apocalypse*, 85–86.
271. Kramer, "The Darkness that Enters the Home," 373.
272. De Bevoise, *Agents of Apocalypse*, 88; Charles Everett MacDonald, "Memo of Life of Charles Everett MacDonald," MacDonald Papers, Box 1, USMHI; Wood Diary, entry for August 24, 1924, Box 22.

273. W. H. Taft to the Secretary of War, January 17, 1901, Taft Papers, Reel 32; W. H. Taft to Dr. David D. Thompson, April 12, 1902, Taft Papers, Reel 35; Devins, *An Observer in the Philippines*, 179.
274. Pronouncement of Maj. Gen. Chaffee, 1901, Taft Papers, Reel 33.
275. Reynaldo C. Ileto, "The Philippine-American War: Friendship and Forgetting," in Shaw and Francia, eds., *Vestiges of War*, 15–16.
276. Wood Diary, entry for August 13, 1924, Box 22; "JIN" to L. R. Wilfley, n.d., Taft Papers, Reel 36; Alfred W. McCoy, *Policing America's Empire: The United States, the Philippines, and the Rise of the Surveillance State* (Madison, WI, 2009), 113.
277. De Bevoise, *Agents of Apocalypse*, 43. Americans who married Filipinas and stayed on in the islands were known derogatorily as "squawmen"; see Friend, *Between Two Empires*, 36.
278. Cannell, *Power and Intimacy*, 99.
279. Hilda Bourne, "It Was Like This," J. M. Bourne Papers, CSAS.
280. R. C. C. Hunt, "Innocents in India," R. C. C. Hunt Papers, CSAS.
281. Reheja, "Caste, Colonialism, and Speech of the Colonized," 499.
282. Lopez-Rizal and Gabriel, "Some Factors," 132.
283. De Bevoise, *Agents of Apocalypse*, 95–96; Worcester, *The Philippines Past and Present*, 330.
284. Stephen Tyler, *India: An Anthropological Perspective* (Prospect Heights, IL, 1986), 129–38; Devins, *An Observer in the Philippines*, 125.
285. Calderon, "Obstetrics in the Philippine Islands," 255–56.
286. Mridula Ramanna, "Perceptions of Sanitation and Medicine in Bombay, 1900–1914," in Fischer-Tiné and Mann, *Colonialism as Civilizing Mission*, 221.
287. Memorandum by the Army Sanitary Commission on the Report of the Sanitary Commissioner of Burma for 1898, May 25, 1900," *Proceedings of the Home Department—Sanitary* (Calcutta, 1902), 335–36.
288. Quoted in Kumar, *Medicine and the Raj*, 197.
289. J. L. H. Williams Memoir.
290. Clements, "Medical Survey of the Town of Taytay," 254. See also Ileto, "Cholera and the Origins," 67; Buckland, *Land of the Filipino*, 237–38.
291. Arnold, *Colonizing the Body*, 6; Kumar, *Medicine and the Raj*, 68; Deepak Kumar, "Unequal Contenders, Uneven Ground: Medical Encounters with British India, 1820–1920," in Cunningham and Andrews, eds., *Western Medicine as Contested Knowledge*, 176.
292. Scriven, "An American in Bohol."
293. Scott, *An Indian Journal*, 114–15.
294. King, *Diary of a Civilian's Wife*, Vol. I, 81–82.
295. E. Valentine Daniel, "The Pulse as an Icon in Siddha Medicine," in Howes, ed., *The Varieties of Sensory Experience*, 100–01.
296. Madhuri Sharma, "Knowing Health and Medicine: A Case Study of Benares, c. 1900–1950," in Kumar and Basu, eds., *Medical Encounters in British India*, 169.
297. Arnold, *Colonizing the Body*, 211, 219, 284.
298. Wagner, *The Great Fear of 1857*, 65.
299. J. L. H. Williams Memoir.
300. Ramanna, "Perceptions of Sanitation and Medicine," 211.
301. Bhattacharya, Harrison, and Worboys, *Fractured States*, 27, 210, 221; Sharma, "Knowing Health and Medicine," 171.
302. James, *Raj*, 424, 524.
303. Memorandum by the Army Sanitary Commission on the Report of the Sanitary Commissioner of Bombay for 1898, May 25, 1900, in *Proceedings of the Home Department—Sanitary* (Calcutta, 1902), 361.
304. Mariano Crisóstomo to W. H. Taft, December 18, 1901, Taft Papers, Reel 34.
305. Worcester, *The Philippines Past and Present*, 278–79.
306. Cannell, *Power and Intimacy*, 81.
307. Heiser, *Annual Report of the Bureau of Health for the Philippine Islands, July 1, 1908—June 30, 1909*, 39–40.

308. Gerald D. Berreman, "Stratification, Pluralism and Interaction: A Comparative Analysis of Caste," in de Reuck and Knight, eds., *Ciba Foundation Symposium on Caste and Race*, 45–73; Tyler, *India*, 147–48.
309. Complaint of the Anglo-Indian Association, Calcutta, Against the Working of Disinfection Rules at Bombay and Ceylon Ports, August 12, 1902, *Proceedings of the Home Department—Sanitary* (Calcutta, 1903), 665.
310. Rules concerning inspection for plague, *Proceedings of the Home Department—Sanitary* (Calcutta, 1904), 813.
311. Bhattacharya, Harrison, and Worboys, *Fractured States*, 65.
312. MacMillan, *Women of the Raj*, 8; Collingham, *Imperial Bodies*, 177.
313. C. E. Tyndale-Biscoe, "The Imperial Touch: Schooling Male Bodies in Colonial India, Part I," in Classen, ed., *The Book of Touch*, 168–69.
314. Freer, *Philippine Experiences*, 198.
315. Conger, *An Ohio Woman*, 115.
316. Julian Go, *American Empire and the Politics of Meaning: Elite Political Cultures in the Philippines and Puerto Rico during U.S. Colonialism* (Durham, NC, 2008), 201.
317. Moses, *Unofficial Letters*, 72.
318. Forbes Journal, Vol. II, n.d. [early 1910].
319. Col. Van Schaik's Journal, April 12, 1932, Theodore Roosevelt Jr., Papers, Box 17, Private Papers, MD, LC.
320. Moses, *Unofficial Letters*, 89–90, 191.

Chapter 7

1. Quoted in Roy, *Alimentary Tracts*, 69.
2. Sidney W. Mintz, *Tasting Food, Tasting Freedom: Excursions into Eating, Culture, and the Past* (Boston, 1996), 48, 67.
3. Lisa Heldke, "But Is It Authentic? Culinary Travel and the Search for the Genuine Article," in Korsmeyer, ed., *Taste Culture Reader*, 386. Of durian, one British correspondent in Burma wrote: "If one is brought into a room the whole house will smell of it for many hours afterwards, and anybody who has partaken of it can be recognized at once as having done so if he goes to another house." "The Smells of Burma," *Times of India*, June 28, 1919.
4. Donna R. Gabaccia, *We Are What We Eat: Ethnic Food and the Making of Americans* (Cambridge, MA, 1998), 6.
5. Deborah Lupton, "Food and Emotion," in Korsmeyer, ed., *Taste Culture Reader*, 322–23; Hoganson, *Consumers' Imperium*, 125.
6. Harriet Martineau, *British Rule in India: A Historical Sketch* (London, 1857), 228; Kramer, *Blood of Government*, 207; Vergara, *Displaying Filipinos*, 19.
7. Quoted in De Viana, *The I Stories*, 116.
8. See, for example,Mark Padoongpatt, "Food and Empire," in Wise and Wallach, eds., *The Routledge History of American Foodways*, 353–69.
9. Sidney W. Mintz, *Sweetness and Power: The Place of Sugar in Modern History* (New York, 1985).
10. Smith, *Sensing the Past*, 82.
11. Arnold, *The Tropics and the Traveling Gaze*, 143; Allen, *Plain Tales from the Raj*, 150; Macmillan, *Women of the Raj*, 161–63; Helen Pike Bauer, "Eating in the Contact Zone: Food and Identity in Anglo-India," in Wagner and Hasan, eds., *Consuming Culture in the Long Nineteenth Century*, 101.
12. Margaret Visser, *Much Depends on Dinner: The Extraordinary History and Mythology, Allure and Obsessions, Perils and Taboos of the Ordinary Meal* (New York, 1986), 222.
13. Collingham, *Curry*, 176.
14. Rachel Laudan, *Cuisine and Empire: Cooking in World History* (Berkeley, 2013), 263.
15. Conger, *An Ohio Woman*, 83; Robert Carter to his mother, August 16, 1899, Shay, *A Civilian*, 132; Gabaccia, *We Are What We Eat*.
16. Sumangala Bhattacharya, "Badly Boiled Potatoes and Other Crises," in Wagner and Hasan, eds., *Consuming Culture*, 3–7.

17. Johnson, *The influence of tropical climates*, 314–15, 433, 440, 442; David Arnold, "Dietetics, Mimesis, and Alterity: Food in Asian Medical Traditions and East-West Exchanges," in Kumar and Basu, eds., *Medical Encounters in British India*, 86.
18. Collingham, *Curry*, 89, 110.
19. Allen, *Plain Tales from the Raj*, 56.
20. David Burton, *The Raj at Table: A Culinary History of the British in India* (London, 1993), 3.
21. William Makepeace Thackeray, *Vanity Fair* (New York, 1994 [1848]), 29.
22. Collingham, *Curry*, 85; Arnold, *Tropics and the Traveling Gaze*, 144.
23. Jayanta Sengupta, "Nation on a Platter: The Culture and Politics of Food and Cuisine in Colonial Bengal," in Ray and Srinivas, eds., *Curried Cultures*, 77; Hutchins, *Illusion of Permanence*, 63–64.
24. Allen, *Plain Tales from the Raj*, 150.
25. Collingham, *Curry*, 158–59.
26. "Wyvern" (Colonel Arthur Robert Kenney-Herbert), *Culinary Jottings for Madras* (Totnes, UK, 2007 [1885]), 1.
27. "India," *Times of London*, December 22, 1858.
28. Quoted in Arnold, *Tropics and the Traveling Gaze*, 144.
29. Collingham, *Curry*, 163–64; Hibbert, *The Great Mutiny*, 29.
30. Allen, *Plain Tales from the Raj*, 91; Mary Chenevix Trench, "A Child's Experience of Gilgit, 1934–37," Mary Chenevix Trench Papers, MSS Eur F226/33, Private Papers, IOR, BL, London; Ghose, *Memsahibs Abroad*, 240; Atkinson, *Curry and Rice*, 147.
31. Anne Bremner Memoir, Bremner Papers, MSS Eur 226/4, Private Papers, IOR, BL; H. D. H. Rance Memoir, Rance Papers, MSS Eur F226/23, Private Papers, IOR, BL.
32. Carol Hyde to her parents, December 20, 1932, Hyde Papers, CSAS.
33. Steel and Gardiner, *Complete Indian Housekeeper*, 55.
34. Hilda Bourne, "It Was Like This," J. M. Bourne Papers, CSAS.
35. J. L. H. Williams Memoir, Williams Papers, MSS Eur C796/12, Private Papers, IOR, BL.
36. Collingham, *Curry*, 173–74.
37. Atkinson, *Curry and Rice*, 112, 118.
38. Evelyn Beeton Memoir, Beeton Papers, CSAS.
39. Lady Chapman, "British India Recollected," Chapman Papers, CSAS.
40. Collingham, *Curry*, 202.
41. Steel and Gardiner, *Complete Indian Housekeeper*, 11, 14, 78–79, 223–25.
42. "Chota Mem," *The English Bride in India*, 40.
43. Atkinson, *Curry and Rice*, 129.
44. Ghose, *Memsahibs Abroad*, 127.
45. Allen, *Plain Tales from the Raj*, 125; Margery Hall, "Autobiography: 'And the Nights Were More Terrible Than the Days,'" Margery Hall Papers, MSS Eur F226/11, Private Papers, IOR, BL.
46. Gilmour, *The Ruling Caste*, 107.
47. Burton, *The Raj at Table*, 61.
48. Marryat quoted in Ghose, *Memsahibs Abroad*, 237.
49. Macmillan, *Women of the Raj*, 128.
50. Macfarlane, *Daughters of Empire*, 112.
51. Buettner, *Empire Families*, 52.
52. Mrs. M. E. (Mary) Gueritz Memoir, MSS Eur 226/9, Private Papers, IOR, BL; Ernest Walter Saxton to Rose Sophia Goldswain, n.d. [1896], MSS Eur B261, Private Papers, IOR, BL.
53. Collingham, *Curry*, 170.
54. E. M. Forster, *Passage to India* (London, 1924), 48–49.
55. Macmillan, *Women of the Raj*, 147.
56. Burton, *The Raj at Table*, 40.
57. Collingham, *Imperial Bodies*, 70; Gilmour, *The Ruling Caste*, 299–300.
58. King, *Diary of a Civilian's Wife in India*, Vol. I, 164.
59. Ibid., 33–34.
60. K. T. Achaya, *Indian Food: A Historical Companion* (Delhi, 1994), 177–78.
61. Burton, *The Raj at Table*, 27–28.

62. Bourne, "It Was Like This."
63. Collingham, *Imperial Bodies*, 72.
64. "Chota Mem," *The English Bride*, 14–16; Bauer, "Eating in the Contact Zone," 96–97, 101.
65. Burton, *The Raj at Table*, 27–28. See also Collingham, *Imperial Bodies*, 68–69.
66. Kasson, *Rudeness and Civility*, 186.
67. Ibid., 200.
68. Ibid., 182, 193, 208–09.
69. Duffy, *The Sanitarians*, 208.
70. Hoyt, *Frontier Doctor*, 205; George Telfer to "Daughter Grace," July 18, 1898, Telfer to Lottie [his wife], August 27, 1898, in Bunnett, *Manila Envelopes*, 30, 43; Ernest R. Tilton to Julia S. Tilton, March 16, 1900, Rollin N. Tilton Papers, Box 43, USMHI. While the British spoke of food as "tinned," Americans preferred to call it "canned."
71. Robert Carter to his father, March 23, 1899, in Shay, *A Civilian*, 47.
72. Anderson, *Colonial Pathologies*, 43.
73. Dawn Bohulano Mabalon, "As American as Jackrabbit Adobo: Cooking, Eating, and Becoming Filipina/o American before World War II," in Ji-Song Ku, Manalansan IV, and Mannur, eds., *Eating Asian America*, 149.
74. René Alexander Orquiza Jr., "*Lechon* with Heinz, Lea & Perrins with *Adobo*," in Ku, Manalansan, and Mannur, eds., *Eating Asian America*, 178.
75. Worcester, *The Philippines Past and Present*, 281.
76. Ruth Meyer to her mother, March 24, 1920, in Meyer, *Letters Home*, 124; Freer, *Philippine Experiences*, 62.
77. Conger, *An Ohio Woman*, 96–97; Freer, *Philippine Experiences*, 62.
78. Freer, *Philippine Experiences*, 204–05; William Cameron Forbes Journal, Vol. III, entry for December 29, 1909, William Cameron Forbes Papers, Harvard University Library.
79. Dr. Charles MacDonald, "With the U.S. Troops to the Philippines," lecture to the Salem, NJ, Grange, *Salem Sunbeam*, June 9, 1911, Charles E. MacDonald Papers, Box 1, USMHI.
80. Charles H. Brent Diary, 1903, entries for January 28, April 29, and May 8, Box 1, Brent Papers, MD, LC, Washington, DC.
81. Heiser, *American Doctor's Odyssey*, 138; Mayo, *Isles of Fear*, 270–71; Kramer, *Blood of Government*, 266.
82. Letters from Fred W. Atkinson, Mr. Tompkins, Sydney Hopson, and R. J. Fanning to W. H. Taft, in memo "The Commissary Privilege," nd [late 1901], William Howard Taft Papers (microfilm), Reel 34, Cornell University Library.
83. Benjamin E. Neal Diary, entry for October 18, 1901, Box 1, Neal Papers, Syracuse University Library.
84. Freer, *Philippine Experiences*, 50.
85. Woods Hutchinson, "Some Diet Delusions," *McClure's Magazine* 26, no. 6 (April 1906), 620.
86. H. E. Barber to the Acting Civil Governor [Luke Wright], February 21, 1902, Taft Papers, Reel 30.
87. George Telfer to Lottie, August 27, 1898, in Bunnett, *Manila Envelopes*, 44. Rations received by US soldiers in Puerto Rico in 1898 were described by a medical officer as having "an odor similar to that of a dead human body after being injected with preservatives." Quoted in Adam D. Shprintzen, "The Nineteenth Century," in Wise and Wallach, eds., *Routledge History of American Foodways*, 43–44.
88. Robert Carter to his mother, September 19, 1899, in Shay, *A Civilian*, 144.
89. W. H. Taft to Col. O. F. Long, January 9, 1901, Taft Papers, Reel 31; Fred W. Carpenter to Caldbeck, Macgregor, and Co., August 3, 1901, Taft Papers, Reel 33.
90. Menu, September 8, 1902, Taft Papers, Reel 35.
91. Orquiza, "*Lechon* with Heinz," 178.
92. Craig and Craig, *Farthest Westing*, 90; Roosevelt, *The Philippines*, 234.
93. Conger, *An Ohio Woman*, 98; Sonnichsen, *Ten Months a Captive*, 91.
94. Moses, *Unofficial Letters*, 118.
95. Robert Carter to father, March 23, 1899; to father, August 1, 1899; to mother, August 16, 1899; to father, September 20, 1899; in Shay, *A Civilian*, 41, 118–19, 132, 148.
96. Williams, *Odyssey*, 56.

97. Conger, *An Ohio Woman*, 56, 75, 83.
98. Heiser, *American Doctor's Odyssey*, 112–13.
99. Victor C. Heiser, "Diary of Leper-collecitng Trip," 1912, entry for May 18, Victor C. Heiser Papers, Box 99, APS.
100. Frank C. Laubach, "Notes taken in the Dansalan Market," September 25, 1933, Frank C. Laubach Papers, Box 130, Syracuse University Library.
101. Moses, *Unofficial Letters*, 224.
102. Robert Carter to mother, September 19, 1899, in Shay, *A Civilian*, 144; Kramer, *Blood of Government*, 395; *Philippines Herald*, May 8, 1934.
103. Sonnichsen, *Ten Months a Captive*, 58; C. H. Brent letter to Edith Brent, March 21, 1903, Brent Papers, Box 63.
104. Freer, *Philippine Experiences*, 59.
105. Ruth H. B. Hunt Travel Diaries, entry for March 12, 1929, Hunt Papers, Box 1, Syracuse University Library.
106. Moses, *Unofficial Letters*, 317.
107. Buckland, *Land of the Filipino*, 55–56, 64–66.
108. Burton, *The Raj at Table*, 34.
109. Tracey Rizzo and Steven Gerontakis, *Intimate Empires: Body, Race, and Gender in the Modern World* (New York, 2017), 163. India subsequently became Osler's largest market outside of Britain, selling glass, crockery, and kerosene and electric lights. See *Thomas Cook's Oriental Travellers' Guide*, January 1892, 4; Arun Chaudhuri, *Indian Advertising 1780 to 1950 A. D.* (New Delhi, 2007), 122.
110. Angma D. Jhala, "Cosmopolitan Kitchens: Cooking for Princely Zenanas in Late Colonial India," in Srinivas and Ray, *Curried Cultures*, 67.
111. Steel and Gardiner, *Complete Indian Housekeeper*, 162.
112. Wilson, *The Chaos of Empire*, 318.
113. Amartya Sen, "Public Action to Remedy Hunger," Arturo Tanco Memorial Lecture, London, August 2, 1990; Mike Davis, *Late Victorian Holocausts: El Niño Famines and the Making of the Third World* (London, 2001), 299, 332–34, 338.
114. David Arnold, *Famine: Social Crisis and Historical Change* (Oxford, 1988), 132.
115. King, *Diary of a Civilian's Wife*, Vol. I, 101.
116. MacMillan, *Women of the Raj*, 231.
117. Linn, *Philippine War*, 302, 310.
118. Leonard Wood Diary, January 1–December 31, 1925, entry for January 1, Leonard Wood Papers, Box 23, MD, LC; Heiser, *American Doctor's Odyssey*, 206; Government of the Philippine Islands, *Elementary Home Economics: A Textbook for Girls in the Intermediate Schools of the Philippine Islands* (Manila, 1925), 42.
119. Worcester, *The Philippines Past and Present*, 356.
120. "Manila's Pioneer Pure Food Establishment," *Philippine Magazine* (October 1908), 78.
121. Orquiza, "*Lechon* with Heinz," 178–79.
122. Fuller, *Housekeeping and Household Arts*, 48.
123. Wood Diary, January 1–December 31, 1926, May 3, Box 23.
124. Alice Magoon, "Domestic Science," *Philippine Teacher* II, no. 2 (July 1905), 23.
125. Government of the Philippine Islands, *School and Home Gardening: A Manual for Teachers of Gardening in the Elementary Schools* (Manila, 1931), 184–85.
126. L. F. Brown to W. H. Taft, July 5, 1901; Taft to Brown, September 20, 1901, Taft Papers, Reel 33.
127. Heiser, *American Doctor's Odyssey*, 117.
128. *Elementary Home Economics*, 38–39.
129. Brown, Russell, and Cariño, *Health Through Knowledge and Habits*, 219, 228–31.
130. Jack Goody, "The High and the Low: Culinary Culture in Asia and Europe," in Korsmeyer, ed., *Taste Culture Reader*, 64.
131. Achaya, *Indian Food*, 61.
132. The gods were offered food through their stone or wood manifestations, but, as a priest told John Scott, "the god only smells" the food "We eat it." Scott, *An Indian Journal*, 85.
133. Eck, *Darśan*.

134. Sylvain Pinard, "A Taste of India: On the Role of Gustation in the Hindu Sensorium," in Howes, ed., *The Varieties of Sensory Experience*, 224.
135. Goody, "The High and the Low," 64.
136. David Arnold, "Dietetics, Mimesis," 89, 93.
137. Bhattacharya, Harrison, and Worboys, *Fractured States*, 148–49.
138. Pinard, "A Taste of India," 222.
139. B. N. Goswamy, "*Rasa*: Delight of the Reason," in Korsmeyer, ed., *Taste Culture Reader*, 216–19.
140. R. S. Khare, *The Hindu Hearth and Home* (Delhi, 1976), 44, 54, 83, 96, 98, 26; Achaya, *Indian Food*, 63–64; Roy, *Alimentary Tracts*, 62; Arjun Appadurai, "How to Make a National Cuisine: Cookbooks in Contemporary India," *Comparative Studies in Society and History* 30, no. 1 (January 1988), 10–11.
141. Rudolph and Rudolph, *Reversing the Gaze*, 236.
142. Scott, *An Indian Journal*, 157.
143. Monier Williams, "A Traveller's Impression of India," *Times of London*, April 17, 1874.
144. Quoted in Bauer, "Eating in the Contact Zone," 103.
145. Jhala, "Cosmopolitan Kitchens," 52.
146. King, *Diary of a Civilian's Wife*, Vol. I, 35–36.
147. Burton, *The Raj at Table*, viii; "The New India: Eastwards or Westwards?" *Times of London*, May 9, 1924.
148. Allen, *Plain Tales from the Raj*, 202.
149. Collingham, *Curry*, 230.
150. Irene Bose, "Unwoven Carpet of Hindustan," Bose Papers, Box 1, CSAS.
151. Hussain, *Hints on Indian Etiquette*, 26–27.
152. Collingham, *Curry*, 19.
153. James, *Raj*, 252.
154. Quoted in Sen, *Feasts and Fasts*, 223.
155. Sengupta, "Nation on a Platter," 79.
156. M. K. Gandhi, *Gandhi's Autobiography: The Story of My Experiments with Truth* Transl. Mahadev Desai. (Washington, DC, 1948), 55–56, 67, 256–60; Roy, *Alimentary Tracts*, 80–81, 95; Sengupta, "Nation on a Platter," 83–86.
157. Doreen G. Fernandez, "Food and War," in Shaw and Francia, eds., *Vestiges of War*, 237.
158. Go, *American Empire*, 127.
159. Doeppers, *Feeding Manila in Peace and War*, 291.
160. Karnow, *In Our Image*, 246.
161. Rosa Balunsat, "Nursing Tuberculosis Patients in a Sanatorium," *Proceedings of the First National Congress on Tuberculosis, Manila, December 13–18, 1926* (Manila, 1927), 576.
162. Doeppers, *Feeding Manila in Peace and War*, 125–27, 135, 158, 189, 266, 279.
163. Cannell, *Power and Intimacy*, 20.
164. Heiser, *American Doctor's Odyssey*, 143.
165. Ibid., 138.
166. Quoted in Arnold Molina Azurin, *Reinventing the Filipino Sense of Being and Becoming: Critical Analyses of the Orthodox Views in Anthropology, History, Folklore and Letters* (Quezon City, 1995), 25.
167. Padoongpatt, "Food and Empire," 358.
168. Wolfgang Schivelbusch, "Spices: Tastes of Paradise," in Korsmeyer, ed., *Taste Culture Reader*, 128.
169. Akhil Gupta, "A Different History of the Present: The Movement of Crops, Cuisine, and Globalization," in Srinivas and Ray, *Curried Cultures*, 41
170. Burton, *The Raj at Table*, 1–4.
171. Sen, *Feasts and Fasts*, 218.
172. Gabaccia, *We Are What We Eat*, 10–11.
173. Bhattacharya, "Badly Boiled Potatoes," 3, 6–7.
174. Richard Terry, *Indian Cookery* (London, 2011 [1861]).
175. James, *Raj*, 518.

176. Sen, *Feasts and Fasts*, 228.
177. Bourne, "It Was Like This."
178. Collingham, *Curry*, 182; Lady Reynolds Memoir, MSS Eur F226/25, Private Papers, IOR, BL.
179. Burton, *The Raj at Table*, 45.
180. Hoganson, *Consumers Imperium*, 211.
181. Gabaccia, *We Are What We Eat*, 65–67, 227.
182. Sonnichsen, *Ten Months a Captive*, 91.
183. Scriven, "An American in Bohol."
184. Wilcox, *Through Luzon*, 122.
185. Williams, *Odyssey*, 106.
186. Fee, *A Woman's Impressions*, 50; Moses, *Unofficial Letters*, 23.
187. Wood Diary, May 1–June 25, 1921, May 18, May 23, Box 19.
188. Taft, *Recollections*, 257–58.
189. Anderson, *The Spell of the Hawaiian Islands*, 249.
190. Moses, *Unofficial Letters*, 147.
191. Halili, *Iconography of the New Empire*.
192. Craig and Craig, *Farthest Westing*, 24.
193. Laudan, *Cuisine and Empire*, 193.
194. Mabalon, "As American as Jackrabbit Adobo," 150.
195. Freer, *Philippine Experiences*, 29–30, 77.
196. Forbes Journal, Vol. II.
197. Williams, *Odyssey*, 148.
198. Kramer, *Blood of Government*, 188.
199. Moses, *Unofficial Letters*, 65, 79, 171.
200. Ibid., 132–33.
201. Mary Douglas, *Implicit Meanings: Essays in Anthropology* (London, 1975), 255.
202. Gabaccia, *We Are What We Eat*, 271.

Conclusion

1. Mary Chenevix Trench memoir, Mary Chenevix Trench Papers, MS Eur F226/33, Private Papers, IOR, BL.
2. Allen, *Plain Tales from the Raj*, 225; Erica Farquharson, "Indian Idyll," J. M. Bourne Papers, CSAS.
3. Collingham, *Imperial Bodies*, 201.
4. Bernard Norling, *The Intrepid Guerrillas of North Luzon* (Lexington, KY, 1999); R. W. Volckmann, *We Remained: Three Years Behind the Enemy Lines in the Philippines* (New York, 1954), 52–55.
5. Benito J. Legarda Jr., *Occupation: The Later Years* (Quezon City, 2007), 59.
6. Karnow, *In Our Image*, 322, 327.
7. Anand A. Yang, *The Limited Raj: Agrarian Relations in Colonial India, Saran District, 1793–1920* (Berkeley, 1989), 6.
8. Moon, *British Conquest*, 668–69.
9. Wilson, *The Chaos of Empire*, 398–403, 422; Metcalf, *Ideologies of the Raj* 225–26; Visram, *Ayahs, Lascars and Princes*, 114–39; Moon, *British Conquest*, 982–85.
10. Cavaliero, *Strangers in the Land*, 208.
11. Ibid., 214.
12. Wilson, *Chaos of Empire*, 450.
13. Cavaliero, *Strangers in the Land*, 211.
14. James, *Raj*, 567.
15. Scott, *An Indian Journal*, 78–79.
16. James, *Raj*, 597.
17. Karnow, *In Our Image*, 241–45; H. W. Brands, *Bound to Empire: The United States and the Philippines* (New York, 1992), 112–16; Frank Hindman Gorlay, *Face of Empire: United States-Philippine Relations, 1898–1946* (Madison, WI, 1998), 201–03.

18. Stanley, *A Nation in the Making*, 259–60; Leonard Wood to Sergio Osmeña, December 6, 1921, Leonard Wood Diary, Vol. I, January 1–June 30, 1922, Leonard Wood Papers, Box 19, MD, LC.
19. Karnow, *In Our Image*, 254–56; Brands, *Bound to Empire*, 154–57; Memorandum for the Governor-General by J. R. Hughes, January 22, 1934, and "By the Governor-General of the Philippine Islands—A Proclamation," June 14, 1935; both Frank Murphy Papers, Bentley Historical Library, University of Michigan (microfilm), Reel 99; George H. Dern to the President, November 23, 1935, BIA, General Records Relating to More Than One Island Possession, Confidential File, 1914–1935, Box 1, [R]ecord [G]roup 350, NAII.
20. Wolfgang Schivelbusch, "The Railway Journey: Panoramic Travel," in Edwards and Bhaumik, eds., *Visual Sense* , 287-95.
21. Karnow, *In Our Image*, 211–12; Paulino Santos to Governor-General Murphy, October 29, 1934, Murphy Papers, Reel 99.
22. MacMillan, *Women of the Raj*, 229.
23. *Graphic*, November 28, 1935.
24. Mrs. E. Tollinton Memoir, Tollinton Papers, MSS Eur F226/31, Private Papers, IOR, BL.
25. H. Otley Beyer, "Social and Racial Unity of the Philippines," November 1936, Murphy Papers, Reel 102.
26. "Message of His Excellency, Governor-General Frank Murphy to the Philippine Legislature in its Final Session, November 14, 1935, Murphy Papers, Reel 103.
27. Abinales, "Progressive-Machine Conflict in Early-Twentieth-Century U.S. Politics," 171.
28. Trench memoir; R. A. Duckworth-Ford to Nicholas Roosevelt, September 27, 1930, Nicholas Roosevelt Papers, Box 10, Syracuse University Library.
29. Trench memoir; untitled paper by Frank Murphy, n.d. [1934], Murphy Papers, Reel 98. Brass bands in India soon evolved from their service to military units or status symbols for the princes into essential performers at weddings. On the morning of the wedding day, they raucously accompany the groom to the bride's house. See Venus Upadhyaya, "How Indians Have Turned British Military Bands into Indian Wedding Bands," *The Epoch Times*, January 7, 2015.
30. William Cameron Forbes Journal, entry for September 17, 1904, Forbes Papers, Harvard University Library.
31. Alasdair Pinkerton, "Radio and the Raj: Broadcasting in British India (1920–1940)," *Journal of the Royal Asiatic Society* Series 3, 18, no. 2 (2008), 167–91. The widespread use of radios by all classes by the mid-1940s could mean increased noise, as Indian elites defined it. A letter to the *Times of India* complained that "it has become a fashion in Poona amongst restaurant keepers to open their wireless sets at the highest pitch and to multiply the noise by the help of loudspeakers. This nuisance has become a menace to the people in the vicinity." The letter was signed, "TORTURED." *Times of India*, February 22, 1946.
32. Untitled paper by Murphy; Anderson, *The Philippine Problem*, 315–16.
33. Concert program, September 21, 1934, Murphy Papers, Reel 99.
34. Sarvepalli Gopal, "The English Language in India since Independence, and its Future Role," Twelfth Jawaharlal Nehru Memorial Lecture, Cambridge, November 3, 1988.
35. Manuel L. Carreon, *Philippine Studies in Mental Measurement* (Yonkers, NY, 1926).
36. Murphy to Philippine Legislature, November 14, 1935, Murphy Papers, Reel 103.
37. Constantino, "The Miseducation of the Filipino," 188.
38. Cavaliero, *Strangers in the Land*, 201.
39. C. Carkeet James, *Drainage Problems of the East* (Bombay, 1906); Report of the Commissioner of Health and Welfare, November 1935, Murphy Papers, Reel 102.
40. Memorandum for the Governor-General by G. C. Dunham, October 26, 1935, Murphy Papers, Reel 101.
41. Sir Frank Pearson, "Reminiscences of an Indian Political Officer," MSS Eur 226/21, Private Papers, IOR, BL.
42. Lady Chapman, "British India Recollected," Lady Chapman Papers, CSAS.
43. Frank Murphy, "In Manila I Have Noticed That," n.d. [1934], Murphy Papers, Reel 98.
44. W. Cameron Forbes, "The Philippine Carnival, February 21–28, 1911" (Manila, 1911), AHC.

45. "Annual Report of the Bureau of Health, for the Year Ending 1935," Murphy Papers, Reel 102; Arnold, "Malaria and Race," 123–43; Michael Worboys, "Tuberculosis and Race in Britain and its Empire, 1900–1950," in Ernst and Harris, eds., *Race, Science, and Medicine, 1700–1960*, 144–66.
46. Arnold, *Colonizing the Body*, 294; Anderson, *Colonial Pathologies*, 227–28.
47. McKenna, *American Imperial Pastoral*, 166–67.
48. Mathur, *India By Design*, 33–42.
49. Cohn, "Cloth, Clothes, and Colonialism," 334–41.
50. Mathur, *India By Design*, 46–49.
51. H. H. Bandholtz to Mr. I. Beck, March 11, 1909, Harry Hill Bandholtz Papers, Bentley Historical Library, University of Michigan (microfilm), Reel 2.
52. Anderson, *The Philippine Problem*, 142.
53. 'Bernyece,' "Milady Goes Shopping," *Philippine Touring Topics* (August 1933), 98.
54. "The Meaning of a Handshake," *Philippines Herald*, May 1, 1936.
55. Appadurai, "How to Make a National Cuisine," 3–9; Jill Gibson to her parents, March 8, 1939, in Jack Gibson, "As I Saw It," Jack Gibson Papers, Box 3, CSAS.
56. Mrs. H. A. Barnes Memoir, MSS Eur F226/1, Private Papers, IOR, BL.
57. Elizabeth Buettner, "'Going for an Indian': South Asian Restaurants and the Limits of Multiculturalism in Britain," in Ray and Srinivas, eds., *Curried Cultures*, 149.
58. Fernandez, "Food and War," 239.
59. Orquiza, "*Lechon* with Heinz," 177, 180–81.
60. T. H. Pardo de Tavera to William Howard Taft, February 9, 1904, William Howard Taft Papers, Cornell University Library (microfilm), Reel 42.
61. G. C. Dunham memorandum for Governor-General Murphy, September 14, 1934, Murphy Papers, Reel 99.
62. Roosevelt, *The Philippines*, 223.
63. Menus for the *S. S. Mayon*, June 28–30, 1934, Murphy Papers, Reel 99; menus for official lunches and dinners, November–December, 1934, Murphy Papers, Reel 100.
64. Macfarlane, *Daughters of the Empire*, 139.
65. Karnow, *In Our Image*, 198.
66. Hutchins, *Illusion of Permanence*, 141–42, 201.
67. James, *Raj*, 516–17.
68. Winston Churchill, "Our Duty in India," speech at Albert Hall, London, March 18, 1931; Madhusree Mukerjee, *Churchill's Secret War: The British Empire and the Ravaging of India during World War II* (New York, 2010), 106.
69. Churchill to Attlee, May 21, 1947, National Archives, www.nationalarchives.gov.uk/education/resources/the-road-to-partition/churchill-pm-attlee/.
70. Collingham, *Imperial Bodies*, 198.
71. Roosevelt, *The Philippines*, 273, 275.
72. L. P. Hammond to Nicholas Roosevelt, September 7, 1928, Roosevelt Papers, Box 9; Dr. Heiser Diary, entry for May 12, 1928, Series V, Box 80, Victor C. Heiser Papers, APS.
73. Paul McNutt radio address on NBC, March 14, 1938, BIA, General Records Relating to More Than One Island Possession, Confidential File 1914–1935, Box 5, RG 350, NAII.
74. "Report of the Special Mission to the Philippine Islands to the Secretary of War, 1922," BIA, General Records Relating to More Than One Island Possession, Confidential File 1914–1935, Box 9, RG 350, NAII.
75. Address by Frances B. Sayre before American Chamber of Commerce, Manila, November 13, 1939, in E. C. Ross, "Office report of the U.S. High Commissioner for the period July 26, 1939 to January 1, 1940," BIA, General Records Relating to More Than One Island Possession, Confidential File 1914–1935, Box 5, RG 350, NAII.
76. See Nandy, *The Intimate Enemy*, 3.
77. Fisher, *Counterflows to Colonialism*, 15.
78. Mathur, *India by Design*, 63.
79. Alex Sutherland to W. H. Taft, October 24, 1903, Taft Papers, Reel 41.
80. Mabalon, "As American as Jackrabbit Adobo," 147, 154–55.

81. Martin F. Manalansan IV, "Immigrant Lives and the Politics of Olfaction in the Global City," in Drobnick, ed., *The Smell Culture Reader*, 46.
82. Harald Fischer-Tiné, "National Education, Pulp Fiction and Contradictions of Colonialism: Perceptions of an Educational Experiment in Early-Twentieth Century India," in Fischer-Tiné and Mann, eds., 230.
83. Kennedy, *Magic Mountains*, 203, 219, 229.
84. Wilson, *Chaos of Empire*, 424.
85. Amrith, "Health and Sovereignty in the New Asia," 103.
86. James, *Raj*, 593.
87. M. J. Akbar, *Nehru: The Making of India* (London, 1988), 49–50.
88. John Gunther, *Inside Asia* (New York, 1939), 417–19.
89. Akbar, *Nehru*, 349.
90. Major H. D. H. Rance, "A Grandfather's Tale," MSS Eur F226/23, Private Papers, IOR, BL.
91. Which the Americans welcomed: as Julian Go has written, "they leaned heavily on the very Filipino 'oligarchs' and 'caciques' whom they had initially derided." Julian Go, "Introduction: Global Perspectives on the U.S. Colonial State in the Philippines," in Go and Foster, eds., *Colonial State in the Philippines*, 14.
92. Anderson, "Cacique Democracy in the Philippines," 13.
93. Chester A. Horne, "Bi-Weekly Summary of Intelligence, May 1–15, 1935, BIA, General Records Relating to More Than One Island Possession, Confidential File, 1914–1935, Box 7, RG 350, NAII; Report by Manuel Alba from Zamboanga, Mindanao, September 16, 1931, Box 11.
94. W. Cameron Forbes, "Notes on the Early History of Baguio," *Manila Daily Bulletin* (1943).
95. Brands, *Bound to Empire*, 230.
96. H. H. Bandholtz to Col. J. G. Harbord, October 7, 1906, Bandholtz Papers, Reel 1.
97. Craig and Craig, *Farthest Westing*, 130; Gunther, *Inside Asia*, 287–301.
98. "Report by the High Commissioner to the Secretary of War, covering the period Nov. 15–December 31, 1935," BIA, General Records Relating to More Than One Island Possession, Confidential File, 1914–1935, Box 4, RG 350, NAII.
99. H. Ford Wilkins, "Philippine Republic Is Born As U.S. Rule Ends in Glory," *New York Times*, July 4, 1946.
100. Karnow, *In Our Image*, 256, 323.
101. "New Republic is Born in the Philippines," *Life*, July 22, 1946, 19–25.
102. Dean J. Kotlowski, *Paul V. McNutt and the Age of FDR* (Bloomington, IN, 2015), 393.
103. Robert Trumbull, "India and Pakistan Become Nations; Clashes Continue," *New York Times*, August 15, 1947.
104. Trench memoir.
105. "Delhi Bedecked for Independence Day," *Times of India*, August 13, 1947.
106. Akbar, *Nehru*, 421–22; Trumbull, "India and Pakistan"; "Birth of India's Freedom," *Times of India*, August 15, 1947.
107. "Delhi Bedecked for Independence Day."
108. Rotter, *Comrades at Odds*, 52.
109. Lord Gladwyn, *The Memoirs of Lord Gladwyn* (New York, 1972), 208.
110. Karnow, *In Our Image*, 334–36.
111. Williams, *Keywords*, 59–60.
112. Anderson, *Colonial Pathologies*, 183.
113. Frank Costigliola, "Culture, Emotion, and the Creation of the Atlantic Identity," in Lundestad, ed., *No End to Alliance*, 21–36.
114. Samuel P. Huntington, "A Clash of Civilizations?" *Foreign Affairs* 72, no. 3 (Summer 1993), 24. The sitting American president has found this analysis of civilization persuasive; see Peter Beinart, "The Racial and Religious Paranoia of Trump's Warsaw Speech," *The Atlantic*, July 7, 2017.
115. Nandy, *The Intimate Enemy*, 31–32.
116. Classen, Howes, and Synnott, *Aroma*, 165.
117. O. Mannoni, *Prospero and Caliban* (New York, 1956), 18.

BIBLIOGRAPHY

Archival Sources

NATIONAL ARCHIVES II (NAII), COLLEGE PARK, MD, RECORD GROUP 350

Records of the War Department, Bureau of Insular Affairs (BIA)
Quotations from Speeches and Statements by the President of the U.S. Concerning the Philippine Islands, 1900–1904
Correspondence of the Philippine Commission Confidential File, 1914–1935

MANUSCRIPT DIVISION (MD), LIBRARY OF CONGRESS (LC), WASHINGTON, DC

Papers of Charles Henry Brent, Burton Harrison, Theodore Roosevelt Jr., Leonard Wood

NATIONAL ARCHIVES OF INDIA (NAI), NEW DELHI

Proceedings of the Home Department—Sanitary
Proceedings of the Home Department—Medical

ATANEO DE MANILA UNIVERSITY LIBRARY, MANILA

American Historical Collection

CENTRE OF SOUTH ASIAN STUDIES, UNIVERSITY OF CAMBRIDGE (CSAS)

Papers of The Anglican Missions of India, Viola Bayley, W. A. Barnes, Evelyn Beeton, V. M. L. Bogle, Irene Bose, J. M. Bourn, Sir Ernest Bradfield, Lady Chapman, M. L. Darling, Gallwey Family, Jack Gibson, Carol Hyde

BRITISH LIBRARY (BL), LONDON

India Office Records (IOR)
Additional Manuscripts (Add MS): Aden (A), Departmental Records (L), Public (P), and Judicial (J).

LONDON SCHOOL OF HYGIENE AND TROPICAL MEDICINE

Papers of Sir Leonard Rogers

WIDENER LIBRARY, HARVARD UNIVERSITY, CAMBRIDGE, MA

William Cameron Forbes Papers

SPECIAL COLLECTIONS, BIRD LIBRARY, SYRACUSE UNIVERSITY, SYRACUSE, NY

Papers of Ruth H. B. Hunt, Frank C. Laubach, Benjamin E. Neal, Nicholas Roosevelt

UNITED STATES MILITARY HISTORY INSTITUTE (USMHI), CARLISLE, PA

Papers of Matthew A. Batson, William C. Brown, Walter L. Cutter, George D. DeShon, Halstead-Maus Family, Guy V. Henry, Charles E. MacDonald, Clenard McLaughlin, Dana True Merrill, William and Grace Paulding, Richie Routt, Rollin N. Tilton, Simeon Villa, Samuel B. M. Young

DOE LIBRARY, UNIVERSITY OF CALIFORNIA-BERKELEY, BERKELEY, CA

Papers of David P. Barrows, Eli Lundy Huggins

AMERICAN PHILOSOPHICAL SOCIETY (APS), PHILADELPHIA, PA

Victor G. Heiser Papers

MUDD LIBRARY, PRINCETON UNIVERSITY, PRINCETON, NJ

L. M. Garrison Papers, Arthur Poillon Papers

Microfilm

CORNELL UNIVERSITY LIBRARY, ITHACA, NY

William Howard Taft Papers

BENTLEY HISTORICAL LIBRARY, UNIVERSITY OF MICHIGAN, ANN ARBOR, MI

Henry Hill Bandholtz Papers
Frank L. Murphy Papers

Periodicals

Manila Times

New York Times
Times of India
Times of London

Published Sources

Abinales, Patricio N. "Progressive-Machine Conflict in Early-Twentieth-Century U.S. Politics and Colonial-State Building in the Philippines," in Go and Foster, eds., *Colonial State in the Philippines*, 148–181

Achaya, K. T. *Indian Food: A Historical Companion*. Delhi: Oxford University Press, 1994.

Ackerman, Diane. *A Natural History of the Senses*. New York: Random House, 1990.

Aftel, Mandy. *Essence and Alchemy: A Book of Perfume*. New York: North Point Press, 2001.

Agarwal, Rishi Kumar. "Origin of Spectacles in India." *British Journal of Opthalmology* 55, 2 (1971), 128–29.

Ahuja, Ravi. "'The Bridge Builders': Some Notes on Railways, Pilgrimage and the British 'Civilizing Mission' in Colonial India," in Fischer-Tiné and Mann, eds., *Colonialism as Civilizing Mission*, 95–116.

Akbar, M. J. *Nehru: The Making of India*. London: Penguin, 1988.

Allen, Charles, ed. *Plain Tales from the Raj*. New York: Holt, Rinehart, and Winston, 1985.

Alvarez, Santiago V. *Recalling the Revolution: Memoirs of a Filipino General*. Transl. by Paula Carolina S. Malay. Intro. By Ruby R. Paredes.

Amrith, Sunil. "Health and Sovereignty in the New Asia: The Decline and Rise of the Tropics," in Kumar and Basu, eds., *Medical Encounters in British India*, 98–119.

Anderson, Benedict. "Cacique Democracy in the Philippines: Origins and Dreams," in Rafael, ed., *Discrepant Histories*, 3–47.

Anderson, Benedict. *Imagined Communities: Reflections on the Origin and Spread of Nationalism*. Rev. ed. London: Verso, 1991.

Anderson, Isabel. *The Spell of the Hawaiian Islands and the Philippines*. Boston: The Page Company, 1916.

Anderson, Stuart. *Race and Rapprochement: Anglo-Saxonism and Anglo-American Relations, 1895–1904*. East Brunswick, NJ: Associated University Presses, Inc., 1981.

Anderson, Warwick. *Colonial Pathologies: American Tropical Medicine, Race, and Hygiene in the Philippines*. Durham, NC: Duke University Press, 2006.

Anderson, Warwick. "Excremental Colonialism: Public Health and the Poetics of Pollution." *Critical Inquiry* 12, 3 (1995), 640–669.

Anderson, Warwick. "States of Hygiene: Race 'Improvement' and Biomedical Citizenship in Australia and the Colonial Philippines," in Stoler, ed., *Haunted By Empire*, 94–115.

Anderson, Warwick. "'Where Every Prospect Pleases and Only Man is Vile': Laboratory Medicine as Colonial Discourse." *Critical Inquiry* 18, no. 3 (Spring 1992), 506–29.

Anderson, William H. *The Philippine Problem*. New York: G. P. Putnam's Sons, 1939.

Appadurai, Arjun. "How to Make a National Cuisine: Cookbooks in Contemporary India." *Comparative Studies in Society and History* 30, no. 1 (January 1988), 3–24.

Arnold, David. "'An Ancient Race Outworn': Malaria and Race in Colonial India, 1860–1930," in Ernst and Harris, eds., *Race, Science and Medicine*, 123–143.

Arnold, David. *Colonizing the Body: State Medicine and Epidemic Disease in Nineteenth-Century India*. Berkeley: University of California Press, 1993.

Arnold, David. "Dietetics, Mimesis, and Alterity: Food in Asian Medical Traditions and East-West Exchanges," in Kumar and Basu, eds., *Medical Encounters in British India*, 80–97.

Arnold, David. *Famine: Social Crisis and Historical Change*. Oxford: Basil Blackwell, 1988.

Arnold, David, ed. *Imperial Medicine and Indigenous Societies*. Manchester: Manchester University Press, 1988.

Arnold, David. *The Tropics and the Traveling Gaze: India, Landscape, and Science, 1800–1856*. Seattle: University of Washington Press, 2006.

Aron, Hans. "Investigation of the Action of the Tropical Sun on Men and Animals." *Philippine Journal of Science* 6, no. 2 (April 1911), 101–32.

Ashenburg, Katherine. *The Dirt on Clean: An Unsanitized History*. New York: North Point Press, 2007.

Atkinson, George F. *Curry and Rice: The Ingredients of Social Life at "Our Station" in India.* Chennai: Rupa and Co., 2001 [1859].

Azurin, Arnold Molina. *Reinventing the Filipino Sense of Being and Becoming: Critical Analyses of the Orthodox Views in Anthropology, History, Folklore and Letters* 2nd ed. Quezon City: University of the Philippines Press, 1995.

Babb, Lawrence. "Glancing: Visual Interaction in Hinduism." *Journal of Anthropological Research* 37, 4 (1981), 387–401.

Bailey, Peter. *Popular Culture and Performance in the Victorian City.* Cambridge: Cambridge University Press, 1998.

Balce, Nerissa S. *Body Parts of Empire: Visual Abjection, Filipino Images, and the American Archive.* Ann Arbor: University of Michigan Press, 2016.

Ballhatchet, Kenneth, and John Harrison, eds. *The City in South Asia: Pre-Modern and Modern.* London: Curzon Press, 1980.

Balunsat, Rosa. "Nursing Tuberculosis Patients in a Sanatorium." *Proceedings of the First National Congress on Tuberculosis, Manila, December 13–18, 1926* (Manila, 1927), 575–578.

Barnes, David S. "Cargo, 'Infection,' and the Logic of Quarantine in the Nineteenth Century," *Bulletin of the History of Medicine* 88, no. 1 (Spring 2014), 75–104.

Barnes, David S. "Confronting Sensory Crisis in the Great Stinks of London and Paris," in Cohen and Johnson, eds., *Filth*, 106–132.

Barnes, David S. *The Great Stink of Paris and the Nineteenth-Century Struggle against Filth and Germs.* Baltimore: Johns Hopkins University Press, 2006.

Barringer, Tim. "Sonic Spectacles of Empire: The Audio-Visual Nexus, Delhi-London 1911–12," in Edwards, Gosden, and Phillips, eds., *Sensible Objects*, 169–198.

Barrow, Ian. *Making History, Drawing Territory: British Mapping in India, c. 1756–1905.* New Delhi: Oxford University Press, 2003.

Bate, Bernard. "'To Persuade Them Into Speech and Action': Oratory and the Tamil Political, Madras, 1905–1919." *Comparative Studies in Society and History* 55, no. 1 (2013), 142–66.

Bauer, Helen Pike. "Eating in the Contact Zone: Food and Identity in Anglo-India," in Wagner and Hasan, eds., *Consuming Culture in the Long Nineteenth Century*, 95–106.

Bayly, C. A. *Indian Society and the Making of the British Empire.* Cambridge: Cambridge University Press, 1998.

Bean, Robert Bennett. "Filipino Ears—A Classification of Ear Types," *Philippine Journal of Science* 4A (January 1909), 27–54.

Bean, Robert Bennett. *The Racial Anatomy of the Philippine Islanders.* Philadelphia: J. B. Lippincott Co., 1910.

Bederman, Gail. *Manliness and Civilization: A Cultural History of Gender and Race in the United States, 1880–1917.* Chicago: University of Chicago Press, 1995.

Bentley, James. *Ritualism and Politics in Victorian Britain: The Attempt to Legislate for Belief.* Oxford: Oxford University Press, 1978.

Berreman, Gerald D. "Stratification, Pluralism and Interaction: A Comparative Analysis of Caste," in de Reuck and Knight, eds., *Ciba Foundation Symposium on Caste and Race*, 45–73.

Bewell, Alan. *Romanticism and Colonial Disease.* Baltimore: Johns Hopkins University Press, 1999.

Bhattacharya, Sabyasachi. *Talking Back: The Idea of Civilization in the Indian Nationalist Discourse.* New Delhi: Oxford University Press, 2011.

Bhattacharya, Sanjoy, Mark Harrison, and Michael Worboys. *Fractured States: Smallpox, Public Health and Vaccination Policy in British India 1800–1947.* New Delhi: Orient Longman, 2005.

Bhattacharya, Sumangala. "Badly Boiled Potatoes and Other Crises," in Wagner and Hasan, eds., *Consuming Culture*, 3–16.

Bijsterveld, Karin. "The Diabolical Symphony of the Mechanical Age: Technology and Symbolism of Sound in European and North American Noise Abatement Campaigns, 1900–1940," in Bull and Back, eds., *Auditory Culture Reader*, 165–189.

Blower, Brooke L., and Mark Philip Bradley, eds. *The Familiar Made Strange: American Icons and Artifacts after the Transnational Turn.* Ithaca, NY: Cornell University Press, 2015.

Boas, Franz. "On Alternating Sounds." *American Anthropologist* 2, no. 1 (January 1889), 47–54.

Bourdieu, Pierre. *Distinction: A Social Critique of the Judgement of Taste*. Transl. by Richard Nice. Cambridge, MA: Harvard University Press, 1984.

Brands, H. W. *Bound to Empire: The United States and the Philippines*. New York: Oxford University Press, 1992.

Bratton, Jacqueline S., Richard Allen Cave, Breandan Gregory, Heidi J. Holder, and Michael Pickering, *Acts of Supremacy: The British Empire and the Stage, 1790–1930*. Manchester: Manchester University Press, 1991.

Brayne, F[rank]. L[ugard]. *Village Uplift in India*. Allahabad: The Pioneer Press, n.d. [1927].

Brody, David. *Visualizing American Empire: Orientalism and Imperialism in the Philippines*. Chicago: University of Chicago Press, 2010.

Brown, Kathleen M. *Foul Bodies: Cleanliness in Early America*. New Haven, CT: Yale University Press, 2009.

Brown, William H., Paul F. Russell, and Clara Palafox Cariño. *Health Through Knowledge and Habits*. Boston: Ginn and Co., 1933.

Buckingham, Jane. *Leprosy in Colonial South India: Medicine and Confinement*. London: Palgrave, 2002.

Buckland, Ralph Kent. *In the Land of the Filipino*. New York: Every Where Publishing Company, 1912.

Buettner, Elizabeth. *Empire Families: Britons and Late Imperial India*. Oxford: Oxford University Press, 2004.

Buettner, Elizabeth. "'Going for an Indian': South Asian Restaurants and the Limits of Multiculturalism in Britain," in Ray and Srinivas, eds., *Curried Cultures*, 143–174.

Bull, Michael, and Les Back, eds. *The Auditory Culture Reader*. Oxford: Berg, 2003.

Bunnett, Sara, ed. *Manila Envelopes: Oregon Volunteer Lt. George F. Telfer's Spanish-American War Letters*. Portland: Oregon Historical Society Press, 1987.

Burton, Antoinette. *Empire in Question: Reading, Writing, and Teaching British Imperialism*. Durham, NC: Duke University Press, 2011.

Burton, David. *The Raj at Table: A Culinary History of the British in India*. London: Faber and Faber, 1993.

Bushman, Richard J., and Claudia I. Bushman. "The Early History of Cleanliness in America," *Journal of American History* 74, no. 4 (March 1988), 1213–38.

Bynum, Helen. *Spitting Blood: The History of Tuberculosis*. Oxford: Oxford University Press, 2012.

Bynum, W. F., and Roy Porter, eds. *Medicine and the Five Senses* (Cambridge: Cambridge University Press, 1993).

Cannell, Fenella. *Power and Intimacy in the Christian Philippines*. Cambridge: Cambridge University Press, 1999.

Carreon, Manuel L. *Philippine Studies in Mental Measurement*. Intro. by Arthur S. Otis. Yonkers, NY: World Book Co., 1926.

Catanach, I. J. "Plague and the Tensions of Empire: India, 1896–1918," in Arnold, ed., *Imperial Medicine and Indigenous Societies*, 149–71.

Cavaliero, Roderick. *Strangers in the Land: The Rise and Decline of the British Indian Empire*. London: I. B. Tauris, 2002.

Chamberlain, Weston P. "Observations on the Influence of the Philippine Climate on White Men of the Blond and of the Brunette Type." *Philippine Journal of Science* 6, no. 6 (December 1911), 427–66.

Chamberlain, Weston P. "The Study of Tropical Diseases in the Philippine Islands." *Journal of the American Medical Association* 58, no. 14 (1912), 998–1002.

Chapman, Ronald Fettes. *Leonard Wood and Leprosy in the Philippines: The Culion Leper Colony, 1921–1927*. Lanham, MD: The University Press of America, 1982.

Chatterjee, Kumkum, and Clement Hawes. *Europe Observed: Multiple Gazes in Early Modern Encounters*. Lewisburg, PA: Bucknell University Press, 2008.

Chaudhary, Zahid R. *Afterimage of Empire: Photography in Nineteenth-Century India*. Minneapolis: University of Minnesota Press, 2012.

Chaudhuri, Arun. *Indian Advertising 1780 to 1950 A. D.* New Delhi: Tata McGraw-Hill, 2007.

Chaudhuri, Nupur, and Margaret Strobel, eds. *Western Women and Imperialism: Complicity and Resistance*. Bloomington: Indiana University Press, 1992.

"Chota Mem" (Mrs. C. Lang). *The English Bride in India*. 2nd ed. London, 1909.

Classen, Constance, ed. *The Book of Touch*. Oxford: Berg, 2005.

Classen, Constance, ed. *A Cultural History of the Senses. Volume Five: In the Age of Empire*. London: Bloomsbury, 2014.

Classen, Constance. *The Deepest Sense: A Cultural History of Touch*. Urbana: University of Illinois Press, 2012.

Classen, Constance. *Worlds of Sense: Exploring the Senses in History and Across Cultures*. London: Routledge, 1993.

Classen, Constance, and David Howes. "The Museum as Sensescape: Western Sensibilities and Indigenous Artifacts," in Edwards, Gosden, and Phillips, eds., *Sensible Objects*, 199–222.

Classen, Constance, David Howes, and Anthony Synnott. *Aroma: The Cultural History of Smell*. New York: Routledge, 1994.

Cleere, Eileen. *The Sanitary Arts: Aesthetic Culture and the Victorian Cleanliness Campaigns*. Columbus, OH: Ohio State University Press, 2014.

Clements, Paul. "Medical Survey of the Town of Taytay." *Philippine Journal of Science* 4B, 4 (August 1909), 247–256.

Cohen, William A., and Ryan Johnson, eds. *Filth: Dirt, Disgust, and Modern Life*. Minneapolis: University of Minnesota Press, 2005.

Cohn, Bernard S. *An Anthropologist Among the Historians and Other Essays*. New York: Oxford University Press, 1987.

Cohn, Bernard. "Cloth, Clothes, and Colonialism: India in the Nineteenth Century," in Weiner and Schneider, eds., *Cloth and Human Experience*, 304–353.

Cohn, Bernard S. *Colonialism and Its Forms of Knowledge: The British in India*. Foreword by Nicholas B. Dirks. Princeton, NJ: Princeton University Press, 1996.

Cohn, Bernard S. "Notes on the History of the Study of Indian Society and Culture," in Singer and Cohn, eds., *Structure and Change in Indian Society*, 3–28.

Cole, Shaun. *The Story of Men's Underwear*. New York: Parkstone Press International, 2010.

Collingham, E. M. *Imperial Bodies: The Physical Experience of the Raj, c. 1800–1947*. Cambridge: Polity Press, 2001.

Collingham, Lizzie. *Curry: A Tale of Cooks and Conquerors*. Oxford: Oxford University Press, 2006.

Commonwealth of the Philippines. *Graded Exercises in Sentence Rhythm and Emphasis Through Inflection*. Manila: Department of Public Instruction, Bureau of Education, 1940.

Conger, Emily Bronson. *An Ohio Woman in the Philippines*. Akron: Press of R. H. Leighton, 1904.

Constantino, Renato. "The Miseducation of the Filipino," in Shaw and Francia, eds., *Vestiges of War*, 177–192.

Cook, James W. "Seeing the Visual in U.S. History." *Journal of American History* 95, no. 2 (September 2008), 432–41.

Cooper, Gail. *Air-Conditioning America: Engineers and the Controlled Environment, 1900–1960*. Baltimore: Johns Hopkins University Press, 1998.

Corbin, Alain. *The Foul and the Fragrant: Odor and the French Social Imagination*. Cambridge, MA: Harvard University Press, 1986.

Corbin, Alain. *Time, Desire, and Horror: Towards a History of the Senses*. Transl. by Jean Birrell. Cambridge: Polity Press, 1995.

Corbin, Alain. *Village Bells: Sound and Meaning in the 19th-Century French Countryside*. Transl. by Martin Thom. New York: Columbia University Press, 1998.

Costigliola, Frank. "Culture, Emotion, and the Creation of the Atlantic Identity," in Lundestad, ed., *No End to Alliance*, 21–36.

Costigliola, Frank, and Michael J. Hogan, eds. *Explaining the History of American Foreign Relations.* New York: Cambridge University Press, 2016.

Craig, Josephine, and Austin Craig. *Farthest Westing: A Philippine Footnote.* Philadelphia: Dorrance and Company, 1940.

Crosbie, Barry, and Mark Hampton, eds. *The Cultural Construction of the British World.* Manchester: Manchester University Press, 2016.

Cullinane, Michael. *Ilustrado Politics: Filipino Elite Responses to American Rule, 1898–1908.* Manila: Ataneo de Manila University Press, 2003.

Cunningham, Andrew, and Bridie Andrews, eds. *Western Medicine as Contested Knowledge.* Manchester: Manchester University Press, 1997.

Cunnington, C. Willett, and Phillis Cunnington. *The History of Underclothes.* With revisions by A. D. Mansfield and Valerie Mansfield. London: Faber and Faber, 1951.

Daniel, E. Valentine. "The Pulse as an Icon in Siddha Medicine," in Howes, ed., *The Varieties of Sensory Experience,* 100–110.

Darwin, John. *Unfinished Empire: The Global Expansion of Britain.* London: Bloomsbury, 2012.

David, Saul. "Greased Cartridges and the Great Mutiny of 1857: A Pretext to Rebel or the Final Straw?," in Kaushik, ed., *War and Society in Colonial India,* 82–113.

Davis, Mike. *Late Victorian Holocausts: El Niño Famines and the Making of the Third World.* London: Verso, 2001.

De Bevoise, Ken. *Agents of Apocalypse: Epidemic Disease in the Colonial Philippines.* Princeton, NJ: Princeton University Press, 1995.

Dendooven, Dominiek. "Trench Crap: Excremental Aspects of the First World War," in Saunders and Cornish, eds., *Modern Conflict and the Senses,* 183–95.

de Reuck, A. V. S., and Julie Knight, eds., *Ciba Foundation Symposium on Caste and Race: Comparative Approaches.* London: Churchill, 1967.

De Viana, Augusto V., ed. and compiler. *The I Stories: The Events in the Philippine Revolution and the Filipino-American War as told by Its Eyewitnesses and Participants.* Manila: University of Santo Tomas Publishing House, 2006.

Devins, John Bancroft. *An Observer in the Philippines, or, Life in Our New Possessions.* Foreword by William Howard Taft. Boston: American Tract Society, 1905.

Doeppers, Daniel F. *Feeding Manila in Peace and War, 1850–1945.* Madison: University of Wisconsin Press, 2016.

Douglas, Mary. *Implicit Meanings: Essays in Anthropology.* London: Routledge and Kegan Paul, 1975.

Douglas, Mary. *Leviticus as Literature.* Oxford: Oxford University Press, 2000.

Douglas, Mary. *Purity and Danger.* London: Routledge, 1966.

Drobnick, Jim, ed. *The Smell Culture Reader.* Oxford: Berg, 2006.

Duffy, John. *The Sanitarians: A History of American Public Health.* Urbana: University of Illinois Press, 1990.

Eck, Diana L. *Darśan: Seeing the Divine Image in India.* 3rd ed. New York: Columbia University Press, 1998.

Edensor, Tim. "The Social Life of the Senses: Ordering and Disordering the Modern Sensorium," in Howes, ed., *A Cultural History of the Senses in the Modern Age,* 31–54.

Edmond, Rod. *Leprosy and Empire: A Medical and Cultural History.* Cambridge: Cambridge University Press, 2006.

Edwards, Elizabeth, and Kaushik Bhaumik, eds. *Visual Sense: A Cultural Reader.* Oxford: Berg, 2008.

Edwards, Elizabeth, Chris Gosden, and Ruth B. Phillips, eds. *Sensible Objects: Colonialism, Museums and Material Culture.* Oxford: Berg, 2006.

Edwards, Ralph T. "A Biological Study of the Water Supply of the Philippine Islands, with a Description of a New Pathogenic Organism." *Philippine Journal of Science* 3B, no. 1 (January 1908), 121–130.

Edwards, Rebecca. *New Spirits: Americans in the "Gilded Age," 1865–1905* New York: Oxford University Press, 2015.

Einolf, Christopher J. *America in the Philippines, 1899–1902: The First Torture Scandal*. New York: Palgrave Macmillan, 2014.

El Edroos, Syed Fakhruddin Aboobaker. *Modern Indian Etiquette*. Surat: The Mission Press, 1922.

Elfers, James. *The Tour to End All Tours: The Story of Major League Baseball's 1913–1914 World Tour*. Lincoln: University of Nebraska Press, 2003.

Elias, Norbert. *The Civilizing Process: The History of Manners*, transl. Edmund Jephcott. New York: Urizen Books, 1978.

Eraly, Abraham. *The Mughal World: Life in India's Last Golden Age*. London: Penguin, 2007.

Ernst, Waltraud, and Bernard Harris, eds. *Race, Science, and Medicine, 1700–1960*. London: Routledge, 1999.

Eyot, Canning, ed. and intro. *The Story of the Lopez Family: A Page from the History of the War in the Philippines*. Boston: James H. West Company, 1904.

Falconer, John. "'A Pure Labor of Love': A Publishing History of *The People of India*," in Hight and Sampson, eds., *Colonialist Photography*, 51–83.

Fanon, Frantz. *A Dying Colonialism*. Transl. by Haakon Chevalier. New York: Grove Press, 1965.

Fanon, Frantz. *Black Skin, White Masks*. Transl. Charles Lam Markmann. New York: Grove Press, 1967.

Fayrer, Joseph. *European Child-Life in Bengal*. London: J. and A. Churchill, 1873.

Fayrer, Joseph. *Tropical Dysentery and Chronic Diarrhea: Liver Abcess—Malarial Cachexia—Insolation with Other Forms of Tropical Disease*. London: J. A. Churchill, 1881.

Fee, Mary H. *A Woman's Impression of the Philippines*. Chicago: A. C. McClurg and Co., 1910.

Feeley, Kathleen A., and Jennifer Frost, eds. *When Private Talk Goes Public: Gossip in American History*. New York: Palgrave Macmillan, 2014.

Feliu', Fernando. "Science, Sight and the Ordering of Colonial Societies," in Edwards and Bhaumik, eds., *Visual Sense*, 121–31.

Fernandez, Doreen G. "Food and War," in Shaw and Francia, eds., *Vestiges of War*, 237–246.

Fischer-Tiné, Harald. "National Education, Pulp Fiction and the Contradictions of Colonialism: Perceptions of an Educational Experiment in Early-Twentieth Century India," in Fischer-Tiné and Mann, eds., *Colonialism as Civilizing Mission*, 229–47.

Fischer-Tiné, Harald, and Michael Mann, eds. *Colonialism as Civilizing Mission: Cultural Ideology in British India*. London: Anthem Press, 2004.

Fisher, Michael H. *Counterflows to Colonialism: Indian Travellers and Settlers in Britain 1600–1857*. Delhi: Permanent Black, 2004.

Flint, Kate. "The Social Life of the Senses: The Assaults and Seductions of Modernity," in Classen, ed., *A Cultural History of the Senses in the Age of Empire*, 25–45.

Forster, E. M. *Passage to India*. London: Harcourt, 1924.

Freer, William B. *The Philippine Experiences of an American Teacher: A Narrative of Work and Travel in the Philippine Islands*. New York: Charles Scribner's Sons, 1906.

Freud, Sigmund. *Civilization and Its Discontents*. Transl. by Joan Riviere. Garden City, NY: Doubleday and Co., 1930.

Friend, Theodore. *Between Two Empires: The Ordeal of the Philippines 1929–1946*. New Haven, CT: Yale University Press, 1965.

Fuller, Alice M. *Housekeeping: A Textbook for Girls in the Public Intermediate Schools of the Philippines*. Bureau of Education. Manila: Bureau of Printing, 1914.

Fuller, Alice M. *Housekeeping and Household Arts: A Manual for Work with the Girls in the Elementary Schools of the Philippine Islands*. Bulletin No. 35, Bureau of Education. Manila: Bureau of Printing, 1911.

Funston, Frederick. *Memories of Two Wars: Cuban and Philippine Experiences*. New York: Charles Scribner's Sons, 1911.

Gabaccia, Donna R. *We Are What We Eat: Ethnic Food and Making of Americans*. Cambridge, MA: Harvard University Press, 1998.

Gaches, Mrs. Samuel Francis, R. N. *Good Cooking and Health in the Tropics*. Published by the American Guardian Association. Manila: Bureau of Printing, 1922.

Gandhi, M. K. *Gandhi's Autobiography: The Story of My Experiments with the Truth*. Transl. Mahadev Desai. Washington, DC: Public Affairs Press, 1948.

Gavin, Hector. *Sketches and Illustrations, of Bethnal Green. A Type of the Condition of the Metropolis and Other Large Towns*. London: John Churchill, 1848.

Geertz, Clifford. *After the Fact: Two Countries, Four Decades, One Anthropologist*. Cambridge, MA: Harvard University Press, 1995.

Ghose, Indira, ed. *Memsahibs Abroad: Writings by Women Travellers in Nineteenth Century India*. Delhi: Oxford University Press, 1998.

Ghosh, Durba. *Sex and the Family in Colonial India: The Making of Empire*. Cambridge: Cambridge University Press, 2006.

Gibbs, H. D. "A Study of the Effect of Tropical Sunlight Upon Men, Monkeys, and Rabbits and a Discussion of the Proper Clothing for the Tropical Climate." *Philippine Journal of Science* 2B, no. 2 (April 1912), 91–114.

Gilman, Sander L. *Difference and Pathology: Stereotypes of Sexuality, Race, and Madness*. Ithaca, NY: Cornell University Press, 1995.

Gilmour, David. *The Ruling Caste: Imperial Lives in the Victorian Raj*. New York: FSG, 2005.

Go, Julian. *American Empire and the Politics of Meaning: Elite Political Cultures in the Philippines and Puerto Rico during U.S. Colonialism*. Durham, NC: Duke University Press, 2008.

Go, Julian. "Introduction: Global Perspectives on the U.S. Colonial State in the Philippines," in Go and Foster, eds., *Colonial State in the Philippines*, 1–42.

Go, Julian. *Patterns of Empire: The British and American Empires, 1688 to the Present*. New York: Cambridge University Press, 2011.

Go, Julian, and Anne L. Foster, eds. *Colonial State in the Philippines: Global Perspectives*. Durham, NC: Duke University Press, 2003.

Goffman, Erving. *Behavior in Public Places: Notes on the Social Organization of Gatherings*. New York: The Free Press, 1963.

Goffman, Erving. *Interaction Ritual: Essays on Face-to-Face Behavior*. New York: Pantheon Books, 1967.

Golay, Frank Hindman. *Face of Empire: United States-Philippine Relations, 1898–1946*. Madison: Center for Southeast Asian Studies, University of Wisconsin-Madison, 1998.

González-Crussi, F. *On Seeing: Things Seen, Unseen, and Obscene*. London: Duckworth Overlook, 2006.

Goody, Jack. "The High and the Low: Culinary Culture in Asia and Europe," in Korsmeyer, ed., *Taste Culture Reader*, 57–71.

Gopal, Sarvepalli. *Jawaharlal Nehru: A Biography. Volume One: 1889–1947*. Delhi: Oxford University Press, 1975.

Goswamy, B. N. "*Rasa*: Delight of the Reason," in Korsmeyer, ed., *Taste Culture Reader*, 215–25.

Gourlay, Jharna. *Florence Nightingale and the Health of the Raj*. Aldershot: Ashgate, 2003.

Government of the Philippine Islands. *Annual Report of the Commissioner of Public Health, September 1, 1903—August 31, 1904*. Manila: Department of the Interior, Bureau of Public Health, 1905.

Government of the Philippine Islands. *Course of Study in Phonics for Primary Grades*. Manila: Department of Public Instruction, Bureau of Education, 1932.

Government of the Philippine Islands. *Elementary Home Economics: A Textbook for Girls in the Intermediate Schools of the Philippine Islands*. Manila: Department of Public Instruction, Bureau of Education, 1925.

Government of the Philippine Islands. *School and Home Gardening: A Manual for Teachers of Gardening in the Elementary Schools*. Manila: Department of Public Instruction, Bureau of Education, 1931.

Grasse, Marie-Christine, ed. *Perfume, A Global History: From the Origins to Today*. Paris: Somogy Art Publisher, 2007.

Greenbie, Sydney. *The Romantic East*. New York: R. M. McBride, 1930.

Greenblatt, Stephen. "Filthy Rites." *Daedalus* 111, no. 3 (Summer 1982), 1–16. Gregory, Breandan. "Staging British India," in Bratton, Cave, Gregory, Holder, and Pickering, eds., *Acts of Supremacy*, 150–178.

Griffith, Charles E. "The Music of the Philippine Islands," *Philippine Education Magazine*, November 1928.

Gunn, Simon. *The Public Culture of the Victorian Middle Class: Ritual and Authority and the English Industrial City, 1840–1914*. Manchester: Manchester University Press, 2000.

Gunther, John. *Inside Asia*. New York: Harper and Brothers, 1939.

Gupta, Akhil. "A Different History of the Present: The Movement of Crops, Cuisines, and Globalization," in Ray and Srnivas, eds., *Curried Cultures*, 29–46.

Gussow, Zachary. *Leprosy, Racism, and Public Health: Social Policy in Chronic Disease Control*. Boulder, CO: Westview Press, 1989.

Halili, Servando D. Jr., *Iconography of the New Empire: Race and Gender Images in the American Colonization of the Philippines*. Manila: University of Philippines Press, 2006.

Hall, Catherine, ed. *Cultures of Empire: Colonizers in Britain and the Empire in the Nineteenth and Twentieth Centuries*. New York: Routledge, 2000.

Halliday, Stephen. *The Great Stink of London: Sir Joseph Bazalgette and the Cleansing of the Victorian Metropolis*. Phoenix Mill, UK: Sutton Publishing, 1999.

Halttunen, Karen. *Confidence Men and Painted Women: A Study of Middle-Class Culture in America, 1830–1870*. New Haven, CT: Yale University Press, 1982.

Hannavy, John, ed. *Encyclopedia of Nineteenth-Century Photography*. New York: Routledge, 2008.

Harris, Marvin. *Good to Eat: Riddles of Food and Culture*. New York: Simon and Schuster, 1985.

Harris, Susan K. *God's Arbiters: Americans and the Philippines, 1898–1902*. New York: Oxford University Press, 2011.

Harrison, J. B. "Allahabad: A Sanitary History," in Ballhatchet and Harrison, eds., *The City in South Asia*, 166–195.

Harrison, Mark. "From Bazaar Medicine to Hospital Medicine: Calomel, India, and the British Empire, c. 1750–c. 1800," in Kumar and Basu, eds., *Medical Encounters*, 61–79.

Heiser, Victor M. D. *An American Doctor's Odyssey: Adventures in Forty-five Countries*. New York: Norton, 1936.

Heiser, Victor M. D. *Annual Report of the Bureau of Health for the Philippine Islands, July 1, 1908–June 30, 1909*. Manila:Bureau of Printing, 1909.

Heiser, Victor M. D. *Annual Report of the Bureau of Health for the Philippine Islands, July 1, 1912–June 30, 1913*. Manila:Bureau of Printing, 1913.

Heiser, Victor G. "Fighting Leprosy in the Philippines." *The World's Work* (January 1916), 310–20.

Heiser, Victor G. "Some Considerations with Regard to the Cause of the Frequent Reappearance of Cholera in the Philippine Islands, with Statistics Beginning with the Outbreak in 1902 to January 1, 1908." *Philippine Journal of Science* 3B, no. 1 (January 1908), 89–106.

Heiser, Victor G. "Unsolved Health Problems Peculiar to the Philippines." *Philippine Journal of Science* 5B, 2 (July 1910), 171–78.

Heldke, Lisa. "But Is It Authentic? Culinary Travel and the Search for the 'Genuine Article,'" in Korsmeyer, ed., *Taste Culture Reader*, 385–94.

Herbert, Trevor, and Margaret Sarkissian. "Victorian Bands and Their Dissemination in the Colonies," *Popular Music* 16, no. 2 (May 1997), 165–79.

Herr, Michael. *Dispatches*. New York: Knopf, 1977.

Herz, Rachel S. "I Know What I Like: Understanding Odor Preferences," in Drobnick, ed., *Smell Culture Reader*, 190–203.

Hibbert, Christopher. *The Great Mutiny: India 1857*. New York: Viking, 1978.

Hight, Eleanor M., and Gary D. Sampson, eds. *Colonialist Photography: Imag(in)ing Race and Place*. London: Routledge, 2002.

Hill, Daniel Delis. *American Menswear: From the Civil War to the Twenty-First Century*. Lubbock, TX: Texas Tech University Press, 2011.

The History of the Men's Wear Industry—1890–1950, 60th Anniversary Issue of *Men's Wear*. February 10, 1950.

Hobsbawm, Eric, and Terence Ranger, eds. *The Invention of Tradition* (Cambridge: Cambridge University Press, 1983.

Hoffenberg, Peter H. *An Empire on Display: English, Indian, and Australian Exhibitions from the Crystal Palace to the Great War*. Berkeley: University of California Press, 2001.

Hoganson, Kristin L. *Consumers' Imperium: The Global Production of American Domesticity, 1865–1920*. Chapel Hill: University of North Carolina Press, 2007.

Hoganson, Kristin L. *Fighting for American Manhood: How Gender Politics Provoked the Spanish-American and Philippine-American Wars*. New Haven, CT: Yale University Press, 1998.

Hopkins, Donald R. *The Greatest Killer: Smallpox in History* Chicago: University of Chicago Press, 1983.

Horn, Florence. *Orphans of the Pacific*. New York: Reynal and Hitchcock, 1941.

Howes, David, ed. *A Cultural History of the Senses, Vol. Six: In The Modern Age*. London: Bloomsbury, 2014.

Howes, David. "Can These Dry Bones Live? An Anthropological Approach to the History of the Senses." *Journal of American History* 95, no. 2 (September 2008), 442–451

Howes, David, ed. *Empire of the Senses: The Sensual Culture Reader*. Oxford: Berg, 2005.

Howes, David, ed. *The Varieties of Sensory Experience: A Sourcebook in the Anthropology of the Senses*. Toronto: University of Toronto Press, 1991.

Howes, David, and Constance Classen. "Conclusion: Sounding Sensory Profiles," in Howes, ed., *Varieties of Sensory Experience*, 257–88.

Howes, Davd, and Marc Lalonde. "The History of Sensibilities: Of the Standard of Taste in Mid-Eighteenth Century England and the Circulation of Smells in Post-Revolutionary France." *Dialectical Anthropology* 16, no. 2 (1991), 125–35.

Hoyt, Henry F. *A Frontier Doctor*. Intro. by Frank B. Kellogg. Boston: Houghton Mifflin Co., 1929.

Huang, Xuelei. "Deodorising China: Odour, Ordure, and Colonial (Dis)order in Shanghai, 1840s–1940s." *Modern Asian Studies* 50, no. 3 (2016), 1092–122.

Hull, Edmund C. P. *The European in India; or, Anglo-India's Vade Mecum*. London: C. Kegan Paul, 1878.

Hume, David. "Of the Standard of Taste," in Korsmeyer, ed., *Taste Culture Reader*, 197–208.

Huntington, Samuel P. "The Clash of Civilizations?" *Foreign Affairs* 72, no. 3 (Summer 1993), 22–49.

Huntington, Samuel P. *The Clash of Civilizations and the Remaking of World Order*. New York: Simon and Schuster, 1996.

Hussain, S. Iftikhar. *Hints on Indian Etiquette, Specially Designed for the Use of Europeans*. Lucknow: Newul Kishore Press, 1911.

Hutchins, Francis G. *The Illusion of Permanence: British Imperialism in India*. Princeton, NJ: Princeton University Press, 1967.

Hyde, Alan. "Offensive Bodies," in Drobnick, ed., *Smell Culture Reader*, 53–58.

Ileto, Reynaldo C. "Cholera and the Origins of the American Sanitary Order in the Philippines," in Rafael, ed., *Discrepant Histories*, 51–81.

Ileto, Reynaldo C. "The Philippine-American War: Friendship and Forgetting," in Shaw and Francia, eds., *Vestiges of War*, 3–21.

Inden, Ronald B. *Imagining India*. Oxford: Basil Blackwell, 1990.

Isaacs, Harold R. *Scratches on Our Minds: American Views of China and India*. New York:John Day, 1958.

Jackson, Thomas W. "Sanitary Conditions and Needs in Provincial Towns." *Philippine Journal of Science* 3B, 5 (November 1908), 431–37.

Jacobson, Matthew Frye. *Barbarian Virtues: The United States Encounters Foreign Peoples at Home and Abroad, 1876–1917*. New York: Hill and Wang, 2000.

James, Allison. "Identity and the Global Stew," in Korsmeyer, ed., *Taste Culture Reader*, 372–84.

James, C. Carkeet. *Drainage Problems of the East*. Bombay: The Times Press, 1906.

James, Lawrence. *Raj: The Making and Unmaking of British India*. Boston: Little, Brown, 1997.

Jay, Martin. *Downcast Eyes: The Denigration of Vision in Twentieth-Century French Thought*. Berkeley: University of California Press, 1993.

Jay, Martin, and Sumathi Ramaswamy, eds. *Empires of Vision: A Reader*. Durham, NC: Duke University Press, 2014.

Jay, Martin, and Sumathi Ramaswamy. "The Imperial Optic," in their *Empires of Vision*, 23–43.

Jebb, Lord Gladwyn. *The Memoirs of Lord Gladwyn*. New York: Weidenfeld and Nicolson, 1972.

Jenner, Mark S. J. "AHR Forum: Follow Your Nose? Smell, Smelling, and Their Histories." *American Historical Review* 116, no. 2 (April 2011), 335–51.

Jenner, Mark S. J. "Tasting Lichfield, Touching China: Sir John Floyer's Senses." *The Historical Journal* 53, no. 3 (2010), 647–70.

Jhala, Angma D. "Cosmopolitan Kitchens: Cooking for Princely Zenanas in Late Colonial India," in Ray and Srinivas, eds., *Curried Cultures*, 49–72.

Johnson, James. *The influence of tropical climates, more especially the climate of India on European constitutions; the principal effects and diseases thereby induced*. London: J. J. Stockdale, 1813.

Jones, J. A. *Manual of Hygiene, Sanitation, and Sanitary Engineering, with Special Reference to Indian Conditions*. Madras: Superintedent, Government Press, 1896.

Jütte, Robert. *A History of the Senses: From Antiquity to Cyberspace*. Transl. by James Lynn. Cambridge: Polity Press, 2005.

Karnow, Stanley. *In Our Image: America's Empire in the Philippines*. New York: Ballantine Books, 1989.

Kasson, John F. *Rudeness and Civility: Manners in Nineteenth-Century Urban America*. New York: Hill and Wang, 1990.

Kaye, Sir John. *Kaye's and Mallenson's History of the Indian Mutiny of 1857–8*. Ed. by Colonel Mallenson. 6 vols. London: W. H. Allen and Co., 1888–1889.

Kelly, Alice M. "The Bua School: A Few Personal Notes," in Pecson and Racelis, eds., *Tales of the American Teachers in the Philippines*, 77-82.

Kennedy, Dane. *The Magic Mountains: Hill Stations and the British Raj*. Berkeley: University of California Press, 1996.

Kern, Stephen. *The Culture of Time and Space*. Cambridge, MA: Harvard University Press, 1983.

Kettler, Andrew. "'Ravishing Odors of Paradise': Jesuits, Olfaction, and Seventeenth-Century North America." *Journal of American Studies* 50, no. 4 (November 2016), 827–52.

Keyes, Sarah. "'Like a Roaring Lion': The Overland Trail as a Sonic Conquest." *Journal of American History* 96, no. 1 (June 2009), 19–43.

Khan, Syed Ahmed. *The Causes of the Indian Revolt*. Oxford: Oxford University Press, 2000 [org. published privately as pamphlet, 1858].

Khare, R. S. "Food with Saints," in Korsmeyer, ed., *Taste Culture Reader*, 156–65.

Khare, R. S. *The Hindu Hearth and Home*. New Delhi: Vikas Publishing House, 1976.

Kidd, Benjamin. *The Control of the Tropics*. New York: The Macmillan Company, 1898.

Kiechle, Melanie. "Navigating by Nose: Fresh Air, Stench Nuisance, and the Urban Environment, 1840–1880." *Journal of Urban History* (March 18, 2015), 1–19.

Kiechle, Melanie. "The Smell Detectives." *Chemical Heritage* (Summer 2011), 33–36.

Kiechle, Melanie A. *The Smell Detectives: An Olfactory History of Nineteenth-Century Urban America*. Seattle: University of Washington Press, 2017.

King, Anthony D. *The Bungalow: The Production of a Global Culture*. New York: Oxford University Press, 1995.

King, Mrs. Robert Moss. *The Diary of a Civilian's Wife in India 1877–1882*. 2 Vols. London: Richard Bentley and Son, 1884.

Kipling, Rudyard. *100 Poems, Old and New*. Ed. by Thomas Pinney. New York: Cambridge University Press 2013.

Kipling, Rudyard. *The City of Dreadful Night*. New York: Alex. Grosset and Co., 1899.

Kipling, Rudyard. *Collected Verse of Rudyard Kipling*. Garden City, NY: Doubleday, Page & Company, 1916.

Kipling, Rudyard. *The Jungle Book*. New York: The Century Co., 1894.

Kipling, Rudyard. *Plain Tales from the Hills*. Garden City, NY: Doubleday, 1924.

Knowles, Adam. "Conjecturing Rudeness: James Mill's Utlilitarian Philosophy of History and the British Civilizing Mission," in Watt and Mann, eds., *Civilizing Missions in Colonial and Postcolonial South Asia*, 37–63.

Konishi, Shino. "Discovering the Savage Senses: French and British Explorers' Encounters with Aboriginal People," in West-Sooby, ed., *Discovery and Empire*, 99–140.

Korsmeyer, Carolyn, ed. *The Taste Culture Reader: Experiencing Food and Drink*. Oxford: Berg, 2005.

Kotlowski, Dean J. *Paul V. McNutt and the Age of FDR*. Bloomington: Indiana University Press, 2015.

Kramer, Paul A. *Blood of Government: Race, Empire, the United States, and the Philippines*. Chapel Hill: University of North Carolina Press, 2003.

Kramer, Paul A. "The Darkness That Enters the Home: The Politics of Prostitution during the Philippine-American War," in Stoler, ed., *Haunted by Empire*, 366–404.

Kramer, Paul A. "Empires, Exceptions, and Anglo-Saxons: Race and Rule between the British and United States Empires, 1880–1910." *Journal of American History* 88, no. 4 (March 2002), 1315–53.

Ku, Robert Ji-Song, Martin F. Manalansan IV, and Anita Mannur, eds. *Eating Asian America: A Food Studies Reader*. New York: NYU Press, 2013.

Kumar, Anil. *Medicine and the Raj: British Medical Policy in India, 1835–1911*. Walnut Creek, CA: Altamira Press, 1998.

Kumar, Deepak. "Unequal Contenders, Uneven Ground: Medical Encounters in British India, 1820–1920," in Cunningham and Andrews, eds., *Western Medicine as Contested Knowledge*, 172–90.

Kumar, Deepak, and Raj Sekhar Basu, eds. *Medical Encounters in British India*. New Delhi: Oxford University Press, 2013.

Kupinse, William. "The Indian Subject of Colonial Hygiene," in Cohen and Johnson, eds., *Filth*, 250–76.

LaFeber, Walter. *The New Empire: An Interpretation of American Expansion, 1860–1898*. Ithaca, NY: Cornell University Press, 1963.

Lamont, Peter. *The Rise of the Indian Rope Trick: How a Spectacular Hoax Became History*. New York: Thunder's Mouth Press, 2004.

Laporte, Dominique. *History of Shit*. Transl. by Nadia Benabid and Rodolphe el-Khoury. Cambridge, MA: The MIT Press, 2000.

Largey, Gale, and Rod Watson. "The Sociology of Odors," in Drobnick, ed., *Smell Culture Reader*, 29–40.

Laudan, Rachel. *Cuisine and Empire: Cooking in World History*. Berkeley: University of California Press, 2013.

Le Bon, Gustave. *The Crowd: A Study of the Popular Mind*. London: T. Fisher Unwin, 1903.

Legarda, Benito Jr. *Occupation: The Later Years*. Quezon City: Vibal Publishing House, 2007.

Lévi-Strauss, Claude. *Tristes Tropiques*. Paris: Librairie Plon, 1955.

Levine, Philippa. "Naked Natives and Noble Savages: The Cultural Work of Nakedness in Imperial Britain," in Crosbie and Hampton, eds., *The Cultural Construction of the British World*, 17–38.

Levine, Philippa. *Prostitution, Race, and Politics: Policing Venereal Disease in the British Empire*. London: Routledge, 2003.

Linn, Brian McAllister. *The Philippine War, 1899–1902* Lawrence: University Press of Kansas, 2000.

Lowe, Donald M. *The History of Bourgeois Perception*. Chicago: University of Chicago Press, 1982.

Lui, Mary Ting Yi. *The Chinatown Trunk Mystery: Murder, Miscegenation, and Other Dangerous Encounters in Turn-of-the-Century New York City*. Princeton, NJ: Princeton University Press, 2005.

Lundestad, Geir, ed. *No End to Alliance: The United States and Western Europe, Past, Present and Future*. New York: St. Martin's, 1998.

Lupton, Deborah. "Food and Emotion," in Korsmeyer, ed., *Taste Culture Reader*, 317–24.

Lurie, Jonathan. *William Howard Taft: The Travails of a Progressive Conservative*. New York: Cambridge University Press, 2012.

Mabalon, Dawn Bohulano. "As American as Jackrabbit Adobo: Cooking, Eating, and Becoming Filipina/o American before World War II," in Ku, Manalansan, and Mannur, eds., *Eating Asian America*, 147–76.

Macfarlane, Iris. *Daughters of Empire: A Memoir of Life and Times in the British Raj*. Intro. by Susan Bayly. Oxford: Oxford University Press, 2006.

Mackenzie, John M. "Exhibiting Empire and the Delhi Durbar of 1911: Imperial and Cultural Contexts," in McAleer and Mackenzie, eds., *Exhibiting the Empire*, 194–219.

MacLeod, Roy, and Milton Lewis, eds. *Disease, Medicine, and Empire: Perspectives on western Medicine and the Experience of European Expansion*. London: Routledge, 1988.

MacMillan, Margaret. *Women of the Raj*. London: Thames and Hudson, 1988.

Magoon, Alice. "Domestic Science." *Philippine Teacher* II, no. 2 (July 1905), 20–31.

Majeed, Javed. "What's in a (Proper) Name? Particulars, Individuals, and Authorship in the Linguistic Survey of India and Colonial Scholarship," in Sengupta and Ali, eds., *Knowledge Production*, 19–39.

Manalansan, Martin F. IV. "Immigrant Lives and the Politics of Olfaction in the Global City," in Drobnick, ed., *Smell Culture Reader*, 41–52.

Mann, Michael. "'Torchbearers Upon the Path of Progress': Britain's Ideology of a 'Moral and Material Progress' in India. An Introductory Essay," in Fischer-Tiné and Mann, eds., *Colonialism as Civilizing Mission*, 1–26.

Mannoni, O. *Prospero and Caliban*. New York: Frederick Praeger, 1956.

Margolies, Eleanor. "Vagueness Gridlocked: A Map of the Smells of New York," in Drobnick, ed., *Smell Culture Reader*, 107–17.

Martineau, Harriet. *British Rule in India: A Historical Sketch*. London: Smith, Elder and Co., 1857.

Marx, Karl. *The Economic and Philosophic Manuscripts of 1844*. Transl. by Martin Milligan. Ed. and with an Intro. by Dirk J. Struik. New York: International Publishers, 1964.

Mathur, Saloni. *India By Design: Colonial History and Cultural Display*. Berkeley: University of California Press, 2007.

May, Ernest R. *American Imperialism: A Speculative Essay*. New York: Atheneum, 1968.

May, Glenn Anthony. *Social Engineering in the Philippines: The Aims, Execution, and Impact of American Colonial Policy, 1900–1913*. Westport, CT: Greenwood Press, 1980.

Mayo, Katherine. *The Isles of Fear: The Truth About the Philippines*. New York: Harcourt, Brace and Company, 1924.

McAleer, John, and John M. Mackenzie, eds. *Exhibiting the Empire: Cultures of Display and the British Empire*. Manchester: Manchester University Press, 2015.

McCallus, Joseph P., ed. and intro. *Gentleman Soldier: John Clifford Brown and the Philippine-American War*. College Station: Texas A&M University Press, 2004.

McClintock, Anne. *Imperial Leather: Race, Gender, and Sexuality in the Colonial Contest*. London: Routledge, 1995.

McCoy, Alfred W. *Policing America's Empire: The United States, the Philippines, and the Rise of the Surveillance State*. Madison: University of Wisconsin Press, 2009.

McHugh, James. *Sandalwood and Carrion: Smell in Indian Religion and Culture*. New York: Oxford University Press, 2012.

McKenna, Rebecca Tinio. *American Imperial Pastoral: The Architecture of US Colonialism in the Philippines*. Chicago: University of Chicago Press, 2017.

McKenzie, Dan. *The City of Din: A Tirade Against Noise*. London: Adlard and Son, Bartholomew Press, 1916.

McLaughlin, Allan. "The Suppression of a Cholera Epidemic in Manila." *Philippine Journal of Science* 4B, no. 1 (February 1909), 43–58.

McLuhan, Marshall. *The Gutenberg Galaxy*. Toronto: University of Toronto Press, 1962.

Melosi, Martin V. *Garbage in the Cities: Refuse, Reform, and the Environment*. Rev. ed. Pittsburgh: University of Pittsburgh Press, 2005.

Melosi, Martin V. *The Sanitary City: Urban Infrastructure in America from Colonial Times to the Present*. Baltimore: Johns Hopkins University Press, 2000.

Metcalf, Thomas R. *Ideologies of the Raj*. Cambridge: Cambridge University Press, 1995.

Meyer, Milton Walter. *Letters Home: The Meyers and Capiz 1919–1943*. Claremont, CA: The Paige Press, 2003.

Miller, Stuart Creighton. *"Benevolent Assimilation": The American Conquest of the Philippines, 1899–1903*. New Haven, CT: Yale University Press, 1982.

Miller, William Ian. *The Anatomy of Disgust*. Cambridge, MA: Harvard University Press, 1997.

Minger, Ralph Eldin. *William Howard Taft and United States Foreign Policy: The Apprenticeship Years 1900–1908*. Urbana: University of Illinois Press, 1975.

Minturn, Robert B. Jr. *From New York to Delhi, by way of Rio de Janiero, Australia and China*. New York: D. Appleton and Co., 1858.

Mintz, Sidney W. *Sweetness and Power: The Place of Sugar in Modern History*. New York: Viking, 1985.

Mintz, Sidney W. *Tasting Food, Tasting Freedom: Excursions into Eating, Culture, and the Past*. Boston: Beacon Press, 1996.

Moon, Sir Penderel. *The British Conquest and Dominion of India*. London: Duckworth, 1989.

Morris, Edwin T. *Fragrance: The Story of Perfume from Cleopatra to Chanel*. New York: Charles Scribner's Sons, 1984.

Moses, Edith. *Unofficial Letters of an Official's Wife*. New York: D. Appleton and Company, 1908.

Mukerjee, Madhusree. *Churchill's Secret War: The British Empire and the Ravaging of India during World War II*. New York: Perseus, 2010.

Murail, Estelle. "A Body Passes By: The Flâneur in Nineteenth-Century London and Paris." *The Senses and Society* 12, no. 2 (2017), 162–76.

Myrdal, Gunnar. *An American Dilemma: The Negro Problem and Modern Democracy, Vol. I*. New York: Harper, 1944.

Nair, Janaki. "Uncovering the Zenana: Visions of Indian Womanhood in Englishwomen's Writings, 1813–1940," in C. Hall, ed., *Cultures of Empire*, 224–45.

Nandy, Ashis. *The Intimate Enemy: Loss and Recovery of Self under Colonialism*. New York: Oxford University Press, 1983.

Nanni, Giordano. *The Colonisation of Time: Ritual, Routine and Resistance in the British Empire*. Manchester: Manchester University Press, 2012.

Nelan, Charles. *Cartoons of Our War with Spain*, 2nd ed. New York: Frederick A. Stokes Co. 1898.

Nevinson, Henry Woodd. *The New Spirit of India* London: Harper and Brothers, 1908.

Newsholme, Arthur, ed. *Public Health: The Journal of the Incorporated Society of Medical Officers of Health*, Vol. V: October, 1892 to September, 1893. London: E. W. Allen, 1893.

Newton, Gail. "South-East Asia: Malaya, Singapore, Philippines," in Hannavy, ed., *Encyclopedia of Nineteenth-Century Photography*, 1313–16.

Norling, Bernard. *The Intrepid Guerrillas of North Luzon*. Lexington: University of Kentucky Press, 1999.

Ong, Walter J. *The Presence of the Word*. New Haven, CT: Yale University Press, 1967.

Orquiza, René Alexander Jr. "*Lechon* with Heinz, Lea & Perrins with *Adobo*: The American Relationship with Filipino Food, 1898–1946," in Ku, Manalansan, and Mannur, eds., *Eating Asian America*, 177–85.

Ortner, Sherry B. "Introduction." *Representations* 59 (Summer 1997), 1–13.

Orwell, George. *Burmese Days*. Orlando: Harcourt Inc., 1934.

Orwell, George. *The Road to Wigan Pier*. San Diego: Harcourt, Brace, 1958.

Otis, Laura. *Membranes: Metaphors of Invasion in Nineteenth-Century Literature, Science, and Politics*. Baltimore: Johns Hopkins University Press, 1999.

Our Islands and Their People as Seen with Camera and Pencil. Two vols. Intro. by Major-General Joseph Wheeler, with special descriptive matter and narratives by José de Olivares. St. Louis: N. D. Thompson Publishing Company, 1899.

Padoongpatt, Mark. "Food and Empire," in Wise and Wallach, eds., *Routledge History of American Foodways*, 353–69.

Pal-Lapinski, Piya. "Infection as Resistance: Medical Discourse, Indian Courtesans, and Flawed Memsahibs in Flora Steel's Colonial Fiction." *Ariel: A Review of International English Literature* 30, no. 3 (July 1999), 141–61.

Parascandola, John. "Chaulmoogra Oil and the Treatment of Leprosy." *Pharmaceutical History* 45, no. 2 (2003), 47–57.

Parezo, Nancy J., and Don D. Fowler. *Anthropology Goes to the Fair: The 1904 Louisiana Purchase Exposition*. Lincoln: University of Nebraska Press, 2007.

Pearl, Sharrona. *About Faces: Physiognomy in Nineteenth-Century Britain*. Cambridge, MA: Harvard University Press, 2010.

Pecson, Geronima T., and Maria Racelis, eds. *Tales of the American Teachers in the Philippines*. Manila: Carmelo and Bauermann Inc., 1959.

Pernau, Margrit. "Teaching Emotions: The Encounter between Victorian Values and Indo-Persian Concepts of Civility in Nineteenth-Century Delhi," in Sengupta and Ali, eds., *Knowledge Production*, 227–47.

Peyron, Louis. "Perfumes and Odours during the [French] Revolution," in Grasse, ed., *Perfume, A Global History*, 142–47.

Phalen, James M. "An Experiment with Orange-Red Underwear." *Philippine Journal of Science* 5B, no. 6 (December 1910), 525–47.

The Philippines. "The First Civil Governor," by Theodore Roosevelt, and "Civil Government in the Philippines," by William H. Taft. New York: The Outlook Company, 1902.

Picker, John M. *Victorian Soundscapes*. New York: Oxford University Press, 2003.

Pinard, Sylvain. "A Taste of India: On the Role of Gustation in the Hindu Sensorium," in Howes, ed., *The Varieties of Sensory Experience*, 221-230.

Pinkerton, Alasdair. "Radio and the Raj: Broadcasting in British India (1920–1940)." *Journal of the Royal Asiatic Society* Series 3, 18, no. 2 (2008), 167–91.

Pinney, Christopher. *Camera Indica: The Social Life of Indian Photographs*. Chicago: University of Chicago Press, 1997.

Platt, Kate. *The Home and Health in India and the Tropical Countries*. London: Baillière, Tindall, and Cox, 1923.

Porteous, J. Douglas. *Landscapes of the Mind: Worlds of Sense and Metaphor*. Toronto: University of Toronto Press, 1990.

Prashad, Vijay. "The Technology of Sanitation in Colonial Delhi." *Modern Asian Studies* 35, no. 1 (February 2001), 113–55.

Proust, Marcel. *In Search of Lost Time. Volume I: Swann's Way*. Transl. C. K. Scott Moncrieff and Terence Kilmartin. New York: The Modern Library, 1992.

Rafael, Vicente L., ed. *Discrepant Histories: Translocal Essays on Filipino Cultures*. Philadelphia: Temple University Press, 1995.

Rafael, Vicente L. "Nationalism, Imagery, and the Filipino Intelligentsia in the 19th Century," in his *Discrepant Histories*, 133–58.

Raheja, Gloria Goodwin. "Caste, Colonialism, and Speech of the Colonized: Entextualization and Disciplinary Control in India." *American Ethnologist* 23, no. 3 (August 1996), 494–513.

Raman, Kamya, and Anantanarayanan Raman. "Amoebic Dysentery and Introduction of Ementine Source *Carapichea ipecacuanha* in Indian Subcontinent." *Indian Journal of History of Science* 52, no. 1 (2017), 54–65.

Ramanna, Mridula. "A Mixed Record: Malaria Control in Bombay Presidency, 1900–1935," in Kumar and Basu, eds., *Medical Encounters*, 208–31.

Ramanna, Mridula. "Perceptions of Sanitation and Medicine in Bombay, 1900–1914," in Fischer-Tiné and Mann, eds., *Colonialism as Civilizing Mission*, 205–25.

Ramasubban, Radhika. "Imperial Health in British India, 1857–1900," in MacLeod and Lewis, eds., *Disease, Medicine, and Empire*, 38–60.

Ramaswamy, Sumathi. "Introduction: The Work of Vision in the Age of European Empires," in Jay and Ramaswamy, eds., *Empires of Vision*, 1–22.

Ranger, Terence O. *Dance and Society in Eastern Africa 1890–1970: The Beni Ngoma* Berkeley: University of California Press, 1975.

Ranger, Terence. "The Invention of Tradition in Colonial Africa," in Hobsbawm and Ranger, eds., *The Invention of Tradition*, 211–62.

Rath, Richard Cullen. *How Early America Sounded*. Ithaca, NY: Cornell University Press, 2003.

Ray, Krishnedu, and Tulasi Srinivas, eds. *Curried Cultures: Globalization, Food, and South Asia*. Berkeley: University of California Press, 2012.

Ray, Utsa. *Culinary Culture in Colonial India: A Cosmopolitan Platter and the Middle-Class*. Delhi: Cambridge University Press, 2015.

Reinarz, Jonathan. *Past Scents: Historical Perspectives on Smell*. Urbana: University of Illinois Press, 2014.

Report of the Philippine Commission to the President. Vol. I. Washington, DC: Government Printing Office, 1900.

Report of the Philippine Commission to the President. Vol. II: Testimony and Exhibits. Washington, DC: Government Printing Office, 1900.

Report of the Philippine Commission to the President. Vol. III. Washington, DC: Government Printing Office, 1901.

Report of the Philippine Commission to the President. Vol. IV. Washington, DC: Government Printing Office, 1901.

Rice, G. D. "Art in the Philippines." *The Art Amateur*, February 1902, 68–70.

Richman, Paula, ed. *Many Ramayanas: The Diversity of a Narrative Tradition in South Asia*. Berkeley: University of California Press, 1991.

Riis, Jacob A. *How the Other Half Lives*. Ed. with an Intro. by David Leviatin. Boston: Beford/St. Martin's, 1996 [1890].

Rizal, José. *Noli Me Tangere (Touch Me Not)*. Transl. by Harold Augenbaum. New York: Penguin, 2006 [1887].

Rizzo, Tracey, and Steven Gerontakis. *Intimate Empires: Body, Race, and Gender in the Modern World*. New York: Oxford University Press, 2017.

Robertson, James A. "Notes from the Philippines." *Journal of Race Development* 3, no. 4 (April 1913), 467–90.

Roland, Alan. *In Search of Self in India and Japan: Toward a Cross-Cultural Psychology*. Princeton, NJ: Princeton University Press, 1988,

Roosevelt, Nicholas. *The Philippines: A Treasure and a Problem*. New York: J. H. Sears & Company, 1926.

Rosenfeld, Sophia. "AHR Forum: On Being Heard: A Case for Paying Attention to the Historical Ear." *American Historical Review* 116, no. 2 (April 2011), 316–34.

Ross, Ronald. *Mosquito Brigades and How To Organise Them*. New York: Longman, Green, and Co., 1902.

Rotter, Andrew J. *Comrades at Odds: The United States and India, 1947–1964*. Ithaca, NY: Cornell University Press, 2000.

Rotter, Andrew J. "Empires of the Senses: How Seeing, Hearing, Smelling, Tasting, and Touching Shaped Imperial Encounters." *Diplomatic History* 35, no. 1 (January 2011), 2–19.

Rotter, Andrew J. "The Senses," in Costigliola and Hogan, eds., *Explaining the History of American Foreign Relations*, 317–33.

Rotter, Andrew J. "William Howard Taft's Drawers," in Blower and Bradley, eds., *The Familiar Made Strange*, 46–58.

Rowland, Dr. Henry C. "Fighting Life in the Philippines." *McClure's Magazine* 19 (May–October 1902), 241–47.

Roy, Kaushik, ed. *War and Society in Colonial India, 1807–1945*. New Delhi: Oxford University Press, 2006.

Roy, Parama. *Alimentary Tracts: Appetites, Aversions, and the Postcolonial*. Durham, NC: Duke University Press, 2010.

Roy, Rohan Deb. "Quinine, Mosquitoes and Empire: Reassembling Malaria in British India, 1890–1910." *South Asian History and Culture* 4, no. 1 (January 2013), 65–86.

Roy, Tapti. *The Politics of a Popular Uprising: Bundelkhand in 1857*. New Delhi: Oxford University Press, 1994.

Rudolph, Susanne Hoeber, and Lloyd I. Rudolph, with Mohan Singh Kanota, eds. *Reversing the Gaze: Amar Singh's Diary, A Colonial Subject's Narrative of Imperial India*. Boulder, CO: Westview Press, 2002.

Ryan, James R. *Picturing Empire: Photography and the Visualization of the British Empire*. Chicago: University of Chicago Press, 1997.

Rydell, Robert W. *All the World's a Fair: Visions of Empire at American International Expositions, 1876–1916*. Chicago: University of Chicago Press, 1984.

Sacks, Oliver. "The Dog Beneath the Skin," in Drobnick, ed., *Smell Culture Reader*, 184–86.

Said, Edward. "Criticism/ Self Criticism." *Lingua Franca* (February–March 1992), 39–40.

Said, Edward. *Orientalism*. New York: Panteheon, 1978.

Salman, Michael. "'Nothing Without Labor': Penology, Discipline and Independence in the Philippines Under United States Colonial Rule, 1898–1914," in Rafael, ed., *Discrepant Histories*, 113–29.

Sampson, Gary D. "Unmasking the Colonial Picturesque: Samuel Bourne's Photographs of Barrackpore Park," in Hight and Sampson, eds., *Colonialist Photography*, 84–106.

Saunders, Nicholas J., and Paul Cornish, eds. *Modern Conflict and the Senses*. London: Routledge, 2017.

Schafer, R. Murray. *The Tuning of the World*. New York: Knopf, 1977.

Schivelbusch, Wolfgang. "The Railway Journey: Panoramic Travel," in Edwards and Bhaumik, eds., *Visual Sense*, 287–95.

Schivelbusch, Wolfgang. "Spices: Tastes of Paradise," in Korsmeyer, ed., *Taste Culture Reader*, 123–30.

Schmidt, Eric Leigh. *Hearing Things: Religion, Illusion, and American Enlightenment*. Cambridge, MA: Harvard University Press, 2000.

Schwartz, Hillel. "The Indefensible Ear: A History," in Bull and Back, eds., *Auditory Culture Reader*, 487–501.

Scott, James C. *Seeing Like a State: How Certain Schemes to Improve the Human Condition Have Failed*. New Haven, CT: Yale University Press, 1998.

Scott, Nora. *An Indian Journal*. Ed. by John Radford. London: The Radcliffe Press, 1994.

Scriven, George Percival. "An American in Bohol, The Philippines, 1899–1901." Online Archival Collection, Special Collections Library, Duke University. https://library.duke.edu/rubenstein/scriptorium/scriven/

Sen, Amartya. *Public Action to Remedy Hunger*. The Fourth Annual Arturo Tanco Memorial Lecture, August 2, 1990. London: The Global Hunger Project, 1990.

Sen, Colleen Taylor. *Feasts and Fasts: A History of Food in India*. London: Reaktion Books, 2015.

Sengupta, Indra, and Daud Ali, eds. *Knowledge Production, Pedagogy, and Institutions in Colonial India*. New York: Palgrave Macmillan, 2011.

Sengupta, Jayanta. "Nation on a Platter: The Culture and Politics of Food and Cuisine in Colonial Bengal," in Ray and Srinivas, eds., *Curried Cultures*, 73–87.

Sharma, Madhuri. "Knowing Health and Medicine: A Case Study of Benares, c. 1900–1950," in Kumar and Basu, eds., *Medical Encounters*, 160–86.

Shaw, Angel Velasco, and Luis H. Francia. *Vestiges of War: The Philippine-American War and the Aftermath of an Imperial Dream 1899–1999*. New York: NYU Press, 2002.

Shay, Michael E., ed. *A Civilian in Lawton's 1899 Philippine Campaign: The Letters of Robert D. Carter*. Columbia: University of Missouri Press, 2013.

Shprintzen, Adam D. "The Nineteenth Century," in Wise and Wallach, eds., *Routledge History of American Foodways*, 37–47.

Shridharani, Krishnalal. *My India, My America*. Garden City, NY: Halcyon House, 1943.

Shulman, David. "The Scent of Memory in Hindu South India," in Drobnick, ed., *Smell Culture Reader*, 411–26.

Siebenga, Rianne. "Colonial India's 'Fanatical Fakirs' and Their Popular Representations." *History and Anthropology* 23, no. 4 (December 2012), 445–66.

Simmons, James Stevens, Tom F. Whayne, Gaylord West Anderson, and Harold Maclachlan Horack. *Global Epidemiology: A Geography of Disease and Sanitation*. London: William Heineman, 1944.

Singer, Milton B., and Bernard S. Cohn, eds. *Structure and Change in Indian Society*. Chicago: University of Chicago Press, 1968.

Sinha, Mrinalini. "'Chathams, Pitts, and Gladstones in Petticoats': The Politics of Gender and Race in the Ilbert Bill Controversy, 1883–1884," in Chaudhuri and Strobel, eds., *Western Women and Imperialism*, 98–116.

Sinha, Mrinalini. *Colonial Masculinity: The "Manly Englishman: and the "Effeminate Bengali" in the Late Nineteenth Century*. Manchester: Manchester University Press, 1995.

Smilor, Raymond W. "Cacophony at 34th and 6th: The Noise Problem in America, 1900–1930." *American Studies* 18, 1 (1977), 23–38.

Smith, Bruce R. "How Sound is Sound History?," in Smith, ed., *Hearing History*, 389–94.

Smith, Bruce R. "Tuning Into London c. 1600," in Bull and Back, eds., *Auditory Culture Reader*, 127–35.

Smith, Mark M., ed. *Hearing History: A Reader*. Athens, GA: University of Georgia Press, 2004.

Smith, Mark M. *How Race Is Made: Slavery, Segregation, and the Senses*. Chapel Hill: University of North Carolina Press, 2006.

Smith, Mark M. "Listening to the Heard Worlds of Antebellum America," reprinted in Smith, *Hearing History*, 365–84.

Smith, Mark M. *Sensing the Past: Seeing, Hearing, Smelling, Tasting, and Touching in History*. Berkeley: University of California Press, 2007.

Smith, Mark M., ed. "The Senses in American History: A Roundtable." *Journal of American History* 95, no. 2 (September 2008), 378–451.

Smith, Mark M. *The Smell of Battle, the Taste of Siege: A Sensory History of the Civil War*. New York: Oxford University Press, 2015.

Smith, Richard Saumarez. *Rule by Records: Land Registration and Village Custom in Early British Panjab*. Delhi: Oxford University Press, 1996.

Smith, Virginia. *Clean: A History of Personal Hygiene and Purity*. Oxford: Oxford University Press, 2007.

Sonnichsen, Albert. *Ten Months a Captive Among Filipinos: Being a Narrative of Adventure and Observation During Imprisonment on the Island of Luzon, P. I.* New York: Charles Scribner's Sons, 1901.

Stallybrass, Peter, and Allon White. *The Politics and Poetics of Transgression*. Ithaca, NY: Cornell University Press, 1986.

Stanley, Peter W. *A Nation in the Making: The Philippines and the United States, 1899–1921*. Cambridge, MA: Harvard University Press, 1974.

Steel, Flora Annie, and Grace Gardiner. *The Complete Indian Housekeeper and Cook*. Ed. by Ralph Crane and Anna Johnston. Oxford: Oxford University Press, 2010 [1888].

Stein, Burton. *A History of India*. Malden, MA: Blackwell Publishers, 1998.

Sterne, Jonathan. "Medicine's Acoustic Culture: Mediate Auscultation, the Stethoscope and the 'Autopsy of the Living,'" in Bull and Back, *Auditory Culture Reader*, 191–217.

Stoddart, Brian. *A People's Collector in the British Raj: Arthur Galletti*. New Delhi, Readworthy Publications, 2011.

Stokes, Adrian. "Strong Smells and Polite Society." *Encounter* (September 1961), 50–56.

Stoler, Ann Laura, ed. *Haunted By Empire: Geographies of Intimacy in North American History*. Durham, NC: Duke University Press, 2006.

Stradling, David. *Smokestacks and Progressives: Environmentalists, Engineers, and Air Quality in America, 1881–1951*. Baltimore: Johns Hopkins University Press, 1999.

Strong, Dr. R. P. "Comment on Dr. McLaughlin's Paper." *Philippine Journal of Science* 4B, no. 1 (February 1909), 65.

Subrahmanyam, Sanjay. "On the Hat-Wearers, Their Toilet Practices, and Other Curious Usages," in Chatterjee and Hawes, eds., *Europe Observed*, 45–81.

Sudan, Rajani. *The Alchemy of Empire: Abject Materials and the Technologies of Colonialism*. New York: Fordham University Press, 2016.

Sullivan, Rodney. "Cholera and Colonialism in the Philippines, 1899–1903," in MacLeod and Lewis, eds., *Disease, Medicine, and Empire*, 284–300.

Sullivan, Zohreh T. *Narratives of the Empire: The Fictions of Rudyard Kipling*. New York: Cambridge University Press, 1993.

Suri, Jeremi. *Liberty's Surest Guardian: American Nation-Building from the Founders to Obama*. New York: The Free Press, 2011.

A Survey of the Educational System of the Philippine Islands: 1925. Manila: Bureau of Printing, 1925.

Süskind, Patrick. *Perfume: The Story of a Murderer*. Trans. John E. Woods. New York: Knopf, 1986.

Sutherland, John. *Orwell's Nose: A Pathological Biography*. London: Reaktion Books, 2016.

Sutton, David E. "Synesthesia, Memory, and the Taste of Home," in Korsmeyer, ed., *Taste Culture Reader*, 304–16.

Taft, Mrs. William Howard. *Recollections of Full Years*. New York: Dodd, Mead & Company, 1914.

Talusan, Mary. "Music, Race, and Imperialism: The Philippines Constabulary Band at the 1904 St. Louis World's Fair." *Philippine Studies* 52, no. 4 (2004), 499–526.

Teltscher, Kate. "The Floating Lexicon: *Hobson-Jobson* and the *OED*," in Sengupta and Ali, eds., *Knowledge Production*, 41–57.

Terry, Richard. *Indian Cookery*. London: Oriental Society of London, 2011 [1861].

Thackeray, William Makepeace. *Vanity Fair*. New York: W. W. Norton, 1994 [1848].

Thompson, Emily. *The Soundscape of Modernity: Architectural Acoustics and the Culture of Listening in America, 1900–1933*. Cambridge, MA: The MIT Press, 2002.

Tomes, Nancy. *The Gospel of Germs: Men, Women, and the Microbe in American Life*. Cambridge, MA: Harvard University Press, 1998.

Tuan, Yi-Fu. *Passing Strange and Wonderful: Aesthetics, Nature, and Culture*. Washington, DC: Island Press, 1993.

Tunick, Mark. "Tolerant Imperialism: John Stuart Mill's Defense of British Rule in India." *Review of Politics* 68, 4 (2006), 568-611.

Tyler, Stephen. *India: An Anthropological Perspective*. Prospect Heights, IL:Waveland Press, 1986.

Tyndale-Biscoe, C. E. "The Imperial Touch: Schooling Male Bodies in Colonial India, Part I," in Classen, ed., *The Book of Touch*, 168–70.

Van Heyningen, Elizabeth. "The Social Evil in the Cape Colony 1868–1902: Prostitution and the Contagious Disease Acts." *Journal of South African Studies* 10, no. 2 (April 1984), 170–97.

Vergara, Benito M. Jr. *Displaying Filipinos: Photography and Colonialism in Early 20th Century Philippines*. Quezon City: University of the Philippines Press, 1995.

Visram, Rozina. *Ayahs, Lascars and Princes: Indians in Britain 1700–1947*. London: Pluto Press, 1986.

Visser, Margaret. *Much Depends on Dinner: The Extraordinary History and Mythology, Allure and Obsessions, Perils and Taboos of the Ordinary Meal*. New York: Grove Press, 1986.

Viswanathan, Gauri. *Masks of Conquest: Literary Study and British Rule in India*. New York: Columbia University Press, 1989.

Volckmann, R. W. *We Remained: Three Years Behind the Enemy Lines in the Philippines*. New York: Norton, 1954.

Wagner, Kim A. *The Great Fear of 1857: Rumours, Conspiracies and the Making of the Indian Uprising*. Oxford: Peter Lang, 2010.

Wagner, Tamara S., and Narin Hassan. *Consuming Culture in the Long Nineteenth Century: Narratives of Consumption, 1700–1900*. Plymouth, UK: Lexington Books, 2007.

Walsh, Judith E. *Domesticity in Colonial India: What Women Learned When Men Gave Them Advice*. Lanham, MD: Rowman & Littlefield, 2004.

Walsh, Judith E. *Growing Up in British India: Indian Autobiographers on Childhood and Education Under the Raj*. New York : Holmes and Meier, 1983.

Warboys, Michael. *Spreading Germs: Disease Theories and Medical Practice in Britain, 1865–1900*. Cambridge: Cambridge University Press, 2000.

Watt, Carey A., and Michael Mann, eds. *Civilizing Missions in Colonial and Postcolonial South Asia: From Improvement to Development*. London: Anthem Press, 2011.

Weaver, John C. *The Great Land Rush and the Making of the Modern World, 1650–1900*. Montreal: McGill-Queen's University Press, 2003.

Weiner, Annette B., and Jane Schneider, eds. *Cloth and Human Experience*. Washington, DC: Smithsonian Institution Press, 1989.

West-Sooby, John, ed. *Discovery and Empire: The French and the South Seas*. Adelaide: University of Adelaide Press, 2013.

Wickberg, Daniel. "What Is the History of Sensibilities? On Cultural Histories, Old and New." *American Historical Review* 112, no. 3 (June 2007), 660–84.

Wilcox, Marrion, ed. *Harper's History of the War in the Philippines*. New York: Harper and Brothers, 1900.

Wilcox, Willis Bliss. *Through Luzon on Highways and Byways*. Philadelphia: Franklin Book Company, 1901.

Williams, Daniel R. *The Odyssey of the Philippine Commission*. Chicago: A. C. McClurg & Co., 1913.

Williams, Raymond. *Keywords: A Vocabulary of Culture and Society*. Rev. ed. New York: Oxford University Press, 1983.

Wilson, Anne C. *Hints for the First Years of Residence in India*. Oxford: Clarendon Press, 1904.

Wilson, Jesse R. *Through Shining Archway*. New York: American Baptist Missionary Society, 1953.

Wilson, Jon E. *The Chaos of Empire: The British Raj and the Conquest of India*. New York: Public Affairs Press, 2016.

Wise, Michael D., and Jennifer Jensen Wallach, eds. *The Routledge History of American Foodways*. New York: Routledge, 2016.

Worboys, Michael. "Tuberculosis and Race in Britain and its Empire, 1900–1950," in Ernst and Harris, eds., *Race, Science, and Medicine*, 144–66.

Worcester, Dean C. *The Philippine Islands and Their People*. London: The Macmillan Co., 1898.

Worcester, Dean C. *The Philippines Past and Present*, with Biographical Sketch and Four Additional Chapters by Ralston Hayden. New York: The Macmillan Co., 1930.

Wright, Lawrence. *Clean and Decent: The Fascinating History of the Bathroom & the Water Closet and of Sundry Habits, Fashions & Accessories of the Toilet Principally in Great Britain, France, & America*. New York: Viking, 1960.

"Wyvern" (Colonel Arthur Robert Kenney-Herbert). *Culinary Jottings for Madras, or, A Treatise in Thirty Chapters on Reformed Cookery for Anglo-Indian Exiles*. Intro. by Leslie Forbes. Totnes, UK: Prospect Books, 2007 [1878].

Yang, Anand A. *The Limited Raj: Agrarian Relations in Colonial India, Saran District, 1793–1920*. Berkeley: University of California Press, 1989.

Yates, Nigel. *Anglican Ritualism in Victorian Britain 1830–1910*. Oxford: Oxford University Press, 1999.

Zastoupil, Lynn. *John Stuart Mill and India*. Stanford: Stanford University Press, 1994.

Zealley, Alfred Edward, and J. Ord Hume. *Famous Bands of the British Empire: Brief Historical Records of the recognised leading Military Bands and Brass Bands in the Empire*, with "Historical Sketch of the Evolution of the Military Band" by Colonel J. A. C. Somerville, Late Commandant Royal Military School of Music. London: J. P. Hull, 1926.

Zimmermann, Francis. *The Jungle and the Aroma of Meats: An Ecological Theme in Hindu Medicine*. Berkeley: University of California Press, 1987.

INDEX

For the benefit of digital users, indexed terms that span two pages (e.g., 52–53) may, on occasion, appear on only one of those pages.

Page references followed by *f* refer to figures respectively.